MENOPAUSE
A Guide for Women  and Those Who Love Them

REVISED EDITION

MENOPAUSE

Revised Edition

A Guide for Women
and Those Who Love Them

WINNIFRED B. CUTLER, Ph.D.

CELSO-RAMÓN GARCÍA, M.D.

W·W·NORTON & COMPANY   NEW YORK·LONDON

First published as a Norton paperback 1993

The text of this book is composed in Galliard with the display set in Baker Signet.
Composition and manufacturing by the Haddon Craftsmen, Inc.
Book design by Charlotte Staub.

Library of Congress Cataloging-in-Publication Data

Cutler, Winnifred Berg.
    Menopause, a guide for women and the men who love them. —Rev.
ed. / Winnifred B. Cutler, Celso-Ramón García.
        p.   cm.
    Includes bibliographical references and index.
    ISBN: 0-393-30995-9
    1. Menopause—Popular works.   I. García, Celso-Ramón. 1921–
II. Title.
RG186.C93   1992
618.1'75—dc20   91-30149
                                                         CIP

W. W. Norton & Company, Inc., 500 Fifth Avenue, New York, NY 10110
W. W. Norton & Company Ltd., 10 Coptic Street, London WC1A 1PU

4 5 6 7 8 9 0

CONTENTS

ILLUSTRATIONS

by Caroline Meinstein
and Pamela Sinkler Todd

FIGURES

TABLES

PLATES

PREFACE

By 1975, Winnifred Cutler, then a graduate student in biology at the University of Pennsylvania, had completed an intriguing pilot study: it showed possible and striking relationships between the pattern of sexual behavior of young women and their pattern of menstruation. Since she needed a mentor, her faculty in biology advised her to find a professor in gynecology to supervise her studies. Dr. Celso-Ramón García, professor of gynecology, one of the "fathers" of the oral contraceptive, a scholar and an educator, was interested in the pilot work and agreed to become involved in its development.

Throughout a seven-year tutelage, Dr. García helped Dr. Cutler locate the classic, often-forgotten works that had laid the foundation for the development of modern reproductive endocrinology. He listened to her ideas and provided critical feedback that helped to direct and enhance the growth of her work—a process that still continues. As their collaborative studies of sexual behavior and fertility, ovarian physiology, clinical practice in gynecology, and biology took shape, a number of startling discoveries emerged. It was while presenting those discoveries at scientific meetings that Dr. Cutler met Dr. Julian Davidson and decided to shift her focus temporarily from young women to more mature women.

Dr. Davidson, then an associate professor of physiology at Stanford University, was working on aging and sexual function in rats and in men and invited her to work with him at Stanford. She wanted to study neuroendocrinology; he wanted to learn the rigorous methods of conducting large-scale prospective human studies that she and Dr. García had developed.

In the fall of 1979, after having secured funds from the National Institutes of Health, the Stanford Menopause Study was established at Stanford University jointly by Dr. Davidson and Dr. Cutler. The study was the first of its kind in the United States and was designed to evaluate normal, healthy women as they passed through the menopause. To recruit subjects, Dr. Cutler appeared on a television news show and explained that a study of menopause was getting under way. She described to the audience the need for subjects—that is, for healthy women who were approaching their menopause—and asked these women to get involved in the project so that the process of menopause could be carefully studied.

The response was immediate: for two weeks, the phones rang continuously with offers of help. Several hundred women were enrolled—twenty of them as research assistants, the rest as subjects. Although Dr. Cutler has since returned to her work in Pennsylvania as founder and president of the Athena Institute for Women's Wellness, a biomedical research and service corporation, the project continued under the direction of Dr. Davidson and Dr. Norma McCoy. And some of the original participants in the project are still being studied as they advance deeper into their menopause.

During the study, many of the subjects described to Dr. Cutler the details of their personal search to understand what was happening to them as they approached the menopause. They felt frustrated as they sought, but were unable to find, books from libraries and stores that would provide accurate, comprehensible information on the menopause. Many of them joined the study in hopes of finding answers to their questions, answers that were not in books. They also described their despair and frustration at the treatment (or lack of treatment) offered by the medical establishment when they sought help or information about their hot flashes, loss of a sense of well-being, sagging skin, or vaginal distress during coitus. Because of these experiences, the women who participated in the project asked Dr. Cutler to write a book for people like themselves as well as for others who, as part of the human family, would find such information important in helping them to understand, aid, and live with the women they love.

Now, as the revised edition of this book takes shape, the substance of the original has been confirmed. A great deal of new information has expanded the possibilities for women as they approach the menopause and beyond. For the woman in her mid-thirties through her menopausal onset, hormonal therapies are a sensible option—a phenomenon not yet as extensively researched when the first edition was written. Likewise, for a woman in the more advanced stages of menopause—her sixties and older—a large amount of biomedical data are available to help her lead a long, healthy, vigorous life.

We bring to the book a sense of mission: to offer to our female readers the detailed information that they will need to understand the menopause and to maximize health care. Here, male readers will also find important information about their own changes in sexuality as well as information that will help them comprehend the uniquely female experience of the menopause.

We hope that this book will be helpful. If you find it too simple or too complicated, please understand that each reader brings a different educational background to the reading. We tried to write it for those with inquiring minds but no scientific background. In some cases, we have provided scientific detail that may interest only the more sophisticated reader.

After you finish the book, you may discover that some of your questions remain unanswered. There is still a lot to be learned about the menopause, and we encourage you to share your questions as well as your reactions to the book. Please write to us care of Dr. Winnifred Cutler, President, The Athena Institute for Women's Wellness, Inc., 30 Coopertown Road, Haverford, PA 19041. We would like to hear from you; and although we may be unable to answer all mail personally, we will use your comments to guide us in planning future research.

WINNIFRED B. CUTLER
CELSO-RAMÓN GARCÍA

PREFACE FOR MEN

If you are like most men, the term *menopause* probably has little objective meaning beyond the fact that it marks the end of a woman's reproductive years. You may even think that this is a specifically female subject and have avoided becoming informed about it. Even so, if you are living with a woman going through her menopausal transition, the chances are good that you will have had some firsthand exposure to menopausal symptoms before much time has passed. Although some people use the term *male menopause* to describe parallel changes that men undergo, such a term is misleading. Male and female reproductive physiology are critically different. While men produce a fresh supply of sperm each day, often into advanced age, *women are born with all the eggs they will ever have.* These eggs get used up through time. Menopause describes the end (pause) of the egg-releasing menstrual years. (Other details of male gonadal changes are described in Chapter 8; the changes in a woman's gonadal physiology are described in Chapters 1, 2, and 3.)

Does the woman in your life start sweating suddenly without apparent cause? Drenched with sweat, she may wake you up in the night, needing to change the linen to get dry again. Sexually she may not seem responsive to you. She may appear to have lost interest in sex; and when you do have intercourse, she may have pain. If so, what you are seeing are symptoms commonly experienced by women going through the change of life. And there are other symptoms, too (described in Chapter 3). If your partner's symptoms are distressing to you, imagine what they must be like for her.

Menopausal distress can affect the quality of a relationship between a man and a woman. *How informed you are makes a difference.* Consider this scenario. A woman is distressed because she is experiencing profound physical and emotional discomforts (hot flashes, night sweats, sexual discomfort, etc.). She complains. Her partner is upset because he doesn't understand what is happening. The stable routine of a middle-aged couple is shattered. The more upset he becomes, the more defensive she becomes. He accuses. She reacts. She feels doubly oppressed—first, by the profound physical experience she is going through and, second, by the sinking sense of betrayal by her unaware and unhelpful man. Even a good relationship can suffer under such conditions. Here is what one fifty-four-year-old woman had to say after thirty-seven years of marriage:

I tire easily; hot flashes night and day; sweating and headaches. . . . Sexual activity occurs once a week if I really make myself for my husband's sake though we had a great sex life before and I was always very receptive. . . . Maybe this has no bearing on anything, but I must admit my husband was extremely unsympathetic about my whole problem. The last two or three months he has tried to understand my feelings. He felt the hot flashes and feelings that went with them were pure figments of my imagination. Because I suppose he knew how loving I had always been in the past, but he just couldn't or wouldn't understand. He was certain that I was "holding back." . . . My doctor finally decided I should try these pills for a couple of months to see if some of my discomfort would leave. I do find that the flushes are less. . . . I had hoped to find out why or if it is possible for this menopause to mess up, what was before, a lovely life—it is very distressing to me and it infuriates my husband.

Although a woman's menopausal difficulties can seem to come from nowhere, they are *not* imaginary. They are real. They herald the menopausal transition. And she may not even know what is happening or that these upsets are as natural and as predictable for the vast majority of women as the changing of the seasons are in nature. She may not appreciate how others perceive her. She may look normal but behave strangely because of how she feels. As you become informed, you will be alert to her distress and can help her overcome difficulties. At least she will have you on her side.

As a woman passes through her forties, her physiology changes (as described in Chapter 1). In large part, the symptoms of the change of life are the result (Chapters 2 and 3). Although menopausal symptoms are a natural part of the aging process for most women, you should not assume that you and she are helpless. In fact, appropriate medical treatment can alleviate or prevent those menopausal symptoms that have their roots in a woman's changing physiology.

You do have some control. With knowledge, you can materially affect the process, shorten it, and turn it around from distress to comfort. If you understand what is happening, your assistance can be critically important. Your emotional support has the power to provide a climate for correcting some of the difficulties of this period. With awareness, you can help her seek out effective medical aid. Your efforts during this time of stress can help your relationship to grow. You can turn this major life experience into a marvelous opportunity to understand her and to enrich her appreciation of you. The woman who is blessed with an understanding and emotionally supportive partner—one who takes the trouble to become informed—is likely to give back far more than she was given.

This book is designed to help people become informed about the menopause. In it, you will find chapters that explain what the change of life is and how hormone changes during this period produce a cluster of distressing symptoms. You will find a chapter about bones and osteoporosis, a very serious bone disease that develops in about 50 percent of women over the age of sixty and at any age two years after severe lack of estrogen. Osteoporosis is related to the hormone changes of menopause. You will find out how hormone treatment alleviates menopausal symptoms and prevents the development of osteoporosis, and you will find information about the risks of hormone treatment and how these risks can be reversed. The woman in your life may one day have to decide about whether or not to have a hysterectomy. You will find a chapter that describes the surgery and some of the problems that can result from it.

Taking responsibility for one's health is critically important to a well-lived and happy existence. Both the man and the woman need to maintain their health and to be supportive of each other in order to enjoy the fruits of their life after fifty.

In this book, facts about the menopause have been drawn from our intense study of the scientific and biomedical literature. Throughout the book, two related perspectives are presented: the data from the biomedical studies, and *the actual words of women who have experienced these situations* and who are describing how they felt at the time. If you consider both, you can better understand the menopausal experience.

This uniquely feminine phenomenon affects all women and those who love them.

FOREWORD

Due to the combined efforts of scientists, physicians, and consumers during the past century, there has been an unprecedented and explosively complex expansion in services and health benefits that enhance the quality of women's well-being as well as their longevity. In large part, this expansion comes from the numerous technological advances that have been made in the biological sciences. So rapidly have these advances appeared, and so encompassing their applications, that they have simultaneously produced impressive benefits and unease. Their use often requires an intrusion into the personal self of the user. As a result, many women are concerned about whether the new technologies should be accepted, especially in the treatment of cancer, sexually transmissible diseases, fertility, and the menopause. Ethical-oversight committees and other established medical-evaluation structures assure us that these rapidly occurring changes can be applied in a stable, supportive manner, one guaranteeing security rather than chaos.

These advances have also changed the way in which health care to women is delivered. Doctors have had to become both more specialized in their own field as well as more knowledgeable outside their specialties in order to serve their patients properly. While the family physician is often that family's primary medical professional, in most nonrural areas the obstetrician-gynecologist serves as family physican for women. This person will guide the woman through her reproductive years, not only supervising the care of her pregnancies and the regulation of her fertility, but attending to other, more general health-care needs. Today's gynecologist is not only obstetrically trained, but is also knowledgeable about reproductive endocrinology, general medicine, and modern reproductive surgery, as are many other medical specialists; women should seek out those physicians who possess such coordinated skills, skills that are so meaningful to the well-being of women.

Most important in the changing health-care environment is the impact of the consumer. Coalitions of people combining their energies to improve the quality of health care for women have worked—and are still working—arduously to provide up-to-the-minute educational and data-collection resources. Because of their efforts, not only have women, now armed with knowledge, become more active in making decisions about their own health, but physicians have become more willing to work with their patients as together they review options and plan individual strategies.

Menopause: A Guide for Women and the Men Who Love Them offers an opportunity to continue this trend as women approach their menopause and plan for their future.

CELSO-RAMÓN GARCÍA, M.D.
WINNIFRED B. CUTLER, Ph.D.

ACKNOWLEDGMENTS

We wish to thank the many people whose interest and cooperation at various stages of the research for the book enabled us to write it. In the spring of 1979, Minnie Berg, Evelyn Cutler, and Jean Cutler obtained from 25 women anonymous information about personal details of their menopause. The following fall and spring in California, another 300 women, as part of the Stanford Menopause Study, shared their personal experiences. Some came quite a distance to participate: from 30 miles north of San Francisco to 40 miles south of Santa Cruz. To all of you, our thanks.

Three Stanford students—Celeste Wiser, Emily Woo, and Caryn Truppman—are thanked for working so closely with Dr. Cutler in assembling data and readings on the menopause. She is grateful to the following women for having been research assistants: Pat Brick, Nancy Chilton, Diane Cohen, Patricia Congdon, Helen Hill, Barbara Hogue, Elizabeth Hunt, Jacqueline Hyde, Betty Land, Muriel Maverick, Ruth Miles, Barbara Morton, Joan Morton, Ida Murray, Rita Olson, Joan Piccard, Verne Rice, Sonya Urban, and Catherine Whalen.

The authors thank the scholars, scientists, and physicians who so generously shared their knowledge and expressed their perspectives—at Stanford: Dr. Julian Davidson, Dr. Seymour Levine, Dr. Emmet Lamb, Dr. Norma McCoy, Dr. George Feigen, Dr. Fredi

Kronenberg, and Dr. Pat Cross; at the University of Kansas: Dr. Gilbert Greenwald; at the Medical College of Georgia: Dr. R. Don Gambrell; at the University of Pennsylvania: Dr. Santo Nicosia, Dr. David Goodman, Dr. Luis Blasco, Dr. Pedro Beauchamp, and Ms. Karen Mueller; at Abington Memorial Hospital: Dr. David Reese; at Beaver College: Dr. Richard Polis; and at the Monell Chemical Senses Center: Dr. George Preti.

To the individuals who were kind enough to read various versions and sections of the original manuscript and note their critiques we are especially grateful: Dr. Melvin Moore, Sandy Brennan, Tricia and Bruce Weekly, Kathryn Burkhart, Adolph Berg, Dr. Norman Johnston, Dr. Arnold Jerrall, Ann Williams, Sara Bogdanoff, Joanne Hirsh, Martha Mockbee, Dr. Terry Allen, Karen Mayer, Janis Tyler Johnson, Adele Hertz-Gray, Selma Fiel, Helene Cohan, Teresa O'Dowd, and Lisa Biello.

To Scott Grossman, Stanley Fox, and Dr. Erika Friedmann for assistance in retrieving relevant studies Dr. Cutler expresses her appreciation.

We thank the librarians at Beaver College, particularly Marion Green and Joe Charles, and at the Hospital of the University of Pennsylvania, Michael Rissinger, for their inexhaustible good cheer and help in retrieving numerous scientific papers.

The authors are especially indebted to Dr. Julian Davidson for having provided the forum for beginning the study of menopausal women. It has been especially challenging for Dr. Cutler to work with him.

We particularly appreciate the people at W. W. Norton & Company. A consistently high level of professionalism characterizes this publishing company. Mary Cunnane, our editor, was both a pleasure to work with and a significant contributor to the clarity of the text. By her meticulous competence, Carol Flechner, our manuscript editor, has further enhanced the work.

The authors join each other in expressing pleasure and gratification for the opportunity of working together to create this book. Dr. Cutler formulated the idea of writing it through discussions with Dr. García while she was at Stanford. His willingness to continue to guide her studies as he had been doing since 1974 when she approached him as a graduate student in biology encouraged her to undertake the project. His patience and good will, combined with his extraordinary scientific competence, clinical expertise, and medical compassion, have been a continuing inspiration to her.

This very complex subject of menopausal physiology and psychology has offered a fascinating journey for the authors.

ACKNOWLEDGMENTS TO THE REVISED EDITION

We thank the Metabolic Bone Disease Conference members at the Hospital of the University of Pennsylvania—Dr. Frederick Kaplan, chief of metabolic bone disease; Dr. John Haddad, chief of endocrinology; Dr. Maurice Attie, associate professor of medicine; Dr. Jim McLeod, endocrinologist; Dr. Alan Wasserstein, kidney physiologist; and Dr. Michael Fallon, pathologist specializing in bone—for their continuing interaction during the several years that the weekly scientific conference provided a forum for growth and understanding of bone metabolism. Dr. Abass Alavi, chief of nuclear medicine at the University of Pennsylvania, provided the dual-photon recordings of spinal bone for the Women's Wellness program's first group of patients, allowing us to test bone density in these woman. Drs. Joel Karp, physicist, and Robert Stine, statistician, worked with us as well on the bone studies. Dr. Abba Krieger of the Wharton School at the University of Pennsylvania was a significant contributor to our statistical analyses of the original studies we published.

Thanks are also due to Dr. R. Don Gambrell of the Medical College of Georgia, where he serves as a clinical professor of obstetrics and gynecology, physiology, and endocrinology, for his many interactions with us and for permitting us to use his tables in the text.

Thanks to Jerilynn Prior, M.D., FRCP, who is a professor on the faculty of medicine at the University of British Columbia, for sharing her significant prepublication manuscripts on exercise physiology; her works have since been published and are cited in the text.

We thank Pamela Thompson Sinkler Todd for her wonderful drawings, which have appeared in the book since the first edition.

We thank Carol Flechner of W. W. Norton & Company for her magnificent work on the revised edition; her efforts went above and beyond her input on the first edition. She is meticulous, thoughtful, and a true contributor to this manuscript. Rebecca Castillo and Mary Cunnane are acknowledged for their many editorial roles.

We thank Kathy Kelly for her work in retrieving numerous scientific papers that were added to the revised edition.

We thank employees at the Athena Institute for their efforts in bringing the manuscript to publication: Kate Paffett, Suzanne Galloway, and Kate Felmet.

MENOPAUSE
A Guide for Women
and the Men Who Love Them

REVISED EDITION

INTRODUCTION

The ways in which women experience menopause are as varied as women themselves. For some, it is a gentle variation in the rhythms of their lives, its effects minimal. For others, its effects are pronounced, sometimes difficult, but capable of being coped with. For still others, however, "the change" has devastating physical and emotional consequences.

Most women experience menopause "naturally," the first signs usually appearing when the women are in their early forties (although the signs may appear even sooner). For others, though, menopause comes abruptly and prematurely when, in their thirties or even twenties, they undergo hysterectomies.

Throughout this book we will be alternating between the actual voices of menopausal women and those of the authors. First, some women speak.

The onset of irregular periods came in this last year, and the periods I do have are heavy, with some clotting and discomfort. I tend to also have a few days of the "blues," feeling of frustration and some fatigue. My libido has always been healthy, and the only physical symptom that I have noticed is that my hair is starting to turn grey and I must watch my diet more carefully, as the midline seems to take on weight. I consider menstrual cycles a normal part of my life, and I have always been and still am physically very active. I feel exercise is extremely important for me in keeping my whole personality in balance. I swim, hike, ski, skate, play racketball with or without a period. I have noticed some change in my general attitude to life—but I am not sure that it is due to the "change." My life has been so full of "changes" in the last five years that I find it hard to pinpoint one that has more importance than another. The painful divorce, the loss of income, finding my way as a single person at 50, surviving financially in an inflationary market, managing the entire routine of business, home, and property, social life, sex life, and concern about how to stay healthy are challenging and are all possible sources for the feelings of the blahs. I am gregarious with many friends—young and old—and I do not see behavioral changes in myself, except that my sense of humor has increased and I am more critical of events and people who waste my time or spirit.

[I had an] overwhelming feeling of being stifled and suffocating night sweats; couldn't stand to touch my breasts due to tenderness and heaviness; insomnia which remains a problem; leg aches in the night particularly; backache; overwhelming feelings of anxiety which made me feel sick to my stomach; headaches often intense and often accompanied by worse nausea. . . . My life became intolerable and I felt (feel) I had to save myself. [I] have good relationships with friends and co-workers. Adjusting has been (and is, though less) very difficult—and get[s me] very depressed—but consciously keep very busy with work and taking classes and get completely exhausted.
My husband implies he really "never got enough" from me but I don't believe this is true as my remembrances include much tenderness and sexual enjoyment. I do not have much sexual desire right now but I do miss touching and closeness at night.

I am now 62 years old and in fairly good health. My experience with the menopause lasted about 10–12 years. My gynecologist refused to give me any medication during this period. It was a time of uncomfortableness for me, especially through the winters. At several periods from October through January I had "hot flashes" every half hour, day and night. The perspiration ran down my temples and back. . . . My office mates couldn't believe what they saw. But after having what was happening explained thoroughly to me by my doctor I accepted his decision. I feel many times medication is possibly harmful and readily available to women who are so spoiled by conveniences that they just do not want to be annoyed by "Nature's" body changes. The biggest drawback is the sad situation between mothers and daughters who do not "talk" about our body processes at an early age—knowing something as "natural" as a child can form attitudes that last us through our lives and help us through trying times.

About a year ago hot flashes began and grew very severe. Sleep was interrupted continually. Clothes absolutely soaked through. Kept changes of *night clothes by bedside. In August, September and October flashes were almost regularly [coming] every 40 minutes. . . . Knew when the onslaught was approaching and nothing could be done to stop it. Absolutely felt like I would burn up. Beads of moisture would pour out of pores on breast area, around waistline, back of neck, forehead, above lip line. You could actually see droplets standing and running. Anyone touching body would receive reaction that "I was on fire." Flash would last approximately 3 to 5 minutes and moisture would disappear! Did not have odor. Usual places like under-arms were completely free of this flash. . . . Most embarrassing to be in a business conference eyeball to eyeball with executive and suffer through a flash and try to respond normally as if nothing had happened.*

After a highly satisfying sexual life with same partner (husband) it has been rather upsetting and distressing to find my libido is subsiding. My husband is having trouble in holding an erection which he is most concerned about. He has the desire but cannot respond. Also in the past year, hot flashes have been occurring during intercourse—most distressing to both partners. Have been so absorbed in climbing business ladder successfully, I do not have desire for sex as much and this could be because of my husband's problem and concern over his possible feeling of depression and hurt at not being able to perform as usual. We are a very close couple.

My premature change occurred at the age of 42 due to a hysterectomy and I have been taking estrogen ever since. I'm now 60 years of age and still taking estrogen which helps relieve the hot flashes. I still have those occasional sweating periods but not for long periods of time and not too unbearable. Other than these flashes, the changes one talks about aren't such an obvious thing. Certain changes in the pigmentation occur, causing brown spots on the skin. As far as sexual activity, there are not changes as it is the same as always. Certainly as one gets older, there may be less frequency, but no less qualitatively.

I became a widow at the age of 43 just when I began menopause. . . . I have been celibate since my husband's death. I cannot say with certainty my state of mind is due to my body's changes or the many adjustments I have made these past few years. However, for what it's worth, here it is: I often feel cheated because I am a widow. I was looking forward to menopause—then I could relax and enjoy having a relationship with my husband. Until that time I was always a little uneasy about having sex because of the worry of pregnancy (I used only suppositories and/or prophylactics). Having two beautiful children, I did not want any more. I find that I still have a sex drive. Although it has no direct outlet, I channel my energies into other things. I have always had a good rapport with men and I continue to have male friends with whom I go out occasionally. I don't think menopause should interfere with or affect one's sex life. If anything, it should enhance it because one is more experienced, with fewer inhibitions or fears. . . . I must confess that my patience has shortened considerably, especially toward older people, for whom I had endless patience. I wonder if this due to the fact that I am now older.

Before the change superficial conversation was adequate with friends. I liked just skimming over topics at bridge table. Impressing them with desserts I made seemed important or how my home looked or giving that Christmas party, etc. Now bridge-group–type entertainment and conversation is intolerable. Take me as I am is more my style now. I'm more comfortable with myself and no longer need to impress others. Don't like to entertain any more—prefer to just be home or on a drive with my husband. Before, I just wanted to get involved in everything, couldn't seem to say no. Ego played a big part in what I did. Now I can say No! Want to commit myself to less (committee chairmanships etc.). Need time to just let me enjoy and relax more, doing things I like without pressure.

I was two years past my last period and feeling so badly that I had to take a leave from my job. At that point I was desperate for any information on the subject [of menopause]. I was extremely tired most of the time and feeling very nervous. I was experiencing hot flashes six or seven times at night, which interrupted my sleep, and several times each day. In a three-year period, I had been to two family practitioners (one of whom was my family doctor) and two gynecologists. The first three gave me complete physicals which cost upwards of $100 each, and two referred me to a psychiatrist. I saw the psychiatrist three times for a cost of $155, even though I was convinced that my problem was physical. The third gynecologist, a . . . woman . . . , told me to "tough it out." I later learned from another doctor that she frequently told young people that the only way to prevent pregnancy was to refrain from intercourse. The second physician suggested a course in assertiveness training. I cried a lot after the operation [a hysterectomy performed at the age of 38; she is, at the time of this statement, 51] or when I got home from the hospital. It stopped when I went back to my job. I used to have hot flashes only at night but for the last two years I have them day and night. My doctor gave me hormones but they didn't help. It's very hard to be close to people at work when it happens as I feel like I stink. It happens at least 4 or 5 times a day and at night. I wake up at least 3 or 4 times wet and sweaty and then take off the covers and fall asleep and wake up again because I'm cold.

Truthfully I have experienced very little change because of menopause. My energy level is less. Sexually I did not have much desire before so it hasn't changed. I have very little desire now. Flashes that I got only lasted six months. The nights were the worst time for this but I did not ever take anything during the change. I had had no depression. I think being physically active all my life helped during menopause. Your outlook on life means much and [because of] this [menopause] has not made any difference to me.

I started my change five years ago and if it were not that my period stopped I would never know of a change (besides the six months of hot flashes).

Menopause is experienced by more women today than ever before. Had you been born two hundred years ago, you probably would not have lived much past your childbearing years and, therefore, would not have reached a menopause. Until recently, a woman's life span was usually shorter than her reproductive capacity—most women died before reaching menopause. But today, especially with informed self-care, a woman can expect to live thirty or forty vigorous years *after* the first signs of menopause appear. This book is planned to help women understand the process they will go through during those years, including how unpleasant some of the symptoms can be and what women can do about them.

As a woman, you are in a unique position today. Investigators are now publishing studies that show how hormone alterations, hormone replacement therapy, diet, exercise, and sexual behavior all influence the physical and mental processes of women. Until recently it would not have been possible to write a comprehensive book on menopause—not enough was known. But now enough is known. There is an abundance of new information that can be found in many research articles. Each describes a small but critical aspect of menopausal physiology. Now is the time to assemble this information.

Normally, it takes five to six years for the knowledge of new biomedical discoveries to reach the public. First, it takes two years for the results of a research study to be published in the scientific journals. Then, it takes another two years before scholarly review articles appear that can incorporate the findings into their summaries. It is through such predigested review articles that the time-pressured professionals often try to keep abreast of recent advances. A year or two later the information may finally trickle down to you.

The problem of timing is not critical from an intellectual and historical viewpoint. But for you, a woman going through menopause, a five- or six-year delay in obtaining information that may help you to enhance your life can be unfortunate. With this book, it may be possible for you to circumvent the usual delay. It should serve as a basic reference for you, even as new discoveries continue to be made.

To the consternation of many women, some health professionals have hinted that menopause problems are really a mental (neurotic) condition without basis in physiology. Others push hormonal therapies when women fear them. Both attitudes reflect an insensitivity to the complex physiology of women. Menopausal distress is real. While many subtleties remain unexplained, it has been repeatedly shown that hormone levels have certain clear-cut and simple correspondences both to distress and to freedom from distress.

The issues involved in menopausal health care are complex, and the answers are often not simple. For example, you might ask: Should I use hormone therapy to treat my hot flashes? If yes, then how much hormone is "safe," and for what period of time should it be taken? If you do take hormones that have been prescribed for you and your breasts become sore, you might wonder: Am I taking too high a dosage?

A great deal has been written about the menopause. As a layperson, how can you separate fact from fancy when you read sensational claims in the newspapers and in new books? As a layperson, how do you decide whether to believe those who tell you that hormone replacement therapy is the fountain of youth or those who tell you that it is deadly and an unnecessary evil? Some women take vitamin E. As a layperson, how do you decide whether vitamin E treatment will improve your well-being or waste your money?

One answer is to become alert to the biases inherent in much media reporting. Be suspicious of news that presents only one side of an issue and the data that support only one particular perspective. Because a good reporter knows that he or she, as a nonscientist, is incapable of reaching technical/scientific conclusions, good reporting presents all sides. A sophisticated reader can usually identify biased reports by recognizing their sensational approach to topics. If you read that hormone replacement therapy is an elixir of youth and are then provided only with the series of studies proving this, be on your guard. If you read that hormone replacement therapy is an evil thing that has been perpetrated upon innocent women and do not read anything positive about it, again be on your guard. Remember, there are no simple answers to the complex issues of the maturing years. You will need confidence, perceptual skills, and energy.

Once you are alert to the biases, you should develop a health maintenance plan that will most effectively serve your needs through your menopause. You must get in tune with your body to do this. You need to learn how to listen to what it tells you in order to enjoy it and to make changes when it is hurting.

You will need the strength of will to secure the type of health care that *you* decide is best for *you*. You may have to overcome old habits of placing responsibility for yourself in the hands of others. To maximize your health, you must take responsibility for yourself because only *you* can know how you feel: only *you* are experiencing your body's pains; only *you* are feeling its well-being.

In this era of prolonged extension of life, eighty-five years is a common span, while premenopausal symptoms begin in the midforties. You have a lot of years to live after the onset of menopause. It's important to plan for them. To do this you need the facts. In order to prepare this book, thousands of research reports have been evaluated and cross-checked to bring you these facts. In this book you will also find the comments of women who were studied at Stanford as well as those of women from the Philadelphia area. The perspective provided by these women combined with a separate analysis of the relevant biomedical literature bring an unusually broad focus to this text.

This book is the story of the menopause. As the chapters unfold it will describe how

- beginning at around age forty-three (seven years before the last menstrual flow), menstrual cycle lengths and bleeding quantities change and symptoms usually begin. This is due to the aging and shrinking of the ovaries and the consequent decline in blood levels of estrogen and other hormones.
- the symptoms are experienced in varying degrees of severity by about 85 percent of women. Hot flashes, night sweats, insomnia, and a loss of a sense of well-being are common. In addition, for about 50 percent of women a progressive loss of bone begins that, if left unchecked, leads to the disease osteoporosis.
- after menses stop, hormonal levels continue to decline and symptoms may persist for many years.

Following hormones and symptoms, we will then discuss

- how the body's changes in response to hormonal signals include changes in skin, vagina, urinary tract, breast, bone-calcium content, and possibly memory.
- the critical changes that bones undergo as estrogen levels decline, as well as the effects of these changes on general health.

Having considered these basics, we next focus on hormone replacement therapy, which may help certain problems but, due to its inherent nature, may create others.

Then, we will consider your sexuality in the face of your own and your partner's changes.

Surgery of female reproductive organs is discussed. This includes hysterectomy, the operation that is performed on approximately half of all women. We will take up its benefits, risks, side effects, and the arguments for retaining your ovaries even if you agree that your uterus should be removed.

Five new chapters, including one on cardiovascular health (cardiovascular disease accounts for the lion's share of deaths among menopausal women; indeed, this is the leading cause of death among women who are estrogen-deficient, as is characteristic of those who are menopausal without estrogen replacement therapy), have been added in this, the revised edition:

- Cardiovascular Health
- Nutrition
- Overcoming Smoking and Obesity
- Exercise
- Alternatives to Hormone Replacement Therapy

Finally, a checklist is provided at the end of the book to guide you in reviewing the details of your own health care.

At one time, the doctor assumed all the responsibility for a woman's health care. The woman was docile and evinced the unquestioning faith she had in her doctor, probably the most critical factor in promoting health care. Once upon a time, you may have believed that a doctor could cure your ills and optimize your well-being. Were you taught, as a child, that when you were ill (or to maintain your health) your ultimate resource was your doctor? Were you lucky enough to have a doctor who provided the warmth and kindness to cause you to believe this? And how about today? When you seek gynecological help with vaginal dryness, or hot flashes, or menopausally related loss of the sense of well-being, or any other legitimate menopausal complaint, does your doctor provide real help?

Modern science and the pressures of society have created a different attitude toward the health-care field today, yet the illusion of the old-fashioned doctor often persists. It still is long, arduous, and costly to become a physician. In most other respects, however, the medical profession has changed. Today, for each opening in medical school, there still remain three outstanding candidates, despite a reduction in the number of applicants. Lawsuits have been brought and won that insure that entry to medical schools will be based on the objective criteria of excellent academic performance rather than the independent judgment of the admissions committees. Because of this fierce competition and resulting emphasis on academic standing, qualities of humanity, gentleness, patience, and empathy are often not given sufficient consideration in selecting our nation's future doctors. What we have gained in objectivity we may have lost in subjectivity—that is, in our doctors' ability and willingness to offer concerned and kind care. We shouldn't necessarily blame the doctor. The young man or woman who starts out wanting to serve others by becoming a physician very soon learns that the *only* way he or she will have a chance of occupying a seat in medical school is to single-mindedly pursue the highest possible test scores in college. Only the strongest can make it.

We have taught these students as undergraduates and at medical school. They are bright, intelligent, articulate, and hard-working. The system requires them to be self-centered enough to earn very high grades; to do so, they must usually become highly competitive. University faculties can be irritated by hard-driving premed students, but the pique of the faculty members often seems to reinforce a student's idea that he or she must either compete vigorously or else give up the dream of medical school. Those who do manage to be accepted into medical school face another four pressure-filled years in which they must learn to think fast, respond instantly, and repress their natural sensitivities to the large number of often painful human problems with which they are confronted on a daily basis. Those who go on to specialize in gynecology (an obstetrical-surgical subspecialty) train for several more years (the years vary depending on the specialty) in which they must rapidly digest enormous amounts of information. It is little wonder that the training process often teaches the doctors to rush, to ignore their own (and others') feelings, to lack compassion, and in general to be more concerned about plowing through and completing their enormous work load than about being reflective and displaying gentleness. The demands on the physician's time and energy—including the needs of patients, and the necessity of keeping abreast of a constantly expanding body of medical knowledge and alert to the possibilities of malpractice suits—aggravate and intensify the pressures.

This is reflected in the way some doctors make their own time a priority while showing no respect for the value of their patient's time: it is common to see a waiting room filled with patients who have all been scheduled for 9:00 A.M. and who will be seen throughout the course of the next four hours. Fortunately, not all practitioners are so inconsiderate. In fact, the truly caring physician is just as likely to have a full waiting room but for a very different reason. On occasion, your problem may take more time than the scheduled time allotted. If the doctor cares about you, he or she will, to provide good medical care, take whatever time you need. This may cause other patients to be delayed. Many physicians only delay patients when an unavoidable situation (an emergency or extra patient needs) occur. And then there may be time constraints imposed by the various economic-reimbursement systems. The critical question is: Why are you delayed? The answer can guide your decision about your choice of health-care professional.

Many doctors are very well informed scientifically. Often, they know the latest research on risks and benefits of particular treatments. *Take advantage of the times in which we live. There has never been a better time for a woman to maximize her health care.* Make use of what is available to you: (1) the knowledge of a physician who keeps himself or herself up to date; (2) a book like this one that can be a good personal resource volume; and (3) a strong sense of your self-worth (which requires giving up your emotional and intellectual dependency on the medical establishment). Then you can reap a rich harvest in health care. If you focus your energy on learning about your body and searching for a competent physician who will respect and work with you, you can enjoy a level of health unknown to previous generations.

Don't be afraid to ask questions of your doctor. Make a list of questions before you see him or her. Mailing a copy of the list to your doctor before your appointment may be a good idea. Write down his or her answers to your queries. These notes will give you something to study when you get home; study is probably necessary if you are not a scientist because much of the communication problem between doctors and their patients results from the use of a technical vocabulary. Although your doctor is probably busy and he or she is entitled to your consideration when it comes to his or her time, you also have legitimate rights. You are paying for your doctor's services and are entitled to see to it that you have understood his or her comments. Often, your physician's knowledge and terminology is beyond your usual understanding. By writing down what your doctor says and checking with him or her for accuracy, you can later reread what you have written, ensuring that you have completely understood what he or she has told you. Remember, others are waiting for a turn. If you are well prepared and your questions are to the point, a good physician, in a minimal amount of time, will be happy to assure you that you have understood him or her.

This book provides the tools needed to help you work with a physician. You may be fortunate in that your health habits and hormone levels are adequate to maintain vibrant health. Good! More likely, however, you are having some of the symptoms of menopause that were described at the opening of the chapter. To alleviate these symptoms, you may seriously want to consider hormone therapy. It is important to realize that the recent proliferation of medical malpractice suits has put many physicians in the unfortunate position of being defensive about the treatments they are willing to suggest. In many cases, a woman has to *ask* for hormone replacement therapy in order to receive it—not because hormone replacement therapy is bad, but because the beleaguered medical community often tends to feel there is less risk of problems by avoiding any risk. Patient advocate groups sometimes speak emotionally out of concern for the welfare of women, but their advice lacks a sufficient appreciation of the newer scientific bases that are now apparent.

On the other hand, as physicians become increasingly appreciative of the value of hormone replacement therapy, some women are reporting that they are being pressured into using hormones rather than being told enough to become actively involved in the decision-making process. Education is fundamental to good health in these particular years when so much new knowledge that benefits women is being gathered and published. It requires desire, will power, and time to become educated. But there are great rewards.

Let us begin!

1

THE SEX
HORMONES

Menopause is the natural result of age-related changes in ovarian function. It means, literally, the cessation of uterine menstrual cycles. When two years have passed without a menstrual period, you can be 98-percent sure no more will ensue. To understand the menopause and the change of life that precedes it, you should learn about hormones, where they are produced, and how they act. Hormones are very powerful substances: minute concentrations of them will produce enormous effects on both your body and on your brain.

HORMONES

The blood that circulates through your body is like a pot full of gravy. If, when the gravy is simmering, you add water to it and stir it thoroughly, each spoonful will have about the same flavor and content as any other spoonful. Since the blood is continuously recirculating through your body, your heart's pumping action acts like a

Santo V. Nicosia, M.D., M.S. Pathology (formerly associate professor of obstetrics and gynecology and now professor of pathology at the University of South Florida, Tampa), has generously given of his self and his knowledge, and has contributed the illustrative material on ovaries in this chapter.

spoon, mixing and stirring the ingredients. Your glands produce hormones, which are released into your blood stream. Your kidneys and digestive tract control the amount of water added to your blood. And, like gravy in a pot, the blood's ingredients blend and change form as they heat up and are mixed.

Hormones are substances that are produced in parts of the body called glands and are tiny enough to travel in the blood to other parts of the body to exert their action. A hormone is like an itinerant preacher who travels about, influencing receptive others wherever he goes. The blood serves hormones somewhat like the vehicle that transports the preacher. Blood travels everywhere in the body (within the arteries, capillaries, and veins), and the hormones in blood leave the bloodstream when they reach a receptive tissue. The hormones that are most important in understanding the menopause are estrogen and progesterone. These are produced predominantly in the ovaries. An understanding of menopause, therefore, requires an understanding of the ovaries.

THE OVARIES

The ovaries of a woman may be the most remarkable structures in nature. Nowhere else in the human body, male or female, does an organ undergo a monthly cycle in which both the size and the content change from day to day in a regular and repeating pattern. In addition to this repeating monthly pattern, the ovaries change throughout life, too.

In the prepubescent girl, the ovaries are small but already have all the eggs that she will ovulate over her entire lifetime. She is born with her lifetime supply of eggs and will never produce another one. Around each egg (ovum) lies a flat sheet of cells. The entire structure of the egg with its covering sheet of cells is known as a follicle. Plate A shows a magnified slice of an infant's ovary. Hundreds of follicles appear in this slice.

Since you are probably looking at a photograph of a light micrograph for the first time, it is helpful to consider the perspective of the picture. First, a slice is taken from the ovary much as you might slice up a candy Easter egg. This slice is laid on a flat surface, and a piece of the slice is cut out much like you might use a cookie cutter to cut out

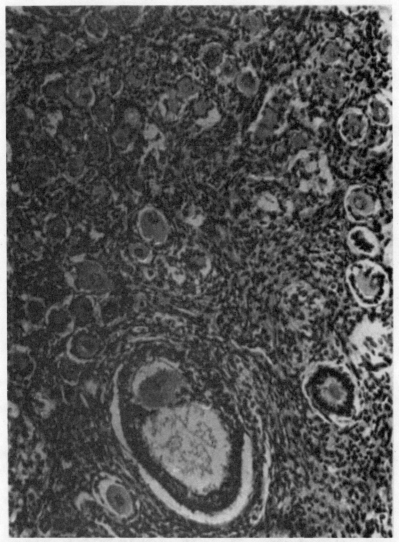

PLATE A   Light Micrograph (Magnified Hundreds of Times) of a Slice of an Infant Ovary

This magnified picture of a slice of ovary shows how some of the cells of the ovary collect into circular groupings called follicles. At the center of each follicle lies a single egg. Note here the one big follicle and the many smaller ones. This picture does not show the outside edges of the ovary—just the more central region.

sections of rolled dough when preparing to bake. All of the photographs in this chapter are mounted on small glass slides that are rectangular in shape. Therefore, when you look at the picture and see a very straight edge, this is the edge formed by the cut from the tissue sample before the ovarian slice was mounted—the ovary itself has no straight edges. Some of the pictures show a curving edge on one or more sides. In that case, you are probably looking at one of the outside edges of the ovary. Much like in the cookie-cutting analogy, you might sometimes cut out a cookie on the edge of the rolled-out dough and, in doing so, fail to get a cookie that is the same shape as the cutter.

THE FERTILE YEARS

THE OVARIAN CYCLE

After puberty (usually around age twelve or thirteen, when pregnancy becomes possible), eight to ten of the follicles begin to mature each month. The cells of the follicular sheet multiply and fill with fluid. These follicular cells start to swell as the fluid, laden with cholesterol, enters them from the surrounding medium of the ovary. After the cholesterol is absorbed into the follicle, the cholesterol is converted into the steroid hormones (predominantly estrogen), and some of these hormones leak out of the follicle back into the ovary. This leaked estrogen works its way into the blood vessels that lie nearby the follicle and gets carried out to the rest of the body through the bloodstream. Usually, only one of each month's crop of follicles matures. The rest die. The one maturing follicle, then, keeps growing until it reaches its time of ovulation. *Ovulation* is the term that describes the release of the egg from its follicle and its escape from the outer surface of the ovary into the Fallopian tube (or oviduct). As an egg begins its journey down the Fallopian tube toward the uterus, the egg is available for a rendezvous with a penetrating sperm; if the egg is fertilized by a sperm, a pregnancy will usually result. Figure 1 shows where the ovaries and the uterus are located.

Each month, after ovulation, the cells that had formed the ruptured follicle reconnect to each other and continue to multiply, swell, and take on a yellowish appearance. What was a follicle now becomes known as a corpus luteum (Latin for "yellow body"). The

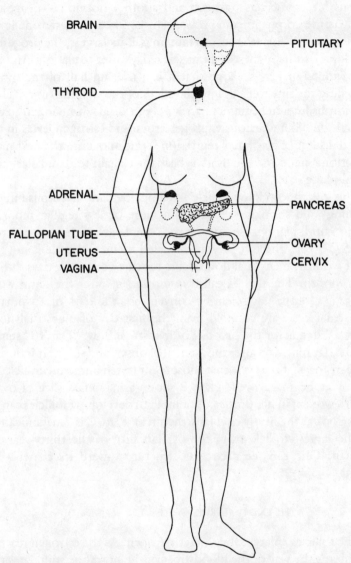

Figure 1   Female Reproductive Anatomy: Endocrine Glands and Sexual Organs

corpus luteum secrets estrogen and another hormone—progesterone. As the corpus luteum grows, estrogen and progesterone levels
in blood rise. When the corpus luteum is at its largest, the progesterone level is at its highest—about seven days after ovulation. And the
corpus luteum gets so large that it can take up half of the ovary,
crowding the tiny follicles into the edges of the swelling ovary. Then
the corpus luteum begins a process of regression, shrinking in size as
its cells die. Simultaneously, progesterone and estrogen levels in the
blood decline. This "luteal regression" continues until the next menstruation occurs and the ovary is back once again to its smaller men-
strual-phase size.

This ovarian cycle of follicle swelling, ovulation, corpus-luteum
swelling, and shrinking repeats in a more or less regular monthly
fashion until menopause. Even if the complexity of the ovarian cycle
is new to you, the fact of your repeated menstrual cycle is not. In
most women, menstrual flow occurs for three to twelve days during
each month. The flow is called *menstruation,* after the Latin word
menses, "month." By scientific convention, the days of a woman's
menstrual cycle are counted from the first day of menstrual flow.
"Day 1" stands for the first day of menstrual flow; "Day 10" stands
for the day nine days after the menstrual onset; and so on. It is during
the early days of the cycle that those eight to ten immature follicles in
the ovary begin to swell. Plate B shows a magnified slice of ovary
from a woman in her thirties. A number of developing follicles can be
seen (look at the neatly circular structures). Plate C is a magnification
of the largest follicle from the ovarian slice of the thirty-year-old
woman. One can see a circular structure toward its center—the
ovum.

THE ENDOMETRIAL CYCLE

As the follicles enlarge, they secret estrogen. As the estrogen reaches
the uterus (by way of the bloodstream), the hormone stimulates the
development of the endometrium of the uterus.

The endometrium is the layer of tissue that lines the inside of the
uterus; it is a composite of glandular (secreting) tissue mixed with
blood vessels and other cells. During the preovulatory portion of the
cycle, endometrial cells increase in number, the endometrial glands
grow in size, and blood vessels grow into them to provide nourish-

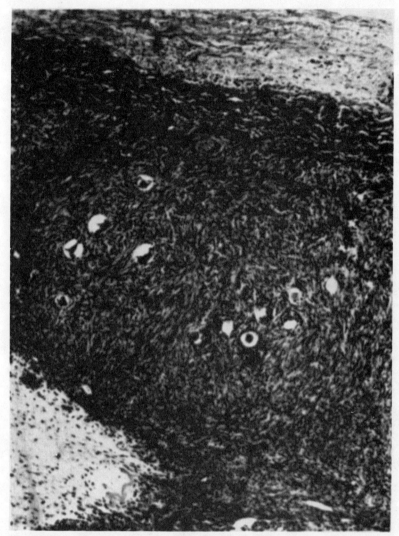

PLATE B Light Micrograph (Magnified) of a Slice of an Ovary of a Thirty-Year-Old Woman

This magnified slice of an ovary from a woman in her thirties shows, at the top, the outer edge (cortex) of the ovary as well as part of the more central region below. It also shows some small follicles that are developing.

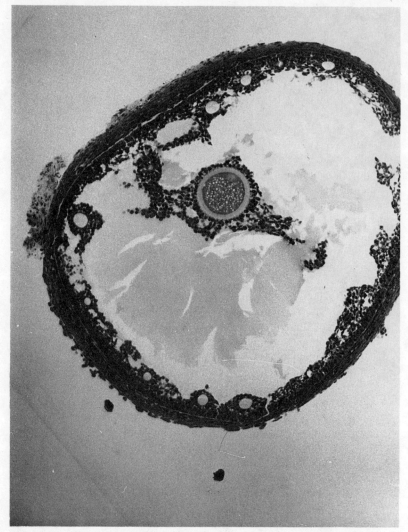

PLATE C Light Micrograph (Magnified) of a Slice of One Ovulatory Follicle from Plate B

This magnified picture shows one follicle that is very large and almost ready to ovulate. The circular structure toward the center of the follicle is the egg that will leave the follicle and the ovary to enter the Fallopian tube.

ment. As a result, the thickness of endometrium greatly increases.

These changes in endometrial composition are shown at the bottom of Figure 2. This chart shows cyclic changes in the ovary, in the lining of the uterus, and in blood levels of several reproductive-system hormones. In the ovary, after the follicle has ovulated its egg, the newly formed corpus luteum secrets both estrogen and progesterone. These two ovarian hormones stimulate even greater growth of the endometrium and endometrial blood supply. If, by fourteen days after ovulation, a fertilization has not occurred, the corpus luteum in the ovary will die. Without a corpus luteum (as well as premenstrually when it is shrinking), estrogen and progesterone levels drop drastically. This sudden withdrawal of hormonal support is followed by a rapid deterioration of the blood vessels in the endometrium. The living cells die without blood to nourish them with oxygen. These dead cells from the endometrial tissue, along with blood and some mucus, form the menstrual fluid, which leaves the body through the vagina. The bleeding soon stops, and the endometrial cycle begins anew.

THE CHANGE OF LIFE

The term *change of life* describes a new pattern. At about age forty-three, the ovaries begin their slow and gradual approach toward menopause. By menopause, the ovary's supply of eggs is almost depleted, although a few may still remain. Developmental processes are beautifully synchronized in nature. It takes about seven years from the first menstrual period until a woman is fully fertile, and it takes about seven years for the reverse process (total infertility) to be complete. During this time, the ovaries gradually lose their ability to ovulate a follicle. The cycle of follicle swelling continues to occur, but the ovulation and subsequent corpus-luteum development increasingly fail to occur. Without ovulation, there cannot be conception. Pregnancy after unprotected intercourse becomes rarer as women move through their forties and may have fewer ovulatory cycles. And any pregnancy that does occur is more likely to result in a child with birth defects.

Why the menopause occurs when it does is probably related to the gradual loss of eggs throughout life. But there must be other factors

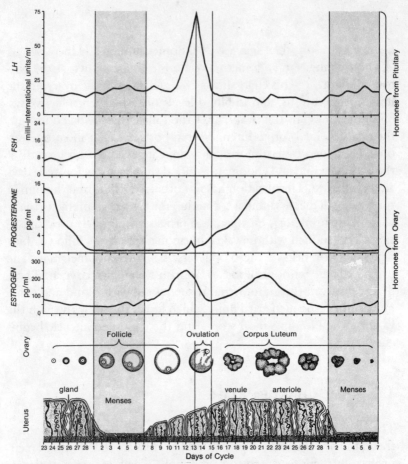

FIGURE 2 The Menstrual Cycle: Monthly Changes in Hormones, Ovarian Tissue, and the Endometrium

This chart shows what is happening in different places at different times of the monthly cycle. For example, select day 2 of the cycle (see bottom line). Then look up in a straight line to see all the things recorded for day 2. (1) The uterus is menstruating, and the lining of the womb is, therefore, thinner than on any other day of the month. (2) The ovary contains a swelling follicle surrounding the tiny egg. (3) The blood levels of hormones from the ovary are shown: first estrogen, then progesterone. Both are at relatively low levels compared to how high the levels of each will become on other days of the cycle. (4) Blood levels of the reproductive hormones produced in the pituitary are also shown. On day 2 of the cycle, both follicle stimulating hormone (FSH) and luteinizing hormone (LH) are rising. Although the units in which hormones are measured (picograms per milliliter of blood, nanograms per milliliter of blood, or milli-international units per milliliter of blood) may be unfamiliar, the essential point is to notice how the levels change from day to day until one cycle is complete. Then the levels repeat that cycle to form the rhythmic ebb and flow of hormone concentration that circulate in the blood.

involved because a few eggs do remain, even after menstrual flows have ceased. Several other, seemingly unrelated pieces of information are also known, and many investigators are trying to figure out the rest of the puzzle. Surprisingly, there is no clear relationship between the age at which a woman has her first menstrual period and her age at menopause.[3, 23] Mothers of twins begin menopause about a year earlier than other mothers,[27] but why this is so is not yet understood. In addition, a woman who smokes is likely to begin menopause sooner than one who does not, and the more she smokes, the sooner it will happen.[4, 10] We do not yet know how it happens, but it appears that smoking affects your reproductive system—it speeds the aging process.

HOW HORMONES CHANGE

As your ovary ages, its follicular tissue content decreases; and, with this, the luteal phase level of estrogen and progesterone also decreases.[17, 20, 22] Since the corpus luteum is the main source (after ovulation each month) of both progesterone and estrogen, the severe decline in the levels of these hormones in the blood is inevitable. By the time menopause has occurred, clear changes in the ovaries are evident. For one thing, the ovaries have become smaller. Only a few follicles remain, but in their place are large masses of undifferentiated tissue called *stroma* as well as scattered follicle and corpus-luteum residues that look degenerated. You can see how different the ovary of a menopausal woman looks (Plate D) by comparing it to an ovary of an infant (Plate E). The pictures are magnified several hundred times so that you can see the actual follicular sheet, described earlier.

But just because the menopausal ovary no longer ovulates each month, this does not mean that it has stopped working altogether. In fact, the central region of the ovary is filled with some healthy and very active cells that are making hormones. This region continues to work as a busy factory producing two androgens—androstenedione and testosterone—and delivers them into the blood stream.[1, 12, 13, 18] The word *androgen* is derived from the Greek *andro,* "masculine." Androstenedione and testosterone are the "male sex hormones," but women have them, too, although in much lesser quantities than do men. Older ovaries often produce more testosterone than younger

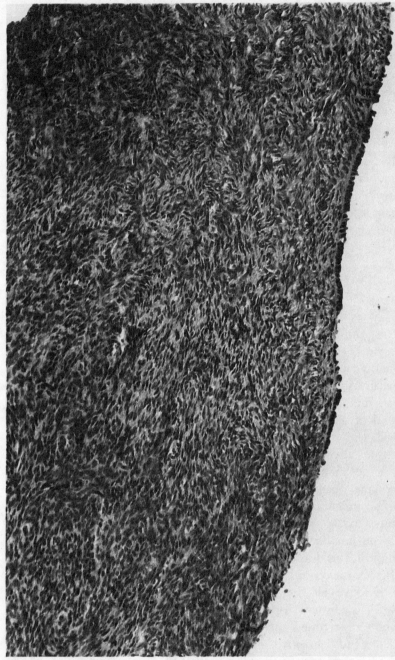

PLATE D   Light Micrograph (Magnified) of a Slice of an Ovary of a
Menopausal Woman

This magnified slice of a menopausal ovary shows part of the edge of the ovary along
the right side. Note the absence of large follicles.

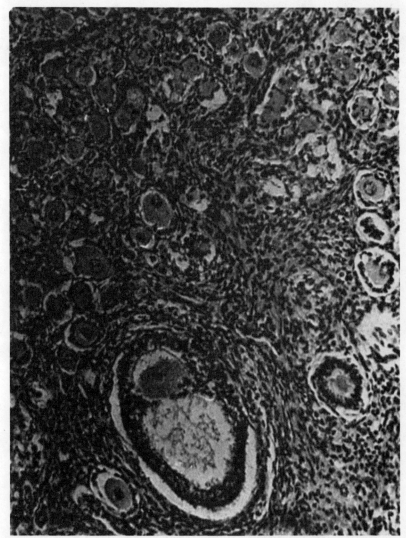

PLATE E   Light Micrograph (Magnified) of a Slice of an Infant Ovary

ones,[11] which probably accounts for the mustache so commonly found in older women.

Just because the ovaries decrease their production of estrogen does not mean that you don't have any female hormones. The cells of fat you have now play a major role in your body's hormonal milieu. The more fat you have, the more estrogen you will have.[26, 25] A fat cell acts as a miniature chemical factory. It takes up the androstenedione and converts it to estrone—a weak estrogen. The estrone is further converted, possibly by cells in the liver, into molecules of estradiol. After menopause, the major source of estrone is supplied this way.[7, 8, 8, 12] These hormones are, among other things, important for well-being, bone health, skin suppleness, and prevention of heart disease. Overall estrogen levels vary enormously among menopausal women;[16] some women have much higher levels than other women.

ESTROGENS AND ANDROGENS

In Figure 3, the two major estrogens—estradiol and estrone—are graphed in order to show how the average levels change with age. Estradiol (E2) plummets at menopause and stays low for the rest of a woman's life unless hormone replacement therapy is administered. Estrone (E1) follows a different pattern: during a woman's fifties, sixties, and seventies, estrone levels decline; after that, estrone levels increase.[2, 15, 21, 24]

When you look at Figure 3, be aware that the numbers are averages of the results of blood tests done on a group of women.[21] For any woman, her own hormonal levels not only fluctuate from day to day, but even within the day. Therefore, if you have undergone hormonal blood tests, the results may not be similar to the graph's if you happen to be at the high or low end of one of your fluctuating secretions.

This is true not only for the hormones graphed in Figure 3, but also for those graphed in Figures 4 and 5. Because of these fluctuations, a woman having her blood tested must have several samples drawn. This means that on the day she supplies blood, she should be giving three or four blood samples at least fifteen minutes apart as well as coming back several times during the month to provide data that will correctly reflect the cyclic variations. Thus, the graphs that are presented here can only be applied in research settings and should not be taken literally by the reader who wants to compare these data to her own circumstances.

The levels of androgens also show changes after the menopause (see Figure 4).[5, 16, 19, 21] And, again, one of them (dehydroepiandrosterone sulfate) continues to decline into old age, while the other (testosterone) has a different pattern: testosterone levels decrease at

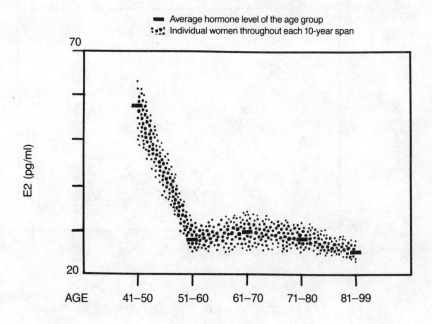

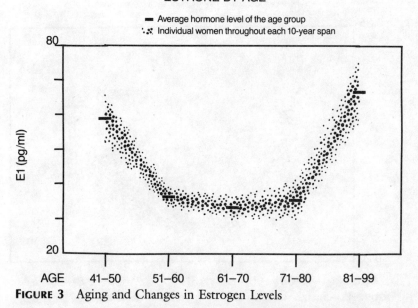

FIGURE 3 Aging and Changes in Estrogen Levels

DHEA-S BY AGE

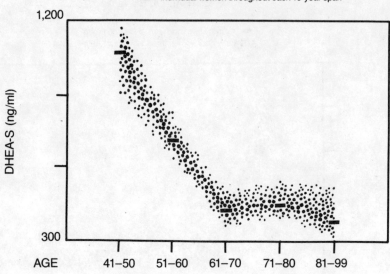

TESTOSTERONE BY AGE

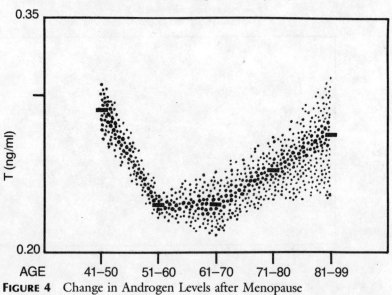

FIGURE 4 Change in Androgen Levels after Menopause

menopause but then, in each decade that follows the menopause, tend to increase.

LH AND FSH LEVELS

The levels of the two hormones from the pituitary gland that influence the ovaries—LH and FSH—also show menopausally related changes. Figure 2 illustrated how these hormones varied throughout the menstrual cycle of a fertile-aged woman. In that figure, the levels of these two hormones was shown to peak each month around the time of ovulation, maintaining relatively lower levels throughout most of the rest of the month. These two hormones also serve as a marker to learn where a woman is with respect to her menopause. In Figure 5, the LH and FSH levels are shown for women between the ages of twenty-three and their late nineties. The pattern is slightly different for each hormone. For LH, a sharp increase is noted around the time of menopause. The hormone tends to stay high for the rest of a woman's life with a mild drop in the last decade. FSH shows a similar pattern except that the increase as menopause approaches can serve to tell you that your menopause is coming. If you look at the FSH changes in women who are entering their forties, you can observe the gradual increase throughout that decade of life.[14, 16, 19, 21]

THE ADRENAL GLANDS

The adrenal glands (two of them, each resting on top of one of the two kidneys) produce a variety of hormones, including cortisol, androgens, and small amounts of estrogens and progesterone. And the central region secretes adrenaline and other substances that have an effect on elements of the nervous and vascular systems. Some of these substances affect our emotions; our emotions, in turn, affect these secretions. You can locate the adrenal glands by looking at Figure 1 (page 51). Both before and after menopause, the adrenal glands contribute small amounts of estrogen to your blood[18] as well as larger amounts of androstenedione and testosterone. But the adrenal glands also change with age, and at around age fifty to fifty-five they decrease their output of androgen (*andrenopause* is the term coined to describe this phenomenon).[6]

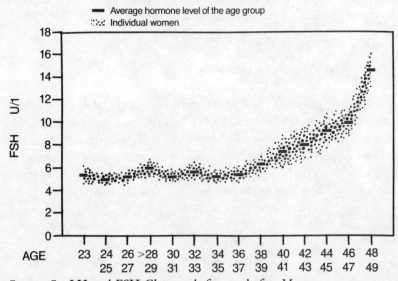

FIGURE 5 LH and FSH Changes before and after Menopause

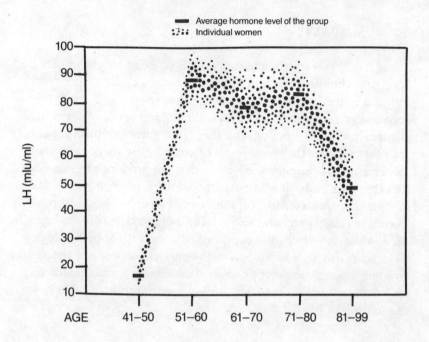

LH AFTER MENOPAUSE TRANSITION BEGINS

— Average hormone level of the group
⋮⦂⋮⋮ Individual women

LH (mIu/ml)

AGE | 41–50 | 51–60 | 61–70 | 71–80 | 81–99

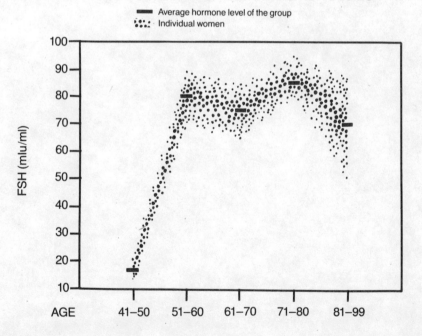

FSH AFTER MENOPAUSE TRANSITION BEGINS

— Average hormone level of the group
⋮⦂⋮⋮ Individual women

FSH (mIu/ml)

AGE | 41–50 | 51–60 | 61–70 | 71–80 | 81–99

SUMMARY

All of this may seem complicated, and it is. Here are the essentials. Sometime during a woman's forties, menstrual cycles become more irregular and eventually cease. Menopause refers to the permanent cessation of menstrual cycles and is the natural result of age-related changes in ovarian function. Another consequence of this change in the ovaries is that the blood levels of estrogen are reduced by about 75 percent—an enormous reduction that can produce a tremendous shock to your body. It is important to understand that the decrease in estrogen characteristic of a premenopausal or perimenopausal woman occurs at precisely the time that menopausal problems begin. Menopausal symptoms also appear to be caused by the body's desperate reaction to its sudden loss of hormonal support. In the next chapter, a complete description of these symptoms is presented as well as an explanation as to why menopausal transition is often called the "change of life."

2

THE CHANGE OF LIFE

I am experiencing hot flashes almost every day. When I do get a period, it seems to take everything out of me. I am beginning to have difficulty coping with people. I find I get my feelings hurt easily. I'm avoiding certain jobs, responsibilities, because I just don't feel like I can handle them well. Sexual activity is infrequent [and] I find myself thinking of it less and less. Never seems to fit into my schedule. Roughly one week before I start a period, I get either terribly irritated at everyone and everything or extremely sensitive and feel like weeping over nothing. I never had the high ups and such low-downs as I have now.

I really haven't had too much discomfort physically but emotionally I have become more and more depressed. It's amazing how much better I feel after I get my period. I feel young again. Maybe I'm afraid of getting old.

I am delighted to no longer have menstrual periods as I always had painful ones—even within 3 periods of the birth of a baby. I am also very happy to have the remote possibility of pregnancy gone from my life. Since I had had the operation [mastectomy] I was never given any hormones and don't feel that I ever needed them. I was given meprobamate as a tranquilizer from my surgery in 1969 till lately. I have stopped refilling the prescription on my own because I feel I can get along just fine with nothing.

I have a general feeling of being old and fat and middle-aged—low self-image.

THE CHANGE

The term *change of life* refers to a process of biological change that takes place in a woman's body over a span of about seven years.[14, 26, 33,]

[50, 56, 57] During this time, her menstrual cycles become increasingly irregular; at the end of this time—usually at around the age of fifty—menopause begins.[30, 34, 56, 57, 58, 59, 60] These menstrual changes vary from woman to woman. Some women experience more frequent menstrual cycles than they had before this change began. Menstruation every twenty days or so is not uncommon. Others menstruate much less frequently, even as rarely as once a year.[58] Some women experience no change in cycle length but find that their flow pattern is different than it had been. You might find that the number of days or the amount of your flow has diminished, or that either or both have increased. Mixed patterns are also common. You might, for example, experience shorter cycles of heavier bleeding or infrequent menses with many days of very light flow. Just as likely, you might have a short cycle followed by a long one and continued unpredictable cycles for several years. If you haven't menstruated for six months, you can be 90 percent sure that you will not menstruate again.[24] But many women oscillate between intervals of no menses and periods of irregular menses for a number of years. The point is that there are no fixed patterns of change. There are wide varieties of changes possible, and they are all normal in healthy women.

The time during which your cycle is changing but before you have reached menopause is called the *premenopause* or the *perimenopause*. The Stanford Menopause Study, mentioned earlier in this book, began with normal, healthy, perimenopausal women. About 20 percent of them found that their menstrual flow had become so heavy or so continuous that dressing fastidiously was difficult for them. If you have these kinds of bleeding problems, seek help from your doctor. But even if your doctor examines you and says "You are okay—there is no disease—you are just approaching menopause," that does not make your problem any easier. Excessive bleeding weakens your system and can leave you feeling fatigued and lethargic. What you must remember is that if you are experiencing long and heavy or erratic bleeding, you can obtain relief through proper medical management.[16] This will usually involve getting some progesterone, either by injection or pill. Ask your doctor about this. It is worth the time to correct the problem.

Oral contraceptives—hormone replacement therapy—if appropriately prescribed in low doses, will probably reduce excessive menstrual bleeding, regulate the menstrual cycle, restore energy, as well as set in motion other positive benefits. It will be critical to determine whether hormones are appropriate for you because not everybody should take them. Until 1989, it was standard medical practice to avoid the use of oral contraceptives after the age of thirty-five (as well as hormone replacement therapies before age fifty) because of their association with myocardial infarction and stroke. We now know better. A number of competent medical scholars believe that it is improper and not justified to withhold routinely either oral contraceptives or other hormonal regimens for all nonsmoking women after the age of thirty-five.[30, 42, 52] We will have more to say about this in Chapters 5, 6, and 7.

If you were premenopausal and experiencing fairly regular menstrual cycles, your estrogen, progesterone, and testosterone levels would be constantly changing from day to day in a predictable and orderly rhythm. The ebb and flow of reproductive hormones during the cycling years is like a well-orchestrated symphony and equally as elegant. But as you enter your menopausal transition years, the new and irregular pattern of menstrual cycling reflects major upheavals in your hormonal milieu, caused at least in part by the decreasing presence of estrogens in your body. Your body is likely to respond to this decrease in a number of ways that generally cause a predictable pattern of physical and emotional distress.[28, 49, 55] These discomforts comprise the symptoms associated with both the perimenopause and the menopause. While many of these discomforts disappear several years after the last menstrual period, the experience of them can be especially unsettling if you do not know what to expect.

PREMATURE MENOPAUSE

Although a woman's average age at her last menstrual period is about fifty years, many women enter menopause as early as age forty-one or forty-two and as late as age fifty-seven or sixty. When menopause occurs before age forty, it is considered "premature" and becomes a source of problems. First, it shortens the childbearing years; and for those who may have waited to have children, the premature menopause may eliminate the chances for a family. Research is now being conducted on treatment methods to facilitate pregnancy in prematurely menopausal women.[1, 5, 40] At this writing, unfortunately, the fertility rate is still very low for prematurely menopausal women who have undergone hormonal therapies and despite efforts to overcome what is now understood to be autoimmune endocrine diseases.[5] Fortunately, less than 1 percent of women are prematurely menopausal naturally—that is, their menopause is not a result of hysterectomy and oophorectomy.[40] But if you are one of these women, it may be years before substantive family-planning help (to promote pregnancy in those who do experience a premature menopause) is readily available—providing your moral or religious values do not preclude this approach. Perhaps the most promising treatment on the horizon uses natural estrogen and progesterone transdermally (applied to the skin for absorption into the blood stream), which seems to produce an endometrial response adequate enough to permit implantation of a fertilized egg.[1, 22]

The other serious problem for women who are undergoing premature menopause is the earlier onset of menopausal symptoms associated with aging. These symptoms—particularly the loss of bone, the increased risk of cardiovascular disease, and the deterioration of the urogenital tract—respond well to hormone replacement therapies and other treatments. The same treatment that a menopausal woman would consider is also appropriate for a prematurely menopausal woman. These hormonal treatments are addressed in Chapters 5 through 7. Alternative treatments are reviewed in Chapters 4, 6, and 14.

THE SYMPTOMS OF MENOPAUSE

HOT FLASHES

What happens during a hot flash? In 1975, actual measurements were recorded.[35] A menopausal woman lay nude on a nylon net bed and was connected to instruments that monitored her physiological changes. Each flash lasted about 3½ minutes. During the flash, there was a sudden rise in her skin temperature of about 1 to 4 degrees Fahrenheit. At the beginning of the flash, her heart would suddenly beat much faster; but as the flash progressed, her heart rate would return to normal. Any time the brain perceives that the body is overheated, whether from fever or another source, a series of reflex changes in blood flow predictably causes the body to attempt to relieve itself from this heat: blood vessels near the skin dilate; blood pours into this path, bringing heat to the skin; the heated skin begins to perspire; and evaporation cools things down. So it is with the hot flash: the brain gets a sudden signal that the body is too hot. We do not yet know what triggers the hot-flash signal since there is no fever, but the reflex response just described occurs anyway.

For the woman whose case study is being detailed, each time a flash started, she reported a sudden shock of intense heat. She showed a rapidly accelerating heartbeat and sweat profusely on her forehead and nose, moderately on her chest and adjacent regions, but not at all on her cheeks. Her water loss from each flash episode was about 1 teaspoon. These changes in temperature were widespread throughout her body. In fact, even the finger and toe temperatures showed a sharp rise at the beginning of a flash. Then they returned to normal several minutes after the flash had ended. This woman's reaction is not unique; other investigators have reported the same general pattern in their studies.

Hot flashes can be alarming, not unlike breaking out into a cold sweat in response to a frightening experience. Here, several women describe what hot flashes feel like:

Since reaching menopause, I have experienced frequent hot flashes where it even seems as though I could feel much more comfortable without my skin.

I perspire profusely with perspiration running down my face and my back. It lasts for a few minutes and then I feel chilled.

Occasional hot flash—feel like a boiled tomato with skin ready to burst— mild perspiration.

The hot flashes are very intense but of short duration. It is mostly my head that feels very hot. Sometimes my ears and my face get red. There also seems to be an increase in pressure in my head at that time. The hot flashes come frequently when I have them but there are long stretches of time when I do not have any. While they are very uncomfortable, except for my fear that other people will notice that my face is getting red, they have not interfered with my life at all.

I always claimed that my thermostat went crazy and even today I go from hot to cold and back again—a little uncomfortable but nothing I cannot live with. A minimum dosage of estrogen has been prescribed.

Hot flashes are experienced by more than 85 percent of women going through menopause, although there is a wide variation in how often the flashes come and how hard they hit.[2, 13, 31, 53] For example, one study of 400 Danish women showed that half of the women who were fifty to sixty years old were currently experiencing hot flashes.[37] For some, only a few mild flashes each week or so will occur. For others (25 percent to 50 percent), flashes can be very troublesome even ten years after the last menstrual period.[6, 23, 48] In severe cases, hot flashes may come as often as six or seven times every hour, and this pattern can last for many years. For two out of three women, hot flashes start well before the last menstruation arrives.[53] Generally, the flashes increase dramatically at menopause and continue to occur, with intermittent flash-free periods (sometimes lasting several months), for about the next five years.[1a] When a woman first begins to experience flashing, the flushes are infrequent and are felt on the face and neck only. Once they start, they tend to get worse before they get better.

Although hot flashes are not dangerous, they are uncomfortable. Moreover, the discomfort is special: it is not the same as being simply overheated. One group of investigators used hot water bottles and blankets in order to learn whether they could induce hot flashes in premenopausal women by making the women very warm. They couldn't. Even when premenopausal women are heated up by external means, they do not show the change in heart rate and blood pressure typical of a menopausal hot flush.[50]

But hot flashes *are* aggravated by hot weather.[36] While hot summer weather probably won't cause hot flashes, it may contribute to your distress if you are having periods of flushing. In one study of several menopausal women conducted during the months of June and July, hot flashes occurred more frequently on hotter days than on cooler days.[11]

We know that hot flashes are caused by a decrease in estrogen, because (1) flashes appear in association with the fall in estrogen that is characteristic of the change of life, and (2) they are eliminated when estrogen is taken. But why does a flash come when it does? What causes it? The onset of a hot flash corresponds to an increase in the blood level of the pituitary hormone called "luteinizing hormone"—LH for short.[9, 51] Significant changes in levels and rhythms of LH secretion are common as menopause nears[41] and appear to be one of the responses the body makes to the shrinking ovary's decrease of estrogen secretion. But other internal secretion surges also occur during hot flashes.[26, 46] Furthermore, just after the flash, other hormonal changes occur. For example, a significant rise in the blood level of some of the adrenal hormones (dehydroepiandrosterone, androstenedione, and cortisol) also occurs at this time.[33] Although there are clear relationships between hot flashes and specific hormone changes, the issues are complex[8] and we don't yet know whether or not these changes actually produce the flash.

NIGHT SWEATS

About a year after I discontinued use of the [oral contraceptive] pill, I started mild menopause symptoms. For the next five years I went through the sudden hot flashes of the skin and the night sweats, etc. But the symptoms weren't consistent enough to alarm me.

Because of flashes up to about 2 months ago, my husband sleeps by himself—so I can have more comfort alone. It is impossible to sleep with anyone as I am wet over most of my body and have to open windows.

Night sweats appear to be the sleep-time equivalent of daytime hot flashes. If you have them, you will be waking up hot and drenched with sweat. Most women who experience night sweats also have daytime hot flashes, but the reverse doesn't always occur. That is, if you have hot flashes during the day, you won't necessarily have night sweats.[53] Night sweats can also be a symptom of emotional distress or medical disease, neither of which has anything to do with the menopause. But if you begin to experience night sweats while you are having daytime hot flashes, they are probably a part of your change of life.

If you are perimenopausal (still cycling, though erratically) or postmenopausal and find yourself awakening in the night a great deal, night sweats may be one reason for this. Sleeplessness in postmenopausal women has been studied and has always been found to be closely linked with night sweats.[53] In the Stanford Menopause Study, women described waking up after they had thrown off their covers to relieve the intense heat of a flash. Often, they had to get up to change their clothing and bed linen because one or both would be drenched with sweat. The most severe cases involved several changes each night.

If you are having a similar experience, you should be aware that polyester and nylon (in nightclothes and bed linen) act like sheets of plastic wrap holding the sweat next to your body, thus intensifying your discomfort. Switching to pure cotton clothing and bed linen should help you find some relief.

What can we conclude about hot flashes? The flash is a real physiological process. An intense, feverlike heat comes suddenly, lasts a minute or two or three, and then disappears. The heart rhythm goes wild. The flash leaves in its wake a sweaty face and chest. A flash is uncomfortable, and the accompanying skin flush and sweating can be embarrassing. Sudden and intense sweating in the middle of a business or social situation can be a disquieting challenge to one's dignity. But a simple remedy does provide rapid, though temporary, relief. Cooling yourself with a fan or cold water splashed on your cheeks ends the flash faster.

A lot of women take vitamin E, thinking it might help. In fact it doesn't, according to carefully controlled studies.[27, 19] What does help, if cooling proves inadequate, is estrogen therapy in a dosage sufficient to compensate for your newly changing ovarian declines.[7, 10, 14] We will say more about this in Chapters 5 and 6. And if you cannot take hormone therapy, Chapter 14 will offer some alternatives.

SKIN AGING

Your skin ages more rapidly at menopause.[38, 39, 43, 44] As the estrogen level declines, the skin gradually loses both its thickness and some of its fluid. As a consequence, it rapidly begins to look older. Your sensitivity to the ultraviolet rays of the sun also increases as you grow older because the number of tanning pigments (melanocytes) decreases the older you get.[32] Therefore, with the approach of the menopause you should take great care to avoid overexposure to the sun.

LOSS OF LIBIDO

A large proportion of perimenopausal and postmenopausal women apparently experience a decline in sexual interest.[25] In the Stanford Menopause Study, 71 percent of the women made comments about changes in their interest in sex since they had noted changes in their menstrual cycles. Forty-eight percent reported a noticeable decline in sexual interest, and most were distressed about this. Twenty-three percent observed an increase in libido. And 29 percent reported that interest in sex was unchanged. Therefore, regardless of your personal experience, a good number of women are experiencing things in pretty much the same way. We will discuss changing sexuality in Chapter 8.

OFFENSIVE MENSTRUAL ODOR

A number of the perimenopausal women in the Stanford Menopause Study described a problem they had that had never happened to them before—an offensive odor when they menstruated. Unfortunately, scientists do not know a great deal about this. The fluid of the vagina normally tends to be acidic, much the way vinegar or lemon juice is. The natural acid provides a hostile environment to most bacteria. Vaginal acidity does change as the estrogen levels decline,[47] and odorous bacteria, without the high acid level to kill them, may begin to flourish in the vaginal tract. Trying an acidic remedy like one of the vaginal pH creams may be sufficient for most simple bacterial infections. More stubborn infections may require more specific aggressive treatment.

MEMORY LOSS

Although this phenomenon has not been carefully documented, a great many Stanford women, as well as women studied by Dr. Barbara Sherwin,[47a, 47b] mentioned that they had recently noticed a memory-loss problem. They made comments like "I forget appointments," "Things which used to be easy to remember now take effort," "I forget where I put things." This could be due to hardening of the arteries, another problem that occurs in estrogen-deficient individuals. If this is happening to you, you might reduce the amount of fatty foods in your diet. This common-sense approach can only enhance your health.

VISUAL DEFICITS

This problem also has not been systematically studied. Many women reported that with the change in their cycles, they had noticed changes in their visual abilities. They had trouble seeing road signs. They needed to change eyeglass prescriptions. Is the problem related to hormone changes at menopause? Only future studies can say.

FORMICATION

Skin tingling or a feeling that unseen insects are crawling across your skin is called formication. It is a symptom of menopausal distress.[23, 27] A study of a group of 5,000 women revealed that the greatest incidence of formication happened within twelve to twenty-four months after the last menstrual period, when 20 percent of the menopausal women reported the problem. About 10 percent of women continued to be annoyed with the formication for more than twelve years after the menopause. Eventually, it disappears, but its cause is still unknown.

BACKACHE

Backache is common. Nonradiating pains (that is, the pains are localized and do not spread outward from the point of origin) begin at the lower back, and these may indicate the beginning of a loss in bone structure. This condition, known as osteoporosis, is discussed in detail in Chapter 4.

EMOTIONAL DISTRESS

Much research is needed in this area but is very difficult to conduct. Consider these comments from women:

Sometimes I get a sort of "trembly" roller coaster ride feeling . . . just a trembly feeling like you'd have after the roller coaster ride. It's so hard to put into words, really. Fluttering; trembling; uneasy. Guess they could all be lumped under the heading of "anxiety." A vague uneasiness.

I have become more aggressive, more outspoken and assertive, less patient. I am easier on myself and less caring about what others think. Sexual activity has become much more enjoyable. My libido is increasing all the time and I look forward to sex. I don't seem to mind aging. I actually enjoy the maturing process.

Never had hot flashes, or other symptoms. Did undergo depression—for which I had to be treated—but doctors were unable to agree on whether or not it was the result of menopause or other factors at the time. My personal feeling is that I did suffer some kind of chemical imbalance which may have triggered depression. Extreme tension and stress since then have not produced another depression (thank God)!

*I am often irritable and cranky without any good reason . . . cry often. I
often feel very depressed for no reason at all and have very little energy. This
all occurred very seldomly before.*

Of course, headache, depression, anxiety, listlessness, insomnia,
and backache also happen to women who are not menopausal. Still,
the fact is that these things are experienced by many menopausal
women. And if you are experiencing them, it may be useful to know
that sleep disturbances do respond well to estrogen therapy[23, 27, 54]
(see Chapter 5).

GENITAL AND URINARY-SYSTEM ATROPHY

Estrogen deficiencies lead to deterioration (thinning) in the urethra,
bladder, vagina, and surrounding labial skin. The cells deteriorate,
dry out, and produce an easily bruised surface. Repeated urinary-tract
infections are common and are frequently accompanied by painful
urination and local vaginal symptoms.[4] These infections are usually
reversed when estrogen therapy is administered.

SLEEPING PROBLEMS

Night sweats can make getting a good night's rest difficult, but hormones may help. In laboratory experiments with menopausal and
perimenopausal women, estrogen users fell asleep faster than women
getting a placebo. Women getting estrogen also spent more time in
the deepest—dreaming—stage of sleep. And they felt better. The
dreaming stage of sleep appears to be particularly important for the
feeling of rest and renewal that comes from sleeping. It is possible
that sleeping problems have a lot to do with the decrease in the sense
of well-being that many menopausal women talk about.[45]

HOW SERIOUS ARE YOUR MENOPAUSAL SYMPTOMS?

The table below, which you may use to calculate your menopausal
distress, will allow you to estimate how mild or serious your situation
is. Although the Kupperman index includes several symptoms that
we have not described—such as nervousness, vertigo, and head-

ache—and omits others that we have mentioned here—such as loss of libido and visual deficits—the scale has been well validated in double-blind placebo-controlled studies. For this reason, we have not modified the table, but have kept it as Kupperman created it.

WHO EXPERIENCES MENOPAUSAL DISTRESS?

Menopausal distress (hot flashes, night sweats, libidinal changes, etc.) affects both healthy and not-so-healthy women, and your general level of health doesn't seem to have much to do with whether you will suffer or escape from menopausal distress.[2] However, some women are more at risk than others. Specifically, according to studies published in the "pre-women's-liberation era" married women experience worse symptoms than single women;[2, 23] those who have given birth have worse symptoms than those who have not,[23] and those who experienced painful menstruation when younger are more likely to experience menopausal distress when older.[2] The facts are clear; at the moment, the reasons are not.

TABLE 1 Calculation of Menopausal Distress[27]

Each menopausal symptom is listed with a given "factor." In the column entitled "Severity," enter the number that reflects the severity of your current experience: 0 for none, 1 for slight, 2 for moderate, and 3 for heavy. Then multiply your severity score by the listed factor to arrive at the numerical conversion.

If, after you have totaled the numerical-conversion column, your score (known as the Kupperman Menopausal Index) is more than 35, you have severe menopausal symptoms; if your score is less than 20, your symptoms are mild.

SYMPTOM	FACTOR	×	SEVERITY (0–3)	=	NUMERICAL CONVERSION
Hot flashes/night sweats	4	×	_____	=	_____
Prickling/burning	2	×	_____	=	_____
Insomnia	2	×	_____	=	_____
Nervousness	2	×	_____	=	_____
Melancholia (depression)	1	×	_____	=	_____
Vertigo (dizziness)	1	×	_____	=	_____
Weakness (fatigue)	1	×	_____	=	_____
Muscle/joint pain	1	×	_____	=	_____
Headache	1	×	_____	=	_____
Palpitations	1	×	_____	=	_____
Formication (itchy feeling on the skin)	1	×	_____	=	_____
Kupperman Menopausal Index (total):					_____

Although some still believe that women with menopausal distress are simply neurotic, a careful and critical review of the literature shows that most menopausal distress is hormonally caused and hormonally cured. Yet even today, some student health professionals are taught that "these [menopausal] symptoms are of sufficient magnitude in approximately 15 percent to warrant treatment. If psychotherapy fails, daily administration of estrogen . . . will reverse the symptoms."[18] The implication of this teaching is that not only are most menopausal symptoms psychologically based, but that psychotherapy is the preferred treatment for these symptoms. However, research shows that psychotherapy is irrelevant; what's important is replacing the hormones whose absence is causing the symptoms.

One investigator reported that there were no appreciable differences in personality traits among women who did and who did not have menopausal distress. Nor were there any detectable personality changes within individuals after successful hormone treatment. Neurosis and menopause troubles were not related. One can imagine how real distress could cause a woman to seek medical help. And if her "help" takes the form of insinuations that she is neurotic, she could begin to lose confidence in her own perceptions, thereby fulfilling this diagnosis while still suffering the real distress associated with menopause. One woman at Stanford illustrated such a case:

Women on both sides of my family have had lots of atherosclerotic heart disease, manifesting itself at menopause. I'm concerned about this for reasons which I consider valid, but most doctors consider neurotic. In some ways, my stress EKG was borderline; i.e., very poor exercise tolerance for a woman of my age (44) and weight (slender)—yet I've been dealt with as a bored housewife (which I am not).

Several studies involving large groups of women have explored possible relationships among roles, behaviors, and a tendency toward menopausal distress. The assumption underlying the questions has been that there must be a large psychological component in the perception of distress and that culturally accepted norms might be at the root of a woman's self-perception. The possibility that women in Western society reach menopause only to find an "empty nest" and suddenly empty days was considered by several investigators. They reasoned that roles which were forced on women had tended to restrict the women to raising children and keeping house.

Many of today's menopausal women have found themselves at the tail end of the women's movement. Even if they agree with its tenets of career rights for women, they may perceive twenty to thirty years of housekeeping as an insurmountable obstacle toward major change in their lives. At this point, they may want a career but feel overwhelmed by difficulties such as little or no career training or knowing how to handle an interview. In short, there can be a general feeling of incompetence due to lack of marketable skills.

Children often leave home or enter adolescence with all its difficulties at just about the time that many women are entering menopause. Could all the complaints of menopause be a simple reaction to a feeling that life has nothing further to offer? Is the reason that unmarried women have less distress simply that they have suffered no sudden loss of meaning coinciding with their menopause? Some health professionals thought so.

Pauline Bart, a well-respected social scientist, described depression problems in middle-aged women. She expressed her belief that our society has robbed women of a place of esteem at menopause.[3] You have only to look at the media, with their adoration of youth and beauty and their advertisements to "hide that gray" or camouflage wrinkles, to see her point.

If menopausal symptoms are the result of society's treatment of women, then we would expect to find no symptoms in those societies that revere their aging women and show this by affording them special privileges and honors. For example, the Hutterites (a culturally isolated sect of North America) automatically relieve the woman of her heavy jobs in agriculture when she reaches forty-five to fifty. They show an increased admiration for their maturing women, which is reflected in the older women's domination of their extended family.[20] Another well-characterized "primitive culture," the Quemant (a pagan Hebraic peasant group of Ethiopia), allows the menopausal woman the special privilege of treading upon normally taboo village sites. Furthermore, only after menopause does a woman reach sufficient status to be allowed to come in contact with ritual food and beverage.[17] Although both cultures revere their aging women, no study has ever evaluated menopausal distress in these societies.

Are there cultures in which women do not have menopausal symptoms? One study[15] of 483 women in one caste in India reported an absence of menopausal symptoms in the women interviewed, none of whom spoke English. No mention of hot flashes or other menopausal distress symptoms was made by any of them, which seemed to suggest to the author of the study that these women did not experience any. If it were true that hot flashes—the major symptom of menopause—are culturally induced, this would provide some extraordinary evidence for the influence of culture on individual hormone processes. However, our careful examination of the details of data collection showed that the research design itself had practically prohibited mention of hot flashes. Each woman in the study was asked a long series of questions about her marital, reproductive, and family history in the public circle of the women of her village. Only one question about menopause was asked, and this had nothing to do with hot flashes: "Any complications of menopause such as hysterectomy or prolapse?" This one question was embedded within a series of other questions that were concerned with nonmenopausal issues. Consider that only the very serious conditions of hysterectomy (surgical removal of the uterus) and prolapse (the dropping of the uterus into or out of the vagina) were mentioned. Even if a woman were suffering from hot flashes, this form of questioning might have obscured that fact. Although this important study has been widely quoted, it has not proved that flashes are a culturally induced pathology.

More recently, a large study of Japanese women[29] did show some cultural differences in the experience of symptoms at menopause. Eleven hundred women were studied as well as physicians in order to learn the Japanese view on the menopause—both by its women and by its medical community. As its authors, experts in Japanese culture, point out, self-control and balance are considered an integral part of health, and healthy people repress physical and psychological symptoms. In this culture, symptoms occur at menopause, but women tend to not want to experience them or to acknowledge them. Although only 10 percent of the women reported experiencing hot flashes, two other symptoms at menopause—"stiff shoulders" and headache—occurred with great frequency: more than half of the women reported having "stiff shoulders" during their menopause, and 27 percent had headaches. It would seem that in Japan, menopausal distress is more likely to be manifest in these symptoms rather than in the symptoms more common to Western women.

Thus, in every culture that has been carefully studied, real physical stresses do emerge at the time of the menopause.

Summary

The "change of life" is a process that women go through as they approach and pass through their menopause. It has many manifestations. Menstrual cycles become more irregular and eventually cease. This reflects the natural life history of the ovaries. One critical result of the changing ovary is a decrease in the amount of estrogen in the body. When your menstrual cycles become irregular, the chances are strong that you will experience some of the symptoms described in this chapter.[9, 11, 14, 17, 25, 26, 31, 33, 50, 56, 57] Hot flashes and some degree of emotional distress are common.

Women tend to suffer alone. However, talking with others who have long since passed through their change of life is likely to be a reassuring experience. You will find that you are not alone and that eventually things will readjust for the better. Comparing notes with other women should not only assure you of the realities of the menopause, but help you to realize that relief is available.

3

BODY CHANGES AT THE MENOPAUSE

I feel that my body is changing but I really can't understand how it is or what is changing.

I had always heard that a shock sometimes stopped periods permanently and this happened to me. At 52, I was still having regular, normal periods although I started slowly the first day. This was happening when I got word my Mother had died. My period never developed and I never had another one.

A woman's body changes in a number of well-understood ways as the menopause approaches.

HOW SKIN AGES

Estrogens decline at menopause, usually accelerating skin aging. Therefore, you need to take special care of your skin after age forty. There is beauty at every age, and since skin is one of the main surface reflections of your beauty, it makes sense to focus on this area first.

With increasing age a number of skin changes occur.[20] These include

- decreased tensile strength (that is, ability to tense up)
- decreased compressibility and mobility

- decreased or general loss of turgor (firmness coming from water-filled cells)
- slight decreases in total skin collagen (one of the main supporting proteins)
- a continual loss of melanocytes (the cells that manufacture melanin, the pigment that causes your skin to tan)

One of the most important things you can do is to guard your skin from the damaging rays of the sun. As the years pass, you will be less protected from exposure to sunlight because the number of melanocyte cells in your skin decreases by 10 percent to 15 percent each decade.[17] Sun screens are relatively new. Those that retard ultraviolet radiation are most helpful for maintaining the vigor and attractiveness of your skin. Since overexposure to sun is bad, it would be most prudent, where possible, to limit your exposure. If you avoid sunbathing or at least limit it to the early and late hours of the day, you will reduce the intensity of your exposure to the aging effects of ultraviolet rays: the rays are less powerful when the sun is less bright.

When you think of skin, you may think of tissue that is on the outside of your body. Similar kinds of cells (epithelia) also line the urinary tract as well as the vagina. So it is not surprising to find changes in both of these areas when skin starts to change.

How Hair Growth Changes

Two kinds of (male pattern) hair-growth changes are common at the menopausal transition and beyond.[24] Some women experience a loss of hair—the medical term is *alopecia*. An excess of androgen appears to be responsible. For those who suffer from alopecia, the average age of onset is about forty.[15] At present, there is no known cure, including the application of estrogen directly to the scalp.

Hirsutism, the growth of excessive dark hair, is another problem that plagues many perimenopausal and postmenopausal women. Generally, both men and women have two kinds of hair: the fine, unpigmented hairs that usually cover most of the body, and the darker, thicker hairs that are responsive to sex hormones. These sex-hormone–responsive hairs are located on the pubis, underarm, back, face, chest, and lower abdomen in women. Androgens circulating in the blood promote the conversion of fine, unpigmented hairs to dark, thick hairs.[24] There are increasing reports that stress can stimulate the adrenal glands to increase androgen secretion at any age, and this may bring about such skin changes as acne and hair growth. The hair grows in cycles: first a stage of growth, then a stage of rest. Estrogens promote the growth phase, and women with higher levels of estrogen probably can grow their hair longer than women with lower levels of estrogen.

Obesity may promote hirsutism. Unfortunately, facial hirsutism gets worse with age, probably due to obesity-induced changes in hormonal metabolism.[27] A small (5 percent) minority of cases of hirsutism is due to the response of one particular disease—congenital adrenal hyperplasia.[1] Table 2 shows the causes of hirsutism in women.

If you suffer from this problem, you must identify the cause before

TABLE 2   Causes of Hirsutism in Women[24]

Estrogen-mediated
Ovarian
   Polycystic ovary syndrome
   Insulin resistance
   Ovarian tumors
Adrenal
   ACTH-dependent Cushing's syndrome*
   Androgen-producing tumors
   Congenital adrenal hyperplasia (classic and attenuated forms)
      11-hydroxylase deficiency
      21-hydroxylase deficiency
      3-β-hydroxysteroid dehydrogenase deficiency
Combined ovarian and adrenal
   Idiopathic hirsutism (mostly ovarian)
   Polycystic ovary syndrome secondary to adrenal hyperandrogenism
Exogenous medications
   Androgens, impeded androgens, or anabolic steroids
   Birth-control pills (uncommon)
Androgen-independent (drug-induced)
   Minoxidil
   Diazoxide
   Phenytoin
   Glucocorticoids
   Cyclosporine

*ACTH = adrenocorticotropic hormone.

an attempt at treatment is made. If no satisfactory treatments are available, you might try a product available in many drug stores and mail-order catalogues that helps you to pluck out the hairs, gradually helping to diminish their regrowth. This product, called Finally Free (manufactured by the Selvac Corporation), sells for about $95.00 and does work. Four problems with electrolysis render Finally Free a better choice:

- The potential for scarring in electrolysis is absent.
- The curved hair shaft can be treated.
- This treatment is less painful than electrolysis.
- This treatment can be done at home by the woman herself.

Although it is tedious to use, it is no more tedious than tweezers and preferable to electrolysis. Each time a hair is removed, what grows in during the next cycle is much thinner and lighter than the hair that was plucked. Eventually, the hairs disappear.

BREAST AND ABDOMINAL CHANGES

As women get older, their breasts tend to flatten and sag. The larger the breasts, the greater the tendency to flatten. There is a physiological reason for this. Breast tissue responds to many hormones, including estrogens, prolactin, oxytocin, and prostaglandins. As the hormone levels change with the progression of the menopause, there is a reduction of estrogen stimulation to all tissue, including the breast. As a consequence, the breasts begin to lose their earlier fullness. Women who take hormone therapy (see Chapters 6 and 8), however, will find some restoration of this fullness, the response lasting as long as hormones are available.

Because breast cancer is among the most common of the female cancers, it is very important for women to examine their breasts regularly. Early detection of a cancerous tumor allows time for treatments that have a high success rate as well as a decreased likelihood of disfigurement. The breasts should be examined two ways: self-examination, which includes seeing and touching (see Appendix 3); and examination by a professional deliverer of health care, which includes visual evaluation, mammography, biopsy, and/or other methods where indicated.

Self-examination is done by standing in front of a mirror in good light and looking for dissimilarities (not in size, but in shape) between the two breasts. For example, flattening, puckering, dimpling of the skin, notable bulges, or any growths of the breast surface that appear suddenly in one breast would be cause for a medical examination. Having completed the visual inspection, the manual inspection (palpation) follows.

The breasts should be palpated periodically (about once a month). If this is being done by a premenopausal woman, the examination should take place immediately after the menstrual flow has stopped. Although some physicians suggest lying down, we feel it can also be done standing up. A sensible time to perform this is while you are showering or bathing. Because moist, soapy fingers can gently slide over the skin of the breast, compressing up and down and side to side, you will be able to feel whether there are any differences between the two breasts. Using a gentle squeezing motion, you should tug the breasts away from the body with your soapy, wet fingers. Do this on both sides, and compare one side to the other, feeling for lumpiness. These examinations should be done in two positions: with your hand at your side, and with your arm elevated and your hand touching the back of your head. Do one breast and then the other in each of the two positions. These actions will place the breasts in position for efficient exploration. As long as they feel similar on both sides, there is no cause for concern.

It is important to know that lumpy breasts and breast pain are common, occurring in about 35 percent of all women. These lumps (or cysts) usually do not bear any relationship to breast cancer. Tumors can feel similar to these lumps, but an expert can distinguish which tissue should be tested and, from the test results, the healthy from the diseased tissue. If anything feels questionable, see your physician for expert advice. Even if you have recently had your breasts checked by your health-care provider, your self-examinations should continue every month. Films and literature on breast self-examination can be obtained by calling or writing the American Cancer Society, 19 West Fifty-sixth Street, New York, NY 10019, (212) 586-8700. For further details about breast cancer and X rays, physical exams, and research, see Chapter 6.

Women who exercise regularly should not notice changes in the size and shape of the abdomen. But women who have stopped having periods and who notice sudden increases in the size of their abdomen should be warned and make an appointment to see their gynecologist. If you feel bloated or distended and your waist has grown in size, this may merely represent dietary indiscretion and inadequate exercise. But it should be noted that of women who have ovarian tumors, the sudden distension of the abdomen may be the first or only warning. So, if you do exercise, the symptom of stomach distension should be promptly reviewed with your physician, who may schedule you for a pelvic examination. And if you do not exercise, you can expect a gradual but increasing loss of abdominal-wall tone. Healthy abdominal muscles form bands of tissue that support the internal organs of the body. The use of a girdle instead of maintenance of proper muscle tone generally provides an unhealthy substitute for exercise. Wearing a girdle will actually promote the development of a lazy musculature and lead to an increase of abdominal bulging. If you have poor abdominal muscle tone, you should take steps to correct the problem. Regular exercise offers many dividends, not the least of which is a better self-image. Good muscle tone makes for attractiveness. You are never too old to begin improving your abdominal muscle tone. But do so under supervision and guidance that will reflect your own rate of exercise tolerance. Inconsistent or overzealous exercising is not beneficial and may actually be harmful. See Chapter 13.

URINARY-TRACT PROBLEMS AND BLADDER TRAINING

Changes in the condition of a woman's urethra and bladder are common (see Figure 6).[2] The urinary tract is composed chiefly of epithelial cells, smooth muscle, and blood vessels. Epithelial cells are the "lining cells" of the body and are found on all internal and external surfaces, including the lining of the urinary tract. With declines in estrogen, the epithelial lining tends to deteriorate, and muscle tone tends to diminish.[2] These changes may lead to some loss of bladder control (urinary incontinence). This may be why some menopausal women are awakened at night with an urge to urinate to a degree that they had not experienced before. Many women report the problem and find it annoying.

Not all urinary problems that women experience are of menopau-

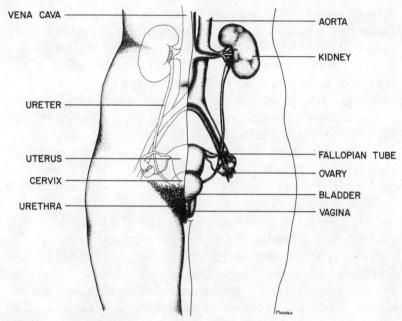

FIGURE 6   The Female Genitourinary System

sal origin. Reports also suggest that some hardening of the arteries may be responsible. When this occurs, the central nervous system undergoes some deterioration, which may lead to an increased urgency to urinate during the night.[2] Whatever the cause, the loss of control of urinary function can be very distressing. Severe problems are rare and tend not to be menopausally related since the condition occurs as often in younger as in older women.[10]

Stress incontinence—the loss of urine when under stress—is relatively more common. Mild stress incontinence involves the loss of a little urine when laughing or coughing or emotionally overwrought. It is quite common among all women and seems to increase slightly with the passing years.

Urge incontinence refers to the sensation that one needs to urinate more often than one would want to or than is reasonable. According to Leslie Talcott, M.S., R.N., who directs the Perineometer Research Institute,* in the facility's experience there is little difference

*Perineometer Research Institute, 242 Old Eagle School Road, Strafford, PA 19087, (215) 254-9412.

between patients who have stress or urge incontinence. She reports that in both cases a weak sphincter component of the pelvic muscles triggers the problem. The difference between the two conditions, then, is how the patient reacts to it. The urinary-stress patient ignores it and then is surprised when she leaks urine after a cough or a sneeze or a laugh. The urinary-urge patient, in contrast, is always thinking about urinating and rushes to the toilet at the first sign of bladder signals; the result is that she forms a habit—the brain quickly learns to stop inhibiting reflex contractions of the bladder to prevent the urge to urinate. In both cases, exercise will help, especially if there is sufficient estrogen circulating throughout the body to maintain physiologic structures.

An exercise regimen, developed in the 1950s by Dr. A. M. Kegel, has been reported to be effective in restoring bladder control. The exercise regimen requires three 20-minute sessions a day and consists of training a woman to tense the pubococcygeal muscles. These muscles form several sheets of contractile tissue in the regions around the vaginal, urethra, and anal structures. Among Dr. Kegel's first 500 reported cases, 75 percent who completed an eight-week exercise program found complete relief.[10] He noted that some of the most gratifying results were achieved among women in their eighties as well as those among who had previously failed to respond to surgery.

If you are having problems with stress incontinence, you could go to a health-care professional who would then place a transducer (pressure gauge) in your vagina and instruct you to contract the vaginal muscles that surround the transducer. He or she would probably find that your muscular function is less than adequate.[10] The fact is, however, that you may not need to undergo such a clinical process. *You* can locate and retrain these muscles in the privacy of your own home.

First, you have to find the pubococcygeal muscles that surround the vagina and anus. If you were to insert a tampon and contract the vaginal muscle (squeeze) around it, you would have located this sheet of muscle. Alternatively, contracting the anal sphincter as one would to prevent a bowel movement will also produce a tightening of these muscles. Don't worry if the first contractions seem weak; with practice, the muscles will get much stronger. Once you have found your pubococcygeal muscles, begin a practice program. One approach is to contract these muscles twenty-five to thirty times, several times each day. Keep at it, and the strength of the contractions will increase.[10] You can do the exercises throughout the day whenever you remember since no one but you need be aware that you are working on toning these muscles: the effort does not show. As the strength of the muscles increases, you will gain conscious control of the necessary muscles for bladder control. In addition, the overall muscle tone of your internal pelvic area will improve greatly. Exercise will improve your pelvic supports. Extensive vaginal relaxations often occur because of childbirth-related tissue plane weaknesses from tears and may require surgical correction if the exercises are not helpful. The simpler approach is always preferable to surgical correction. Persist in your exercise.

If you are having problems with urge incontinence, you might try delaying your trip to the bathroom, if that is feasible. According to recent studies, the reflex responses are thus restrained, and the brain now perceives the need to urinate less often. Do not delay too long, but learn to wait until your bladder is slightly fuller before you head for the bathroom.

If your efforts at exercise and/or bladder training do not work, biofeedback training with a certified biofeedback expert may help.[3] About 90 percent of the time, according to data provided by the Perineometer Research Institute, certified biofeedback experts working with incontinence patients achieve satisfactory results. To locate a certified biofeedback expert, you may want to call or write the Perineometer Research Institute (see page 89 for the address).

If, after having tried these nonsurgical approaches, they all fail, then it may be appropriate to seek medical help. However, before submitting to surgical correction, it is essential to find the specific cause of the urinary leakage.[2] Moreover, if you should opt for surgery, carefully select a gynecologist with expertise in this subspecialty—that is, urogynecology.

VAGINAL AND REPRODUCTIVE-GLAND CHANGES

THE VAGINA

When estrogen levels drop, one of the last symptoms to appear can be vaginal atrophy. To test for this, the physician may take a swab of fluid from the vagina and smear it onto a glass slide, thereby obtaining a "vaginal smear." Estrogenized vaginal smears look different under the microscope than atrophic (regressed) smears. These estrogenized vaginal smears continue to occur for some women well past menopause,[30] and it is clear that not all women lose estrogen stimulation of the vaginal tissue with increasing age. Moreover, contrary to what was formerly assumed, the vaginal skin may not always be a reliable indicator of your overall estrogen blood levels. In fact, in two studies that considered the vaginal maturation index (VMI)—a quantified score of the vaginal smear—both of them showed that estrogen levels could not be predicted by the VMI score.[11, 31]

Estrogen creams are highly effective if vaginal dryness and pain during intercourse occur. Other forms of estrogen, if the dose is sufficiently high, are also effective. But the lowest effective dose will come from a cream because it is applied directly to the site where it is used. Details of routes and dosages are covered in later chapters.

Figure 7 shows the relationships among the vagina, ovaries, uterus, and tubes.

THE OVARIES

As your ovaries mature, two distinct structural changes occur: the ovaries get smaller, and their composition changes. While the meno-

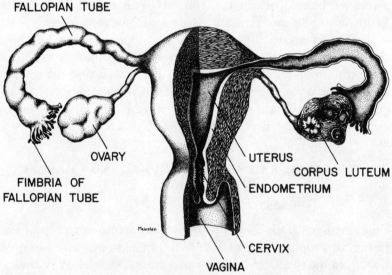

FIGURE 7 Female Reproductive Organs

pausal ovary no longer ovulates an egg each month nor continues the cycle of follicular development, ovulation, corpus-luteum development, and regression,[4] it does perform some vital functions.[12, 13, 20, 21] The idea that an old ovary is useless is incorrect. The cells of the older ovary look different. Look at Plates A through E (pages 49, 53, 54, 58, 59) to see how different they are.

The nonovulating ovary actively participates in the secretion of hormones: chiefly androstenedione.[18] The cortex (outer shell) of the ovary becomes thinner and wrinkled as the entire ovary shrinks.[7] This is to be expected since the cortex contains the primitive cells that give rise to eggs, and by menopause the original lifetime supply of eggs is almost exhausted. The inner part of the ovary (stroma) is quite different. For many women these cells can be actively secreting androgen hormones: androstenedione and testosterone.[4, 7, 14] Older ovaries often produce abundant testosterone.[16, 18, 19] Your ovaries are an important source of the hormones that promote well-being.[8] With age, the adrenal glands appear to produce estrogen in place of the ovary, but at much reduced levels.

THE UTERUS

Your uterus, or womb, is a smooth muscle with a glandular inner surface known as the endometrium. This glandular area, in a younger cycling woman, changes monthly—building up and breaking down with each menstrual cycle. The uterus also appears to produce hormones, called prostaglandins, that seem to have many influences throughout the body. Prostaglandins are produced in many body tissues. Not all of the prostaglandins' functions are completely understood.

In about half of menopausal women, the endometrium begins to regress and become what is known as "senile endometrium."[22] Although all women maintain an endometrium, in some women it may be more atrophic than in others depending on their estrogen levels.

The tip of the womb, called the cervix, resides in the top of the vagina. In surveys of young women at the University of Pennsylvania as well as of perimenopausal women at Stanford University, 30 percent to 50 percent had a definite preference for deep penile thrusting during coitus. It seems, from the women's comments on the questionnaires, that they were aware of and liked direct cervical stimulation. There are sensitive nerves located in the human cervix that are the type that fire impulses to the brain after they are stimulated.[26] As the cervix ages, these nerves gradually disappear. The whole issue of uterine involvement in sexual arousal needs to be examined in light of these and other recent reports.[5, 23, 32] On the subject of the role of the uterus in physiologic functioning, you might want to look at Dr. Cutler's *Hysterectomy: Before and After* (paperback, 1990).

Your uterus is an important part of your body. Future research will probably teach us how important an organ it is—even after the childbearing years are completed.

THE FALLOPIAN TUBES

At the top of your uterus, as an extension of it on either side, rise the Fallopian tubes. During the reproductive years these tubes are vibrant, active, and dynamic organs. Each tube connects the central core of the uterus to the area of the abdominal cavity that is near one of your ovaries. This tube not only picks up the egg through its fingerlike ends, but it is also through this tube that the sperm swim (passing first through the vagina, cervix, and uterus) toward their rendezvous with a waiting egg to start a new life.

At menopause, when estrogen levels decline, the cellular structure of the tubes, like that of the uterus, begin to regress.[9, 25]

OTHER BODY CHANGES

Other body systems also change, and these changes are discussed throughout the book. Specifically, the bones and the cardiovascular system show significant hormone-responsive changes with the maturation of ovarian hormone secretion. These are discussed in the next chapter and in Chapter 10, respectively.

SUMMARY

Major changes occur in skin, hair, breast, abdomen, urinary tract, vagina, and uterus that all begin as the reduced ovarian output of estrogens and progesterone triggers the menopausal years. One of the most critical changes, however, occurs in your bones, and this is dealt with separately in the next chapter.

4

THE BONES
AND HOW
THEY GROW

While the stuff we call bone may look solid, it is not. Actually, bone is composed of countless numbers of molecules that are bound to each other in an ever-changing array of spongy-looking but firm inner matrix and an outer compact, thinner, smooth surface. Blood vessels and nerves travel through the bone tissue just as they do through the rest of the body. Bone is comprised of calcium as well as other structural elements. Each day, calcium leaves bone and enters the blood. Other molecules of calcium, traveling in the blood, are taken up into bone and add to its mass. The different phases of this continuing cycle of bone remodeling (breaking down and building up) are controlled by a variety of hormones, including estrogen.

Figure 8 illustrates how the blood vessels and nerves insert into bone. Figure 9 shows the three kinds of bone that make up the human skeleton: the long bone (for example, an arm), the short bone (a vertebra), and the sesamoid (kneecap).

Muscles also need calcium. If there is not enough calcium in your blood to supply your muscles adequately, your bones—even at the expense of their own strength and health—will give up as much of their calcium as the muscles need. Moreover, a certain amount of calcium is excreted in urine and feces every day, and this loss must be made up in the diet.[34, 54] It is, therefore, very important for you to consume calcium on a daily basis.

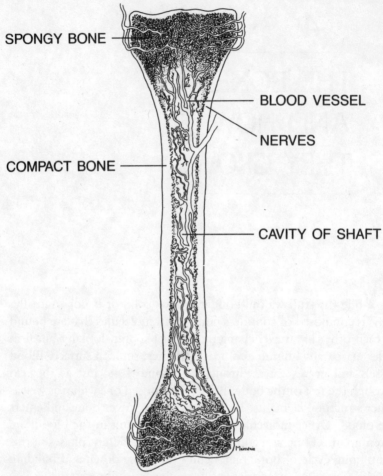

SPONGY BONE

BLOOD VESSEL

NERVES

COMPACT BONE

CAVITY OF SHAFT

FIGURE 8   Bone Structure

YOUR NEED FOR CALCIUM

Studies have shown that when you reach your perimenopausal years, your need for calcium is likely to increase. The reason is complex. Less of the dietary calcium gets absorbed into the body from the digestive tract as people get older.[17, 40, 29] Young people who eat less than the optimal amounts of calcium-rich foods appear to have a "fail-safe system" for increasing the calcium absorption of the foods they do ingest. Vitamin D (specifically the form called $1,25,OH_2D$)

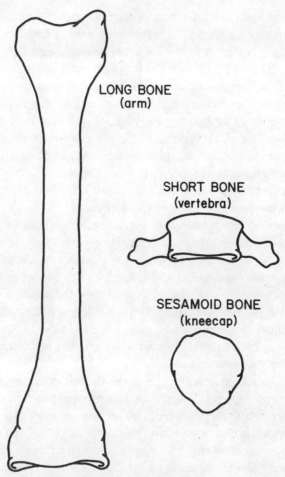

LONG BONE
(arm)

SHORT BONE
(vertebra)

SESAMOID BONE
(kneecap)

FIGURE 9   The Three Types of Bone

comes to the rescue by (so to speak) extracting the calcium passing through the intestines. The vitamin D increases the rate of transfer (uptake) of the calcium from the intestines into the body. Once the calcium passes across the walls of the intestines, it enters the blood stream and travels through the body like hormones do when traveling in blood. When people get older, this fail-safe backup system becomes less efficient.

If you are menopausal, the RDA (recommended daily allowance) for calcium given by the Food and Drug Administration is probably too low for you. Ignore the nutritional charts on the food packages you buy. The information given in percentages rather than in milligrams (mg.), and the percentages may be based on the RDA of 600 mg. per day—too low for a menopausal woman.

Exactly how much calcium you need will vary according to your unique metabolic requirements: the higher the estrogen level, the lower the calcium need. For a woman who is estrogen-rich—characteristic of her younger cycling years—or whose hormone replacement therapy is very high, 650 mg. of calcium a day may be adequate. But by menopause, most women are not estrogen-rich, even if they are taking hormone replacement therapy. To be safe, you should ingest about 1,000 mg. of calcium a day in order to prevent a loss of bone mass due to dietary inadequacy.[19, 54] But do not overdo it. Be sure to stay within a conservative range because excessive calcium could create other problems. People who have excessive blood levels of calcium show a tendency to calcification of arterial areas (promoting arteriosclerosis) and kidney stones. Moderation is the key. You can supply your calcium in an orderly fashion by looking at Table 15 (pages 266–267) to find which calcium-rich foods you prefer. The calorie content of each is also listed to help you plan. Three glasses of skim milk a day will suffice, or any other combination that provides the total needed.

Unfortunately, most women do not consume enough of this essential mineral. Large-scale studies have shown that women, on average, consume less than half of the calcium that they need.[3] One reason some women don't drink enough milk to satisfy calcium requirements is that excessive milk drinking seems to upset their stomach.[7] Skim milk might be better digested; it will be as valuable to your bone. But if you feel this way about all forms of milk, check Table 15 (pages 266–267) for other sources of calcium that you might digest more comfortably. If you find nothing that suits you, take calcium in tablet form. Calcium can be purchased without prescription. Several different brands are available, and some combine calcium and protein within one pill.

However, there have been problems with calcium pills. First, there is a problem about whether or not the pill dissolves once it gets into the stomach. Recent tests have shown that about half of the pills sold in drug stores do not dissolve fast enough to do much good. One way for you to test whether the pill you purchase will dissolve adequately is to place it in a glass of vinegar for about half an hour. You can stir the pill in the glass every now and then. If the pill hasn't disintegrated into fine particles within 30 minutes, it probably won't dissolve adequately in your stomach. Such pills have little value.

A second problem concerns the absorption of calcium. Once the calcium gets past the stomach into the intestine, if it is going to do you any good, it needs to be absorbed across the intestinal walls and into the blood stream. Absorption of some tablets is improved if the calcium pill is taken with a meal. But some forms of calcium are absorbed more easily than others and don't require the presence of a simultaneous meal. These come in the form of calcium citrate. Alternately, taking vitamin C with your calcium should serve the same end.

YOUR NEED FOR EXERCISE AND GOOD POSTURE

Because bone is vital tissue that is constantly building up and breaking down, it is important to know that the way you sit and stand will affect the way your bones shape themselves. If you sit slumped, your bones will grow that way. If you sit straight, your bones will grow that way. If you stand tall and walk with an erect posture, your bones will have a tendency to be straighter than if you slouch. Exercise has profound effects on the strength and integrity of bone. To evaluate your exercise and physical fitness, see Chapter 13.

THE MENOPAUSE AND OSTEOPOROSIS

As we have previously explained, about seven years before menopause your estrogen and progesterone levels are likely to start a long and continuous decline. Since each woman is different, not every woman will have the loss. But the vast majority will. We now know that a combination of estrogen, progesterone, and calcium deficiencies will together accelerate bone deterioration.[59a]

Whenever estrogen and/or progesterone levels fall drastically, whether this is due to natural menopause or surgical removal of the estrogen supply (ovariectomy), bones begin losing mass.[49] Reports have shown this loss of mass to vary from about .5 percent to 3 percent per year.[21, 54] The bones become progressively thinner in the

vast majority of menopausal women not taking replacement estrogen.[30] By the time a woman is eighty, she can easily have lost 40
percent of her bone substance.[50, 53] Although men also suffer some
loss, theirs is not as devastating as that of women.[50] While their loss
of bone mass is as great, breaks occur much less often apparently
because men start out with larger bones. For women, the greatest
declines in bone mass occur between the ages of forty-five and seventy. By age sixty, at least half of all women in every country now
studied show osteoporosis when X-rayed.[30]

Estrogen plays an important role in bone metabolism. Remember
that bone is always exchanging calcium with the blood. Two ways in
which estrogen influences this exchange process are (1) by facilitating
the uptake of calcium from the blood into the bone and (2) by inhibiting the loss of calcium from bone. When estrogen levels fall, bones
begin to disintegrate. *Osteoporosis* means "increased porosity." Think
of the "pores" in Swiss cheese and imagine them enlarging, and you
will have a reasonable analogy to bone porosity. Osteoporosis is the
disease characterized by a decrease in mass so great that as the porosity increases, fractures begin to occur even without severe trauma or
concussion. For a woman with osteoporosis of the spine, a gentle
hug can break her spinal bones.

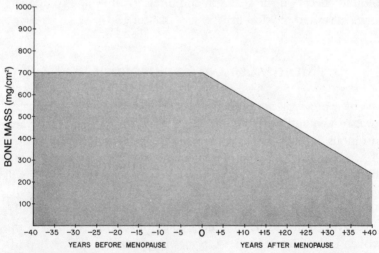

FIGURE 10   Declines in Bone Mass Begin at Menopause and Continue

(From Meema *et al., Obstet and Gynecol* 26:333)

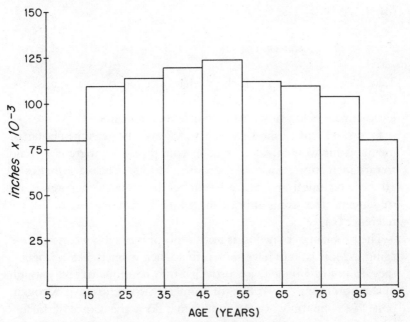

FIGURE 11 Changes in Bone Density with Age: Men

(From Albanese *et al.*, *NY State J Med* [1975]:326–336)

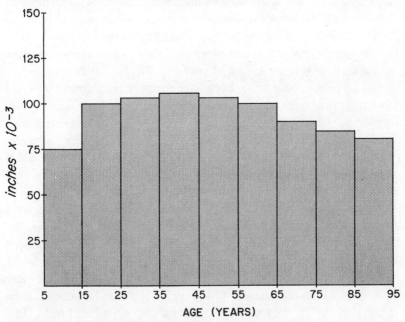

FIGURE 12 Changes in Bone Density with Age: Women

(From Albanese *et al.*, *NY State J Med* [1975]:326–336)

SPINAL FRACTURES

Take a look at Figure 10. It shows that once menopause begins, loss of bone ensues and this loss continues for as long as the estrogen levels remain below bone maintenance requirements.[4, 48, 49, 53]

Figures 11 and 12 show the effect of age on the density of bone for men and for women. Note that in young people, there is a trend toward increasing bone mass each year with age. The scale (inches $\times$ 10^{-3}) is technical and not relevant to the issue of increasing and subsequent decreasing of bone mass with age. (For more detail, see reference 6.)

The problem of bone loss is not simply or inevitably a condition of aging.[65] Most studies have shown that when women take estrogens, they do not lose bone mass, provided they continue to take enough of the hormones.[49, 54, 65] But for women who do not take estrogen, bone loss commonly occurs; and when it does, the degree of the loss occurs in proportion to the degree of the estrogen deficiency. Deterioration of the bone is one of the most critical problems for menopausal women. In fact, it has been estimated that about 50 percent of all women will develop some degree of osteoporosis after menopause.

The earliest warning symptom is a backache in the lower part of the spine—a progressive and persistent pain that seldom radiates.[3] Most aches and pains tend to spread (radiate). If you notice a constant, localized pain in your lower back, take the pain as a warning sign and seek treatment from an orthopedic specialist or a knowledgeable gynecologist.[4] On average, those who do develop the disease begin to notice more severe backaches about $9\frac{1}{2}$ years after their last menstrual period or 13 years after a surgically induced menopause.[18] The spine and pelvic bones are generally, but not always, affected first.[8, 62]

Spinal osteoporosis is rarely diagnosed before spinal bones have broken. The breaks follow a very orderly pattern, which leads to the appearance of the so-called "Dowager's Hump."[76] The Dowager's Hump, that protrusion in the upper back that can give an older woman the appearance of being a hunchback, is one of the clear indications of osteoporosis.[7] On average, at around age sixty, then again at sixty-five and seventy, an afflicted woman suffers breaks. The breaks occur at the places where the spine naturally curves (see Figure 13). These are the weakest points in one's spinal column and are the first to break. After the bones break, the body forms a fat pad over the spine in the region of the fractures to compensate, which adds to the deformity. Figure 14 illustrates the resulting change in posture and height that follow the breakage shown in Figure 13.

HIP FRACTURES

Hip fractures due to osteoporosis occur in 30 percent of all women after age sixty-five who don't take HRT. Figure 15 shows the long hip bone—the femur, on the left, and the iliac crest (pelvis), on the right, which holds this bone. Note that the top rounded region—the hip socket—fits into the pelvic bone. Note also the little notch at the top of the femur, which is shown in both figures. This notched area is the weakest part of this large bone because it is the thinnest and receives the stress of supporting the upper part of the body. When bones become porous and fragile, this spot is vulnerable to fracture. If the bone is thin enough, the mildest bump can break it. As of 1974, 10 percent to 15 percent of those women who suffered a hip

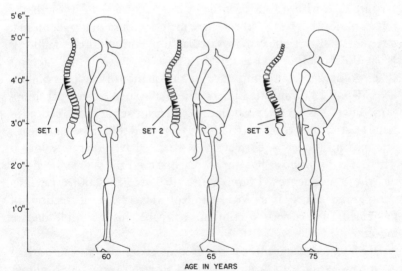

FIGURE 13   Spinal Osteoporosis—Location of Bone Fracture with Resulting Postural Changes

(From Urist, *Clinics Endocrinol Metab* 2:159–176)

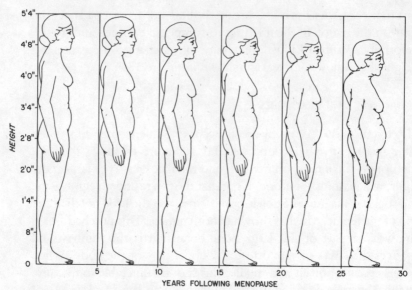

FIGURE 14 Postural Changes Associated with Spinal Osteoporosis and the Dowager's Hump

(From Albanese, *Postgraduate Medecine* 63:167–172)

fracture died within four months of the fracture.[32, 9] Although the causes of death vary, the lion's share includes four: viral pneumonia, myocardial infarction, cerebrovascular accident, and heart failure.[13] What do these four causes of death have to do with hip fracture? Reduced oxygen consumption as a consequence of loss of mobility. See Chapter 13 for information on the vital role of oxygen consumption. There has been a great improvement in surgical correction of bone fracture in the last ten to fifteen years, and this 15 percent death rate may no longer be correct. New studies have not yet evaluated whether the prognosis has improved. But even for those who don't die, the consequences of hip fracture are extremely serious. Life as a cripple in a wheel chair, loss of independence, loss of freedom of movement and travel, all combine to make this a terrible disease indeed.

Hip fractures occur more often in some geographical regions than in others. Women in Scandinavia and England show much higher rates than those in China or South Africa.[18] Whether this variation is due to differences in sunlight (which increases vitamin-D production on one's skin), to physical activity patterns (which promote both

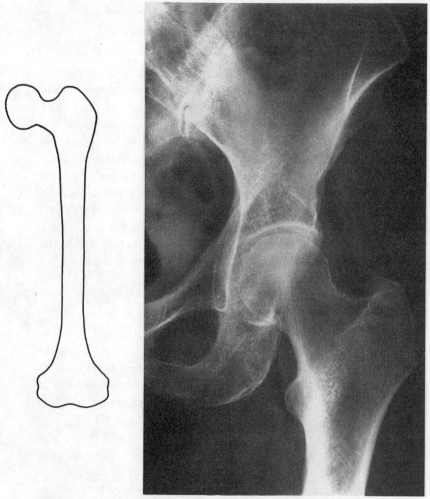

FIGURE 15   The Femur and Its Insertion into the Pelvis

(X ray courtesy of Frederick Kaplan, M.D., Chief of Metabolic Bone Disease, Hospital of the University of Pennsylvania)

stronger bones and better muscle tone, thereby supporting and protecting fragile bones), or to hormonal or other variations among different genetic groups has not yet been resolved. Most likely all three factors contribute.

LOSS OF TEETH

Other effects of a loss of bone mass are found in the mouth. Your teeth are supported by bone; and, not surprisingly, periodontal disease (the loss of tooth-bearing bone) is common in osteoporotic women.[6] In fact, by age sixty, about 40 percent of women will have lost all their teeth, according to one investigator who studied thousands of otherwise healthy women.[7] Whether this dental problem is due solely to osteoporosis or to some interaction with poor dental hygiene is not yet resolved. But daily gum care through flossing and/ or use of a Water Pik or Stim-u-dent is an essential part of fastidious grooming. If you have not been incorporating daily removal of debris from the base of your gums before, it becomes critical that you do so now. A toothbrush cannot retrieve food particles that work their way down below the gum line, and these particles provide the nutrition source for odorous bacteria that will grow in the mouth if the food remains more than twelve hours at a time.

OSTEOPOROSIS BECOMES OBVIOUS

The usual precipitating symptom of osteoporosis that brings a woman to the attention of her doctor is a bone that breaks after a minor jolt. The broken bone causes pain; the woman seeks medical help; and an X ray shows the overall deterioration of her bones.[8] The bones break easily because, through the gradual loss of mass, they have become brittle. Women whose ovaries are removed (regardless of the age) begin to show signs of osteoporosis within two years after the operation if no hormone replacement therapy is instituted.[36] Studies conducted four years after the operation showed that 68 percent of one group of 59 ovariectomized women were suffering from beginning osteoporosis.

Since the loss of estrogen following ovariectomy carries with it an increased risk of osteoporosis, it is not surprising that the estrogen decline of menopause is also likely to lead to the development of osteoporosis. But even after menopause, there is wide variation in blood hormone levels among women. Two studies compared hormone levels of postmenopausal women, some of whom had the disease and some of whom did not have it. Clear differences emerged. Although estradiol and testosterone levels were not different in the two groups, levels of estrone and androstenedione were significantly lower in the women with osteoporosis.[23, 47] In other words, menopausal women with relatively high levels of androstenedione and estrone are less likely to suffer the ravaging effects of osteoporosis. Estrone, therefore, appears to be the estrogen hormone that affects bone health in menopause. Recall that the menopausal ovary secretes both estrone and androstenedione. Some women produce more of these hormones than other women. In some menopausal women, the ovaries are probably quite important in preventing or delaying the onset of osteoporosis. Here is another good reason to keep your healthy ovaries intact even if a hysterectomy (removal of the uterus) for benign disease becomes advisable.

DYNAMIC BONE LOADING AS A PREVENTION

Recently, investigators have been studying the relationship among bone density, the architectural structure of bone, exercise that loads stress onto bone, and the prevention of bone fractures. The results show that women who place weight on bones strengthen those bones, provided that their exercise pattern is gradual, regular, and sensible.[12] This "bone loading" mechanism may help explain why, as women age, those who become less physically active experience a greater incidence of hip fractures while spinal-fracture incidence tends to stabilize. A sedentary life prevents the dynamic "bone loading" on the hip that regular walking and other active life-style motions normally produce. But it does not lower the natural "dynamic bone loading" of the spine; even when we sit still, the weight of the upper body "loads" the spinal bones.[69]

A study was conducted on a group of women in their mid-sixties with osteoporosis.[12] The group was divided in two. One group was assigned a regular exercise program three times a week for 50 minutes each session. The other group (the control) did not exercise. The exercises were specifically structured to impose weight stress ("bone loading") on particular bones. In this experiment, the wrist region was systematically stressed with a series of activities, including hanging from parallel bars and pushing by hand against an opposing force. Within one year, the group who regularly exercised showed an increase of close to 4 percent in bone density in the stressed region. By contrast, the control group had lost about 2 percent of bone mass in the same area. None of these women took hormones, and the only difference between the two groups appeared to be the specific exercise program. Conclusion: those bones that were systematically stressed with dynamic bone loading grew denser.

Other factors also play a role in predicting whose bones will break as they thin out with age. The architectural structure of bones varies from one person to another. Certain kinds of architectural structure appear to cause stronger bones. Genetic differences also count.[56, 78] One thing is clear: bone density by itself is not a complete predictor of whose bones will fracture and whose will not.

DIAGNOSING THE DISEASE

If you suspect that your bones are disintegrating (because your height is shrinking or your back is persistently painful), you can go to a physician for a bone reading. Many different methods are available to check your bone density. Most are painless and quick and involve a form of X-ray visualization of some of your bone. A bone densitometer is a small machine about the size of a typewriter. The technician will guide your arm through a cuff, much as in blood-pressure recording. A small beam of photons that you can neither see nor feel is passed through your arm, and a minicomputer, attached to the machine, calculates how dense your bone is. If you do have the disease, it will be occurring in a number of places simultaneously rather than in just one location. The fingers, spine, lower arm, and hip bones are all affected once osteoporosis is well progressed, and accurate readings can be taken from any of these regions.* Unfortunately, by the time true osteoporosis is detected by X ray or by any other method, the disease has already progressed much further than is healthy.[25]

Recent studies have shown that the single-photon densitometer, which provides a measure that can be taken of the forearm, is probably the most precise diagnostic instrument in terms of its ability to measure bone mass accurately.*, [13, 62, 70] However, most of the bone fractures that take place among women who are osteoporotic do not occur in the arm. Each year in the United States, more than 1 million people suffer from bone fractures, and the distribution of these fractures weighs heavily toward fracture of the spine (538,000 cases).

---

*The newest X-ray densitometer machines have increased the accuracy of spinal readings but are not widely used as of late 1990 due to their high cost.

The hip is the next most vulnerable site, with 227,000 cases per year.[25]

Because the disease is progressive, a number of investigators have suggested that it helps to have bones tested every ½ to 1 year in order to see whether your bones are changing. But there is no universal agreement on this issue. Some specialists advocate a baseline dual-photon absorptionmetry reading (or, better still, the newer densitometry X-ray machines reading) of the lower spine, with repeat evaluations scheduled every ½, 1, or 2 years. But others disagree. Insurance carriers have made this difficult for patients by not covering this cost. Moreover, the institutions find it necessary to charge high fees in order to cover amortization of the costly equipment. So, if you decide to have your bone density monitored, you should be aware that even the question of which bone to measure has not been fully resolved.[24]

By 1988, investigators were looking forward to testing the blood levels of certain substances in order to monitor bone health.[70] In 1989, several European investigators published the first study showing that bone density in the forearm is related to blood levels of a hormone, osteocalcin, that is involved in bone building.[75] For now, these discoveries remain experimental, but we can look toward increasingly sophisticated methods of bone testing. The measurement of bone in the forearm—particularly with the newest equipment— offers the fastest and probably most efficient way to monitor whether your bones are losing density and what you need to do to correct that situation, provided the measurement is taken two or three times a year.

MENOPAUSAL RISK FACTORS

If you are childless, white, small-boned, and slender, your risk of developing osteoporosis is much greater than if you have had children, are black, or large-boned, or chubby.[3, 8, 9, 50] There is enormous individual variation in the ability of the body to maintain its bone density, and about half of menopausal women do not experience any ill effects of menopause on their bones.[50] Even for those in the high-risk categories, estrogens appear to prevent osteoporosis as long as the hormone treatment continues.

SMOKING AND BONE HEALTH

Smoking severely reduces the benefits of hormone replacement therapy to bone health. Smoking also reduces *maximum oxygen consumption*—a measure of how much oxygen your body can take in. Oxygen is needed to promote the healthy functioning of your cells. When maximum oxygen consumption is low, bones tend to be weak. If you want good bones, you must not smoke; if you are smoking, you should stop. In Chapter 12, we discuss what you need to know to stop smoking and to make the withdrawal less painful. Remember this, however: as painful as it is to kick the addiction of smoking, if you do stop, you avoid much greater pain—the pain of life in a wheel chair because of a broken hip or spine.

THYROID TREATMENTS AND BONE HEALTH

Many women take thyroid medications. Recent studies suggest that when the dosage of the prescription is too high, the bones are at increased risk for osteoporosis; when the dose is adjusted downward, the bones are not at increased risk for osteoporosis.

In 1990, the first study of the effects of treating thyroid deficiencies with L-thyroxine showed that when doses got too high, bone loss was accelerated. Women overtreated with thyroxine, as evidenced by low plasma levels of TSH (thyroid-stimulating hormone), were losing hip bone at seven times the rate of women of the same age not on excess doses of the thyroid treatment.[73a] Thus, women who take thyroid treatments should ask to have their blood tested for circulating TSH levels. If the laboratory results indicate that the women are being overtreated (as a low TSH will reveal), these women should have their prescription adjusted and their blood retested. The prescription level will best protect them when the plasma TSH level is in the normal range.

CORTICOSTEROID USE AND BONE HEALTH

Another menopausal risk factor for bone health is now recognized.[25] Certain classes of drugs cause bone to become osteoporotic. The most dangerous of these are the glucocorticoids—or corticosteroids—such as cortisone or prednisone. Many women take these drugs for rheumatoid arthritis or other diseases. If you must take these drugs, ask your physician how to minimize damage to bone.[62] New research indicates that hormone replacement therapy administered in conjunction with corticosteroids can be helpful in lessening bone damage that these latter drugs provoke. Other reports show the limited but beneficial effects of vitamin-D therapy.[63]

PREVENTING AND TREATING OSTEOPOROSIS

As with any disease, the best treatment is prevention. Those who adequately exercise and eat nutritiously will minimize the risk of getting osteoporosis. Moreover, hormone therapy will almost always prevent the disease, provided calcium levels are adequate. Once the disease has been diagnosed, treatment will, optimally, consist of vitamin D, adequate calcium intake (at least 1,500 mg. per day), and some estrogen (most likely with progestin) supplements. Current scientific research is evaluating other approaches such as calcitonin injections and sodium-fluoride treatments. Ultimately, the goal of bone treatment involves controlling the delicate balance between bone formation and bone resorption (breakdown).

Some controversy exists about the nature of treatment. While almost all experts agree that estrogen with or without progesterone is effective, investigations are under way to determine if other agents will also work. In 1988, progestagen* alone was also shown to be effective.[26]

Fluoride treatment appeared effective. When coupled with estrogen, fluoride promotes bone growth.[62, 67] However, the new bone that is formed has been reported to break easily.[19, 66] About 40 percent of the women taking the fluoride developed such severe side effects (rheumatic pains, nausea, and vomiting) that treatment had to be stopped.[67] One recent study evaluated several communities whose water came from deep wells, some with and some without high concentrations of fluoride. Older women who had drunk highly fluoridated water had more osteoporotic bones and twice as many fractures as compared to those who had drunk less fluoridated water.[73] We suggest that you avoid sodium-fluoride treatments at this time.

Some investigators believe that estrogen is the treatment of choice, with or without calcitonin (another bone-related hormone) supple-

*Progestagen, used throughout this book, is the spelling preferred by the authors since etymologically the word is derived from progestational, meaning "pregnancy-like changes."

ments.[20] (Calcitonin is a lesser-known hormone of the thyroid gland and is important in the control of bone function.)[61] This therapy is new; treatment with calcitonin requires frequent injections, and one of the serious objections to this treatment involves antibody reactions that have not yet been worked out.[19, 20] The calcitonin that is used for treatment comes from a nonhuman source and is viewed by the recipients' white blood cells as a foreign invasion; the body response, in this case, is to manufacture antibodies that attack the calcitonin. Some studies show that estrogen therapy increases a woman's natural level of calcitonin,[22] which could be one reason why estrogen is so important for healthy bones. Taking calcitonin directly, either by injection or as an intranasal spray, may one day be demonstrated as beneficial for the treatment of osteoporosis in menopausal women.[33, 38, 59, 74] But the ultimate effectiveness of calcitonin treatments has yet to be clearly demonstrated. Although the early research is promising, potential adverse side effects from the injections have not yet been carefully analyzed in published reports. The nasal spray—as used in Europe—has been reported to produce no adverse side effects.[57] (This nasal route has not been approved by the FDA for use in the United States at this writing.) For the moment, such treatments should still be regarded as experimental.

There are a few investigators who believe that estrogens are irrelevant and that calcium and vitamin-D therapies are sufficient to protect against, or even reverse, osteoporosis.[6] In certain cases, postmenopausal women who have suffered bone fractures can be helped with vitamin-D treatment (the "calcitriol" form). However, if hormone therapy is not contraindicated, hormone therapy is preferable. Then there are the advocates of calcitonin-and-phosphate (a naturally occurring substance) combination therapy.

After considering the available evidence, the sensible approach appears to be one that assures ample exercise as well as adequate calcium levels (800 to 1,000 mg. per day), sufficient vitamin D (400 IU [international units] per day) or 15 minutes of unpolluted sun shining on your skin), and enough estrogen to maintain the retention of bone mass. If you live in a highly polluted area, the necessary wave lengths of solar radiation may not reach your skin. If you have doubts about the quality of the air, a vitamin source or milk (which in the United States contains vitamin-D supplements) is recommended. Be sure to moderate your exposure to the sun. It is better not to go out at noon—particularly if you live in a warm climate, in which case you should get your sunshine either before 10:00 A.M. or after 3:00 P.M.

Estrogen therapy* is particularly important because it reduces the net loss of calcium from the body.[31] In fact, calcium loss can be cut by even very low doses of estrogens. As described earlier, excess calcium (over 2,000 mg. per day) could create problems for the kidneys (stones) or the circulatory system (calcium deposits clogging the arteries).

Several studies have suggested that when progestin is given in opposition to estrogen (but not when low-dose progestin is given alone), bone metabolism responds favorably. The progestins appear to stimulate a small amount of bone formation while the estrogens appear to halt the further loss of bone. In combination, estrogens with progestin opposition in low doses for 10 to 13 days per month seem to optimize bone health.

It has been demonstrated in a number of studies that estrogen therapy helps bone to maintain its mineral strength and mass. Among normal, healthy menopausal women tested for up to eight years, the estrogen-treated women still had as much bone as they had started with years earlier, but the placebo-treated women had lost as much as 9 percent of their bone after eight years.[28, 45, 49] More recent studies provide similar results.[15, 25, 37] But the estrogen effect seems to be dose-dependent: when the dose is high, estrogen appears to be able to increase bone mass a bit in the spine;[22] when the dose is low, the therapy only helps to slow down the natural aging loss. Oral contraceptives contain estrogens and progestins, and tend to be given in higher doses than hormone replacement regimens, and here, too, a dose dependency is found. In fact, a study published in 1988 shows that menopausal women who had formerly taken oral contraceptives for long periods of time had heavier and stronger bones than women who had not taken oral contraceptives.[27]

Estrogens work better than placebos and better than calcium alone. This is graphically illustrated in Figure 16. Note that when these menopausal women took hormones, their bone density either stayed the same or slightly increased. When the women took placebos, their bone density diminished. And that is how it works: when women are estrogen-deficient, as is typical of the menopausal years,

*Descriptions of each kind of estrogen therapy are given in Chapter 5.

their bones lose mass, becoming more and more porous with the years; and when women begin taking sufficient levels of hormones, they stop losing this mass, sometimes even gaining a little.[59a]

In other controlled studies in which women were given placebos, hormones, or calcium, clear differences emerged after two years. The control subjects taking a placebo lost an average of 1.18 percent to 2.83 percent of their bone mass per year (depending on which of two measuring techniques was considered). Calcium (calcium carbonate) was effective in reducing bone loss to about one-fifth that of untreated women. However, the estrogen treatment was the single most effective agent. It reduced bone loss to half that of the calcium-treated group.[19, 21, 35] Estrogen therapy in low doses (for example, .3 or .6 mg. of conjugated equine estrogens per day) does not produce side effects for the vast majority of women. If side effects occur (like a bloated feeling or swollen breasts), this usually indicates that the dose

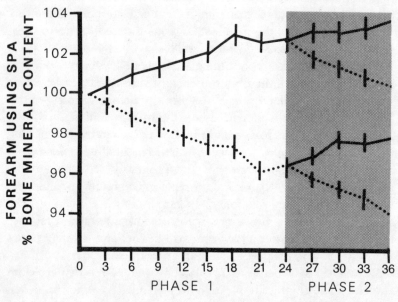

FIGURE 16   Bone Response to Hormone Therapy

of estrogen is too high. Adjustments are made immediately, either by alternating days of therapy (one day on, one day off) or by halving the daily dose.

You will probably find that your choice of a physician will define which treatment for osteoporosis you are offered. Even in 1989, consistent with what we wrote in 1982, the medical community still had not reached a consensus on how best to treat or prevent the condition. In mid-1981, a questionnaire answered by 1,000 specialists showed that only 42 percent used hormone therapy even for treatment of diagnosed osteoporosis.[16] Vitamin D was prescribed by half of those who advocate estrogen treatment for osteoporosis. Dr. Isaac Schiff, professor of obstetrics and gynecology at Harvard Medical School and gynecologist-in-chief at the Massachusetts General Hospital, when presenting his paper at the 1989 meeting of the American Gynecological and Obstetrical Society, reviewed the current attitudes among physicians who were treating menopausal patients. His results in 1989 were similar to what we had discovered in preparing the 1983 version of this book: much education is still needed for the physicians who are treating menopausal patients.

By 1990, the data were beginning to show that not only was the bone response to estrogen therapies dose-dependent, but that bone could actually increase in mass if the hormone doses were sufficient. The first study so far published provides American data on the spine that supports the data illustrated in Figure 16 on the forearm after 12 months of estrogen use. Progestins were not tested. Results show a 2.5 percent increase in spinal density by the end of one year, when women were taking 1.25 mg. of conjugated estrogens a day along with 1,000 mg. of elemental calcium.[30a]

Will these results be sustained in longer-range studies? We will have to await the publication of the research to find out. Moreover, the newer densitometry that uses very low-dose X ray will probably be more accurate and feasible for routine assessment, once the costs come down.

Become informed. You can then increase the scope of your own health care. Here are some guidelines:

1. Develop and maintain good exercise habits. New research indicates that exercise plays a role in preventing osteoporosis. In countries where women are engaged in physical work up to an advanced age, the incidence of age-related bone fractures is significantly re-

duced.[10] The reverse situation—immobilization—has been related to a high incidence of the disease.[6] Total immobility (hospitalized bed rest) produces loss of bone mass.[7, 34] In the opposite condition—extreme activity of a particular limb (as, for example, the throwing arm of a baseball player)—increased bone mass in the heavily used limb occurs.[77] But in two studies that compared the bone mass of active menopausal women to the bone mass of less active individuals, the expected difference was not found.[35, 71]

However, regular physical exercise does help:[41, 42, 58] fit women do better than unfit women. (For details on how to help yourself become fit, see Chapter 13.) Regular exercise will also promote greater muscle tone and mass. This increased muscle will serve to cushion and support the bones, and will be especially beneficial to women whose bone mass is declining.

Of considerable significance in reducing bone fractures is the increased stability of gait that exercise affords. As women age, they have a tendency to fall and trip more frequently. When the muscles are strong and the general level of fitness is good, you are less likely to fall and injure your bones.

2. Maintain an adequate level of calcium—1,000 mg. per day should be enough, unless you have undergone a hysterectomy and ovariectomy or have extremely high Kupperman scores (see page 78). This can be achieved by consuming, for example, 3 glasses of milk or 3 ounces of Swiss cheese per day. (Figure 15, pages 266–267, lists the calcium values of some food sources.) If you must take calcium supplements, be sure that they dissolve in vinegar; and if you use a nonacid form of supplement, take the tablets with your meals (see page 264). Remember, if you are deficient in calcium, increasing your intake will stop that loss of bone mass.

3. Be sure you have a moderate supply of vitamin D. Too little or too much is bad—but for different reasons. If your vitamin-D level is too low, the calcium you ingest won't be absorbed into the body. Instead, it is likely to be lost in the feces.[19] In amounts above 1,000 IU per day, vitamin D promotes an excess release of calcium from bone into the blood.[19, 64] This causes a loss of bone mass. In moderate amounts—that is, 400 IU per day—vitamin D promotes the uptake of the calcium you have eaten from the intestines into the blood stream. You can maintain an adequate intake of vitamin D by either exposing your skin for about fifteen minutes a day to the sun or by

drinking milk (to which vitamin D has been added) or by taking a vitamin pill. Again, moderation is the key. Fifteen minutes of sun exposure with no sunscreen on your skin to block the rays[1] is good in that your skin will manufacture the necessary vitamin D. Excessive sun exposure is destructive to the skin, burning away the melanocyte cells that protect you.

The ability of vitamin D to halt or reverse an osteoporotic condition is limited by the level of estrogen deficiency that is present.[16] If you have too little estrogen in your system, vitamin D won't help. It sounds more complicated than it really is. You need calcium for your bone mass. You need vitamin D to help get the calcium into the body but not so much that the calcium stays in the blood rather than the bone. You need estrogen to keep the calcium inside the bones. Shortages in any of these requirements or excesses in vitamin D can cause your bones to become brittle.

4. Be aware of your height. If you start to shrink, you are probably losing bone. If you are maintaining adequate amounts of calcium, estrogen supplements will help. You don't need a lot of estrogen to do the job of keeping your bones intact. The lowest doses (.3 mg. per day) on the market may be adequate for relief of postmenopausal symptoms and perhaps to keep bones intact. Recently, however, Dr. Robert Lindsay, who is on the faculty of the Columbia University Medical School and its affiliate, Helen Hayes Hospital, and is one of the pioneers in bone-density and hormone studies, presented data to show that among large groups of women, the minimum effective dose to insure adequate bone for all the women would have to be .625 mg. of the conjugated equine estrogen. Therefore, for the individual woman, the dosage might vary. She will have to listen to her body to make sure that the dose she takes is neither too high (causing swollen breasts) or too low (causing hot flashes). See Tables 3 and 4 on pages 132–135 for a list of kinds and dosages of estrogen. Any brand's lowest dose will probably provide as much of the hormone as you need for your bones.

5. If there is risk of bone deterioration, consider hormone replacement therapy as prevention. But be sure your calcium levels are also adequate. And if you already have bone loss, consider hormone therapy to stop further deterioration of your bones.

ESTROGEN THERAPY

Since there is great individual variation in the amount of circulating estrone that different menopausal women show, there is no "proper" dose of estrogen that should be universally prescribed to correct or prevent osteoporosis. Even the lowest doses that are usually prescribed (.3 to .625 mg. of conjugated equine estrogen per day) have been shown to be adequate.[31] Since blood levels of estrone appear to be a critical predictor of bone health and all forms of estrogen treatment lead to significant increases in blood levels of estrone, it is likely that estrogen therapy in any form will be beneficial for bone health. We suggest that you take progesterone if hormone therapy seems advisable and if your uterus has not been removed. Although progesterone is important in preventing adverse effects of estrogen (see Chapter 6), it will not prevent bone loss that is caused by an estrogen deficiency.[28, 46] Androgen is different. It seems to be about as effective as estrogen in halting bone deterioration;[19, 43] but the possibility of masculinizing (for example, causing growth of facial hair) makes this a less desirable hormone treatment than estrogen therapy.

Hormone therapy is generally necessary to halt and reverse the degenerative process of osteoporosis in the presence of adequate levels of vitamin-D intake. Studies confirm this.[19, 21, 45, 52] For example, in one group of 30 women who were beginning to display annual loss of bone mass, those subjects given a placebo showed about 3.6 percent degeneration of their (finger) bones each year. In contrast, the groups given either estrogen therapy or estrogen plus progesterone showed no bone loss; and in some of the women, bone density actually increased slightly at the end of the first year.[46] Another report indicated that women who began taking estrogens within three years after their last menstrual period and who continued taking them for ten years thereafter showed a slight increase in bone mass after the ten years had passed. Those who began estrogens later, after having advanced more than three years into their menopause, stopped losing bone but were not able to regain any of the bone mass lost.[52] Different studies have reported different annual rates of bone degeneration, but all show a clear tendency for bone loss that is progressive when no hormones are taken.

SUMMARY

Osteoporosis is one of the most insidious maladies of the menopausal years. Bones become progressively thinner and more brittle, and are subject to fractures as menopause progresses. Calcium inadequacies and lack of exercise are critical factors in the development of this devastating disease. Smoking stimulates osteoporosis. Thus, smokers should stop smoking in order to prevent its ravaging effects on the bones and the possibility of being permanently crippled. Certain drugs, such as corticosteroids, exacerbate the disease. The relative paucity of estrogen during the menopausal years also appears to play a major role. Hormone therapy with estrogen can prevent the occurrence of osteoporosis and even retard the condition once it has started. There is growing evidence that those who begin taking estrogen early in their menopausal years may even show a slight increase in bone mass over time. If you do take estrogen, you will need to take it as long as you want to prevent further bone loss. As far as your bone health is concerned, the findings are unambiguous: if you are at risk of bone deterioration, estrogen therapy provides a clear benefit.

5

HORMONE REPLACEMENT THERAPY I

Hormone replacement therapy. The words suggest that menopause is a condition of loss. And for most women, this is true. Hormone levels decline as the ovaries shrink with age;[4a] and as the ovaries shrink, the menopausal symptoms discussed earlier begin to appear. But the hot flashes and night sweats are only the most obvious symptoms. They really herald an underlying estrogen deficiency that, if left unchecked, is likely to set in motion the bone-degeneration processes and other body changes that were described in the previous chapters.

Said one woman of sixty:

I approached menopause with a firm determination that this was not going to affect my life! I was sadly disillusioned! I found that the hot flashes did bother me and I was reduced to the emotional level of a young teenager— the least little thing bothered me. I sought the advice of a gynecologist who put me on Premarin [a conjugated estrogen]. That was 10 years ago and I have been fine ever since—feeling good emotionally and physically.

Having a large percentage of menopausal women is natural for a society in which the average life span is seventy years or more. When antibiotics were developed to kill humankind's killers, few said that it was unnatural to promote well-being by killing disease. The drugs ended a common form of death (by infection) that had prevented women from reaching their menopause. As health conditions improved over the last two centuries, few thought it unnatural to improve conditions that lead to longevity, although some suggested that heat and shelter, packaged food and medicine were unnatural. These things increased longevity, and with longevity came menopause.

The development of estrogen therapy is a recent biomedical innovation. The modern study of hormones—how they work, where they are produced, what their benefits are—began in the 1940s. We now know that hormones are natural body secretions that control many of the physiological processes of life. We understand that, after about age thirty-five or forty, women display changes in their patterns of menstruation, and that in the two weeks before menstruation starts, a severe decline in the levels of estrogen and progesterone begins. For women in their forties, compared to their younger years, their preovulatory or mid-cycle levels of estrogen tend to increase while their premenstrual or end-cycle levels of estrogen and progesterone tend to decrease. Consequently, over time, each month the highs get higher and the lows get lower. And for many women, the menstrual flow becomes excessively heavy. Hormone therapies, in either oral-contraceptive form or the lower-dosage hormone-replacement-therapy form, tend to regularize the menstrual flow and put an end to this excessive bleeding.[76]

The development of estrogen replacement therapy began with the use of estrogen alone (that is, unopposed). It is only recently that progesterone has been routinely added to estrogen therapy in an attempt to mimic the natural cyclical pattern of the fertile years. This addition protects the endometrium from developing cancer to which it would otherwise be at risk by the unopposed estrogen therapy. Once progesterone was added to estrogen therapy, the name of the process began to change—from estrogen replacement therapy (ERT) to hormone replacement therapy (HRT). Since the writing of the first edition of *Menopause* in 1981, the composite body of research has convinced us that optimal hormone therapy should include both estrogen and a progesterone in opposition to the estrogen. Whether testosterone should be given remains to be answered by future studies.

The history of HRT shows an ever-increasing refinement in the dosages and types of hormones used. When estrogen therapy was first prescribed, synthetic estrogens were used as often as natural estrogens were. Similarly, as progesterone therapy is more routinely prescribed, synthetic forms predominate. In the case of estrogen, the data clearly indicate that "natural" estrogens are preferable to synthetic ones. These "natural" hormones are widely available and should be used by those women who take estrogen, provided that the women are not concerned about hormonal contracepting (which are only available in synthetic form.) The case for progesterone is not fully resolved. In the United States, most pharmaceutical companies manufacture only synthetic progesterone.

HRT for menopausal symptoms has been praised as well as maligned. Like any other tool of medicine and science, used correctly in the appropriate circumstances its effects are beneficial. The issues involved in HRT—which we will consider—are the following:

- Does HRT relieve the symptoms of menopausal distress?
- What are the side effects of HRT?
- How does one take HRT?
- What constitutes a beneficial dosage of hormones?
- What route of hormonal administration is best (oral pills, vaginal creams, sublingual tablets, subdermal pellets, skin patches, or skin creams)?
- What about progesterone?
- What about testosterone?
- What dosages of hormones are available?
- Who should not use HRT?

HRT AND RELIEF FROM MENOPAUSAL DISTRESS

Too little estrogen appears to be the principal cause of hot flashes, which are usually the first symptom of menopausal distress and often begin as early as seven years before the onset of menopause. Estrogen treatment almost always relieves them—the studies are unambiguous on this point. If you have no symptoms, you are fortunate: your hormone levels are probably adequate enough to maintain the health of your bones as well as your general well-being. Women who have hot flashes, tingling, genital atrophy, or night sweats find relief when they take estrogen regardless of the form in which the hormone is taken.

EXCESSIVE BLEEDING

For women in their late thirties and early forties, too little progesterone in the luteal phase of the ovarian cycle could be responsible for excessive bleeding at menses. What appears to be happening is that in the first two weeks of the menstrual cycle, as estrogen levels rise higher than in former years, this excess estrogen stimulates the endometrium of the uterus and causes it to build up more tissue. When ovulation occurs in women with declining ovarian function (see Figure 3, page 61), the situation changes. Instead of producing high levels of progesterone, the tendency is to decrease production of progesterone as women move from their thirties to their fifties. As a consequence of this unopposed or "less-opposed" estrogen, heavy menstrual bleeding occurs in many women.

Hormone therapies, when appropriately prescribed, tend to solve the problem. Fortunately, we have come to realize that most of the concerns about oral contraceptives were unwarranted. We now have evidence that even for most women past age thirty-five, oral contraceptives—particularly the new low-dose forms—can be used safely by nonsmokers.* Moreover, it should be emphasized that the amount of estrogen and progestin in HRT contains only a small fraction of that of the low-dose oral contraceptives. Consider this: HRT doses approximate—but do not exceed—what the normal body produces. Low-dose oral contraceptives supply at least triple the amount of these hormones. Fortunately, we now know how to provide hormonal support in the form of HRT not only to protect the endometrium, but also to prevent osteoporosis.

HOT FLASHES

The proof that hormone therapy is far superior to placebo, sedatives, or clonidine (an antihypertensive drug) in relieving hot flashes and night sweats is contained in Appendix 1. For a full discussion, please turn there.

---

*Smokers past the age of thirty-five experience unwarranted risks of cardiovascular disease, which is believed to be aggravated by oral contraceptives. See Chapter 12 for help in overcoming the smoking addiction.

Some women take vitamin E to help relieve hot flashes. But according to rigorous scientific studies, this just does not work.[56] Others believe that if a woman exercises regularly, she may be less prone to hot flashes. Exercise, although good for you, does not help to alleviate hot flashes.[18] Even without hormones, hot flashes do diminish with time, although many women continue to experience flashing for ten years or more.

GENITAL SKIN ATROPHY

If you are suffering from hormonal deficits that produce vaginal dryness or painful intercourse, taking estrogen will probably solve the problem.[34, 35] The pressure of a thrusting penis in an inadequately lubricated vagina with a thin epithelial lining can produce abrasions. Abrasions of the vaginal lining lead to inflammation, and this inflammation is commonly seen in women who have estrogen deficiencies. But you will have to continue taking the estrogen to maintain relief. If you stop, your estrogen level will drop and the problems will probably return.

Estrogen can be prescribed in different forms. The effectiveness of a given dose is related to the type of estrogen that is taken. One investigator treated 42 women with atrophic vaginitis (vaginal inflammation with inadequate secretions and a general wasting-away appearance). The study was rigorously carried out in double-blind fashion: neither the patients nor the person evaluating results knew until the study ended who got the hormone and who got the blank (placebo) treatment. A daily dose of .1 mg. of estradiol (the most active form of estrogen) in cream form was sufficient to maintain vaginal normalcy.[35] The necessary dose in pill form probably varies from woman to woman. In two studies, 1.25 mg. (conjugated equine estrogen) or more per day was needed to return the deteriorating vaginal cells to a vigorous state.[16, 34] In another report (1982), .625 mg. per day provided adequate protection.[84] In yet another study (1990), oral estriol, taken in doses of 3 mg. per day for the first 4 weeks and 2 mg. per day thereafter, was also effective.[62a] Moreover, in this study, the hormone reduced the bacteria that cause urinary-tract infections.

In contrast to vaginal atrophy, pelvic tone is usually not restored by hormone therapy.[91] Those women who suffer from vaginal relaxation—a general loss of internal support-structure strength—need other therapy. Loss of vaginal muscle tone is more common in women who have borne many children and apparently is not a reflection of hormonal deficits. Recall that the Kegel exercises (see page 90) not only help restore muscle tone, but you can do them yourself. [54] You might try this before seeking medical help.

FACIAL SKIN

The skin of your face will also respond to estrogen therapy and will, like vaginal skin, benefit with increased tone and glow and thickness.[41, 72, 73, 74] Collagen constitutes a third of the total body mass, and skin collagen and thickness together decline as women age.[10] HRT estrogen opposed with progesterone improves skin collagen.[10] In fact, the more aged the skin is, the greater the degree of collagen increase when hormones are taken.

BACKACHE

Osteoporosis is a common menopausal problem that was described in Chapter 4. It affects in some way about half of the women who do not take HRT. It is progressive (it gets worse) and is prevented by early application and continued maintenance of HRT (see Chapter 4). Backache can be an early warning sign of incipient osteoporosis— that is, thinning out of bone.

EMOTIONAL DISTRESS

Your sense of well-being is likely to improve if you take estrogens. If you have been plagued with hot flashes and other ills, obtaining some relief from them should go a long way toward making you feel better. A sense of well-being is a subtle state. If you have it, there is an internal comfort, a ready smile, and a general feeling of good will toward oneself and others. Estrogen deficits at menopause have been shown to be associated with a loss of this comfortable feeling, and this loss is a menopausal symptom that is quite different from the other distressing symptoms.[51, 85] HRT appears to restore this sense of well-being.[27] It also improves the quality of your sleep.[85] In studies in sleep laboratories in England, it was shown that estrogens changed the proportion of the sleep time spent in the rapid-eye-movement stage, which is characteristic of dreaming. Women dreamed more when they took estrogen and dreamed less when they were estrogen-deficient. As dreams increase, one's general state of peacefulness improves and one feels rested the next morning.[95, 96, 97] We do not yet know exactly why dream deprivation alters the psychological milieu. It may be that dreams serve to change the electrical state of the nervous system for the better. The electrical patterns of brain waves are quite different in dream sleep than in the other (nondream) stages of sleep.

Many menopausal women report headaches, depression, anxiety, and listlessness. These symptoms are experienced by most people at one time or another and are not necessarily related to the hormone changes of the menopause. Still, this cluster of problems tends to vanish within a month or so after hormone therapy begins.[82] Placebos don't work—only the hormones do.[22] In one study, when a psychological treatment program (psychotherapy) was coupled with hormone therapy, women found relief from transient panic attacks and other expressions of anxiety that they had been experiencing.[37]

Thus, if you are suffering from a hormonal deficit and generally feeling down, hormones will work to restore your sense of vigor. But if you are having a severe emotional problem caused by a serious life situation such as the death of a loved one or strains in your marriage, hormones alone probably won't help.[82]

FORMICATION

Formication, a technical term meaning "itching," literally refers to the sensation of ants crawling across the skin. Some patients complain of that sensation, which is associated with estrogen deficiency. About 10 percent of women continue to be annoyed with this itching problem for more than ten years after menopause. Estrogen treatments are the *only* remedy that reliably provides relief.[56]

LIBIDO

By 1982, there was a general impression within the biomedical community that HRT influenced the libido.[6, 92] Until then, the few reports that had been widely quoted were never explained well enough in the scientific journals to allow others to test the results by duplicating them. In the mid-1980s, the first rigorous studies were published, and these showed that women suffer from loss of libido when ovarian function is inhibited. Women who had their ovaries removed tended to have deficient libidos and wanted help. Double-blind placebo-controlled studies showed that when testosterone therapy was added to very low doses of estrogen therapy, these oophorectomized women reported an increase in libido.[86] When the subjects (unknowingly) received placebo, they did not report this improvement. By 1989, the following conclusions could be drawn:

- For women who have had their ovaries surgically removed, some will find their libido restored when low levels of testosterone therapy are prescribed.
- The optimal dosages of testosterone have not yet been defined.
- For women who still have their ovaries, no double-blind placebo-controlled studies have yet allowed us to determine whether testosterone therapy would help or be disadvantageous to other body systems.

"BODY TYPE"

One further benefit of HRT has been reported. It is likely that regular use of estrogen and progestin in a replacement-therapy regimen will alter the body composition toward more lean body mass than toward fat body mass. Estrogen users tend to weigh less than those who don't use hormones.[50] Be cautioned, however: estrogen is not a dietary or weight-control product and should not be used as a substitute for sound nutrition and exercise habits.

WHO SHOULD NOT TAKE HORMONES?

The Food and Drug Administration (FDA) lists contraindications to HRT that, by law, must appear on the package inserts of all HRT prescriptions. This list was developed so that HRT would not be prescribed for women who might be disposed to disease as a result of the therapy. HRT regimens include taking either separately or in combination estrogen, progesterone, and testosterone. Depending on which hormone is formulated, the contraindication list may vary slightly. Four contraindications are listed most often and warn against taking hormone therapy if the following conditions exist:

- venous thrombosis (clots in the veins)
- breast cancer and benign breast disease
- liver intolerance of estrogens, which manifests itself as jaundice (rare)
- gall-bladder disease

Unfortunately, these warnings may damage rather than help women considering hormone therapy. The studies that led the FDA to list these contraindications were not based on HRT in perimenopausal or menopausal women. They were based on experience with higher doses of estrogens—that is, synthetic hormones with dosages that were much higher than dosages used in HRT regimens—and with oral contraceptives. Epidemiologic studies, with their inherent limitations, are all that we have for arriving at these contraindications. Furthermore, the FDA contraindication list does not inform a woman (or her doctor) about the relative risks of taking or not taking hormones when the woman is estrogen-deficient. For example, we know that hormone therapy, as discussed in Chapter 10, protects against cardiovascular disease, heart attacks, and high levels of cholesterol in the blood. We also know that gall-bladder disease is relatively rare. One report that was never replicated claimed an increased incidence of gall-bladder disease in HRT users.[18a] Even if hormone therapy were to increase the risk of gall-bladder disease, the result of, for example, doubling a rare occurrence versus the enormous benefit in reducing a widely occurring disease such as heart disease is not reflected in the contraindication of the FDA. Appropriately prescribed, HRT is estimated to reduce by 40 percent the incidence of cardiovascular disease in women.

Another problem with the contraindication list is the position in which it places physicians when they want to help women. Because we live in a litigious era, physicians must consider the possibility of being sued when they try to help patients. Some doctors, therefore, may elect to do nothing rather than risk helping. We believe that the malpractice suits that are so rampant in America today have changed the kind of health care that women can expect to receive. As a result, women must not only take responsibility for learning about what they want, but must ask for it, or they may not be exposed to all of their treatment options.

The medical community is faced with a difficult problem in prescribing hormones today. Medical knowledge comes from scientific research. We learn about contraindications accurately only when double-blind research studies are conducted in which some women get the hormone and others get the placebo. Scientists then measure the incidence of gall-bladder disease or any other supposed contraindication. Only one such study has been conducted. Previously, no women who have had breast cancer or benign breast disease have entered into a study in which some were given hormones and others were given placebos to see whether there really was an increased risk.

Why has so little research in this area been conducted? First, there are ethical considerations, in addition to the enormous cost of conducting such studies. If an HRT treatment is strongly indicated as beneficial, then denying it (by giving a placebo) produces a dilemma. Likewise, if a treatment might increase the occurrence of disease, a similar ethical problem emerges. What is important for the reader to understand is that definitive studies of breast cancer and HRT have not been done, and, therefore, we do not have all the facts.

And for each woman who is at risk for a disease that hormone therapy may affect, she still needs to make an informed choice based on a delicate balance of competing influences. Even if you know that you are at risk for osteoporosis—which hormone therapy will help— and you know that you have been treated for breast cancer and feel that you are free of this disease at present, there is overwhelming (and inappropriate) bias against the use of estrogen. But if you are also suffering from estrogen deprivation and its attendant hot flashes and other menopausal symptoms (vaginal atrophy, depression, and so forth), you have a tough choice to make. The responsibility for health-care decisions is uniquely yours. One purpose of this book is to provide enough information to help you make choices knowledgeably and intelligently as you weigh an unknown risk against improving the quality of your life.

THE SIDE EFFECTS OF HRT

For women who are beginning HRT, a two to three-month adjustment period is sometimes necessary before full comfort is achieved. Beneficial effects of estrogen may be perceived within two to three days but generally take longer. It is common for women on synthetic progesterone (such as medroxyprogesterone acetate or norgestrel) to feel irritable following administration of the hormone. Fortunately, this irritability tends to evaporate after several months. It appears to be the body's and brain's reaction before they build up the necessary enzyme systems for sufficient metabolism. Except for this temporary irritability, hormones should make you feel good.

Immediate changes for the worse in the way you feel are just as important to consider and should be dealt with promptly. If you feel bad when you are taking hormones to feel good, something is wrong and you should seek an adjustment in your prescription.

Women who take estrogen don't usually experience discomfort. However, if the dose is too high, there may be such side effects as breast tenderness, more vaginal discharge due to increased cervical secretions, weight gain, leg cramps, edema (fluid retention), headache, and unscheduled uterine bleedings.[3, 58, 97] These side effects can continue for as long as the overdose is maintained.[57] With lower doses, side effects disappear. If you take estrogen and experience any of these discomforts, you should work with your doctor to determine the dosage that will make you most comfortable. Generally, there is an ideal level of hormone that is best for each individual. If the dosage is too high, you feel overdose effects; if it is too low, you feel the menopausal distress symptoms. Your body will tell you when you are at the correct dose if you learn to listen to it.

If you take hormones for a year or more, you may need vitamin supplements. Estrogen quickly uses up your vitamin B_6. When vitamin B_6 is depleted, depression can result. This depression is easily cured by supplementing your diet with B_6. The proper dose appears to be 100 mg. per day; you should not exceed this dose level because excessively high doses of this vitamin can produce unpleasant side effects.[13, 39, 40, 78, 95]

One of the reasons that women live longer than men lies in their lower incidence of heart disease before menopause. At the menopause, when estrogen levels decline, the rate of heart disease for women begins to approach the (much higher) rate for men. Although there are some data suggesting that there is an increased rate of heart disease after age forty in menstruating women on oral contraceptives (which contain synthetic hormones), the use of hormones at menopause is clearly different. With few exceptions, menopausal women who take estrogen have less heart disease, no elevation in either systolic or diastolic blood pressure, reduced cholesterol levels, and alterations of blood lipoproteins consistent with reduced risk of heart disease.

To avoid being an exception, you should understand the precautions and take them. (1) You should have your blood pressure monitored to be certain that you are not one of the rare individuals whose blood pressure increases on estrogen (details of the studies of cardiovascular health and hormones are given in Chapter 10). (2) You should confine estrogen therapy to natural estrogen. "Natural estrogens" are those that are chemically identical to the kinds that occur in nature. Some are derived from animal sources; others are made in the laboratory. In contrast, "synthetic estrogens" are those that are dissimilar to the natural ones—perhaps by as little as one atom. The distinction between natural and synthetic estrogen is relevant in the selection of a safe HRT regimen. Natural estrogens appear to be safer than synthetic estrogens. Synthetic estrogens (like ethinyl estradiol) sometimes increase the risk of cardiovascular diseases.[8, 49a, 58a, 65] Moreover, the cardiovascular benefits that accrue to estrogen only apply to the natural estrogens like Premarin, Harmogen (a brand used in Great Britain), and Estrace. For a more extensive list of which hormones are natural and which are synthetic, refer to Tables 3 and 4.

When the first edition of *Menopause* was written, we had not yet learned the importance of regular estrogen opposition with progesterone in a complete hormone regimen. We did know that progesterone needed to be balanced against estrogen in order to prevent endometrial cancer (this subject is reviewed in the next chapter). Since then, research studies have shown that balancing estrogen and progesterone may be beneficial in other ways as well. Beta-endorphins, secretions from the central nervous system, are those substances associated with the general sense of euphoria that runners feel—they call it "runner's high." A series of studies, beginning with rats, progressing to monkeys, and culminating with women, have shown that beta-endorphins rise and fall in response to the estrogen-progesterone cycle. A hysterectomy, a menopause, or any other condition that reduces either the estrogen or the progesterone levels will seriously limit the blood levels of endorphins. Reduced beta-endorphins are associated with depression. We, therefore, believe that hormone replacement regimens are optimized and a woman's general sense of

TABLE 3 HRT Brands Sold in the United States* That Are Cited in This Book (N = natural; S = synthetic)

PRODUCT	CHEMICAL NAME	DOSE (MG.)	MANUFACTURER	METHOD OF DELIVERY
ESTROGENS				
Premarin (N)	Conjugated estrogens	0.3 0.625 0.9 1.25 2.5	Wyeth-Ayerst	Oral
Estrace (N)	Micronized estradiol	1.0 2.0	Mead Johnson	Oral
Estratab (N)	Esterified estrogens	0.3 0.625 1.25 2.5	Reid-Rowell	Oral
Ogen (N)	Estropipate	0.625 1.25 2.5 5.0	Abbott	Oral
Estinyl (S)	Ethinyl estradiol	0.02 0.05 0.5	Schering	Oral
Estrovis (S)	Quinestrol	0.1	Parke-Davis	Oral
Premarin Vaginal Cream (N)	Conjugated estrogens	0.625 mg./gm.	Wyeth-Ayerst	Vaginal cream
Estrace Vaginal Cream (N)	17β-estradiol	0.1 mg./gm.	Mead Johnson	Vaginal cream
Ogen Vaginal Cream (N)	Estropipate	1.5 mg./gm.	Abbott	Vaginal cream
Ortho Dienestrol Cream (S)	Dienestrol	0.01%	Ortho	Vaginal cream
Estragard Cream (S)	Dienestrol	0.01%	Reid-Rowell	Vaginal cream
Diethylstilbestrol Suppositories (S)	Diethyl-stilbestrol	0.1 mg./gm. 0.5 mg./gm.	Lilly	Vaginal suppository
Depo-Estradiol (N)	Estradiol cypionate	1.0 mg./ml. 5.0 mg./ml.	Upjohn	Injection
Delestrogen (S)	Estradiol valerate	10.0 mg./ml. 20.0 mg./ml. 40.0 mg./ml.	Squibb	Injection
Estraval (S)	Estradiol valerate	10.0 mg./ml. 20.0 mg./ml.	Reid-Rowell	Injection
Estrapel (N)	Estradiol pellet	25.0	Bartor, Progynon	Pellet
Estraderm (N)	Transdermal estradiol	0.05 mg./day (4.0 mg./patch) 0.1 mg./day (8.0 mg./patch)	CIBA-GEIGY	Patch
PROGESTAGENS, ANDROGENS, ESTROGEN/ANDROGEN COMBINATIONS				
PROGESTAGEN				
Provera	Medroxyprogesterone acetate	2.5 5.0 10.0	Upjohn	Oral
Curretab	Medroxyprogesterone acetate	10.0	Reid-Rowell	Oral

PRODUCT	CHEMICAL NAME	DOSE (MG.)	MANUFACTURER	METHOD OF DELIVERY
Amen	Medroxyprogester-one acetate	10.0	Carnrick	Oral
Cycrin	Medroxyprogester-one acetate	10.0	Wyeth-Ayerst	Oral
Aygestin	Norethindrone acetate	5.0	Wyeth-Ayerst	Oral
Norlutate	Norethindrone acetate	5.0	Parke-Davis	Oral
Norlutin	Norethindrone	5.0	Parke-Davis	Oral
Megace	Megestrol acetate	20.0 40.0	Bristol-Myers	Oral
Ovrette	Norgestrel	0.075	Wyeth-Ayerst	Oral
Micronor	Norethindrone	0.35	Ortho	Oral
Nor-QD	Norethindrone	0.35	Syntex	Oral
—	Progesterone vaginal supposi-tories	25.0	—	Vaginal suppository

ANDROGENS

PRODUCT	CHEMICAL NAME	DOSE (MG.)	MANUFACTURER	METHOD OF DELIVERY
Oreton	Methyltestosterone	5.0	Schering	Oral
Metandren	Methyltestosterone	5.0	CIBA-GEIGY	Oral
Halotestin	Fluoxymesterone	5.0	Upjohn	Oral
Fluoxymesterone	Fluoxymesterone	5.0	Reid-Rowell	Oral
Depo-Testosterone	Testosterone cypionate	50.0 mg./ml.	Upjohn	Injection
Delatestryl	Testosterone enanthate	100.0 mg./ml.	Squibb	Injection
Testopel	Testosterone pellets	75.0	Bartor	Injection
Oreton	Testosterone pellets	75.0	Progynon	Injection

COMBINATIONS

PRODUCT	CHEMICAL NAME	DOSE (MG.)	MANUFACTURER	METHOD OF DELIVERY
Estratest	Esterified estrogens and methyltestos-terone	1.25 2.5	Reid-Rowell	Oral
Estratest H.S.	Esterified estrogens and methyltestos-terone	0.625 1.25	Reid-Rowell	Oral
Premarin with Methyltes-tosterone	Conjugated estrogens and methyltestos-terone	1.25 and 10.0 0.625 and 5.0	Wyeth-Ayerst	Oral
Depo-Tostadiol	Estradiol cypionate and testosterone cypionate	2.0 and 50.0	Upjohn	Injection
Estrapel	Estradiol pellet (given with testosterone pellets)	25.0	Bartor, Progynon	Pellet

*Generics from animal sources are not included in this table because of the variability in bioavailability. *Bioavailability* refers the amount of biologically active material needed to produce the desired effect. Batches are obtained from animal sources; these have varying levels of the concentration of the hormones. Most generics do not compensate for this variation; when they do, the price is usually higher.

We have excluded combinations of hormones with vitamins and psychotropic drugs.

The brands listed are those that are mainly cited in the text and its review of the literature.

TABLE 4   HRT Brands Sold in Canada*   (N = natural; S = synthetic)

PRODUCT NAME	CHEMICAL NAME	DOSE (MG.)	MANUFACTURER	METHOD OF DELIVERY
ESTROGENS				
Premarin (N)	Conjugated estrogens	0.3 0.625 0.9 1.25	Wyeth-Ayerst	Oral
CES Tab (S)	Conjugated estrogens	0.625 1.25	ICN Canada	Oral
EstroMed (N)	Conjugated estrogens	1.25	Medic Laboratories	Oral
Conjugated Estrogens (N)	Conjugated estrogens	0.625 1.25	Pharmascience	Oral
Oestrogènes Conjugées (N)	Conjugated estrogens	1.25	ProDoc Laboratories	Oral
NeoEstrone (N)	Esterified estrogens	0.625 1.25	Neolab	Oral
Estinyl (S)	Ethinyl estradiol	0.02 0.05 0.5	Schering Canada	Oral
Estrace (N)	Estradiol	1.0 2.0	Bristol Laboratories Canada	Oral
Premarin (N)	Conjugated estrogens	0.625	Wyeth-Ayerst	Vaginal cream
Oestrilin (N)	Estrone	1.0	Desbergers	Vaginal cream
NeoEstrone (N)	Estrone	1.0	Neolab	Vaginal cream
Oestrilin cones (N)	Estrone	0.25	Desbergers	Vaginal suppository
Premarin (N)	Conjugated estrogens	25.0	Wyeth-Ayerst	Injection
Femogen forte (N)	Estrone	5.0	Stickley	Injection
Delestrogen (S)	Estradiol valerate	10.0	Squibb Canada	Injection
Estradiol valerate (S)	Estradiol valerate	20.0	K Line	Injection
Femogex (S)	Estradiol valerate	20.0	Stickley	Injection
Neo-Diol (S)	Estradiol valerate	20.0	Neolab	Injection
Estraderm (N)	Estradiol	0.001 mg./day (2.0 mg./patch) 0.05 mg./day (4.0 mg./patch) 0.1 mg./day (8.0 mg./patch)	CIBA	Patch

PROGESTINS, TESTOSTERONE, ESTROGEN/ANDROGEN COMBINATIONS

PRODUCT NAME	CHEMICAL NAME	DOSE (MG.)	MANUFACTURER	METHOD OF DELIVERY
PROGESTINS				
Provera	Medroxyprogesterone acetate	5.0 10.0	Upjohn Canada	Oral
Colprone	Medrogestone	5.0	Wyeth-Ayerst	Oral
Micronor	Norethindrone	0.35	Ortho Pharmaceutical Canada	Oral
Norlutate	Norethindrone acetate	5.0	Parke-Davis Division, Warner-Lambert	Oral
TESTOSTERONE				
Metandren	Methyltestosterone†	10.0 25.0	CIBA-GEIGY	Oral

PRODUCT NAME	CHEMICAL NAME	DOSE (MG.)	MANUFACTURER	METHOD OF DELIVERY
Metandren	Methyltestos-terone†	10.0 25.0	CIBA-GEIGY	Buccal (under the tongue)
COMBINATIONS				
Premarin Methyl-testosterone	Methyltestosterone and conjugated estrogens	5.0 and 0.625 10.0 and 1.25	Wyeth-Ayerst	Oral
Ortho-Novum 1/35	Norethindrone and ethynil estradiol	1.0 and 0.035	Ortho Pharma-ceutical Canada	Oral
Climacteron‡	Testosterone enan-thate benzilic acid, estradiol dienanthate, and estradiol benzoate	150.0 7.5 1.0	Frosst Division, Merck-Frosst Canada	Monthly injection

*Information courtesy of the Drug Identification Division in Canada, obtained through Dr. Sabine Swieringa.

†These testosterones are not reported on in the HRT studies reviewed here.

‡This is the injectible used by Dr. Sherwin in her study of treatment for libido loss.[86]

well-being increased when progesterone is added to the therapy, opposing the estrogen.[25, 33, 70, 88, 98]

Weight gain and bloating bother some women who take hormone therapy. If you have these problems, several options are available. You might try taking time off from the estrogen—one day a week or perhaps every third day. Or, working with your doctor, you might increase your dose of progestagen to oppose the estrogens better. Alternatively, you might reduce your estrogen dose: pills can be broken in half; creams can be applied in lesser quantities.

HRT AND IMMUNITY

Your ability to withstand infection is largely a function of how efficient your immune system is. There is some evidence that estrogen helps stimulate immunity.[28] Researchers continue to investigate the relationship between sex hormones and immunologic function. A role for these hormones in modulating blood levels of interlukin-1 (an important immune substance) was reported in 1988.[96] Experiments with guinea pigs conducted by Dr. George Feigen, a physiologist at Stanford University, explored relationships between estrogens and antibodies. Antibodies are blood-borne substances that attack

infectious molecules. In guinea pigs, estrogens increase the speed
with which antibodies are produced and also act to lower the speed of
antibody decay. This improves immunity because the antibodies remain around longer to attack infectious molecules. It seems likely
that some kind of increased immune responsiveness might account
for the better health in the menopausal women who take hormones.
This includes lower rates of breast cancer for most groups that have
been studied, as is detailed in the next chapter (immune response is
relevant to cancers), and longer life spans.[15]

Taking HRT

To treat the symptoms of menopause, hormones are usually prescribed by the physician in one of four ways: the hormones can be
swallowed in pill form; applied as a patch (like a Band-Aid), usually
on the buttocks or abdomen; applied as a cream to the vagina; or
placed under the tongue, where it dissolves. When you ingest the
pill, the hormone enters the blood by a different route than when
you use a patch or cream or when you place a wafer under your
tongue. The pill is swallowed, dissolves, and then passes through
your stomach and out into the intestines. Once the dissolved pill
moves through the intestinal tract, normal absorption occurs, and
the hormone crosses the walls of the intestine into the liver and
finally into the blood stream.

Patches and creams are different: the hormone is absorbed
through the cells of the skin and moves directly into the blood
stream. The application of the patch must be carefully controlled. If
you don't place it smoothly on the skin but let it bubble, then the
hormone will not be properly absorbed into the skin. You should
smooth the patch carefully with your fingertips to make sure its entire
surface closely touches your skin to promote even and maximum
absorption.

Hormone administration by vaginal delivery is similar to that of
the patch. The way it works is simple. You apply cream with a
plunger in much the same way as you insert a tampon. The cream
coats the vaginal lining, is absorbed through the walls of the vagina,
and moves into the blood stream. Once absorbed, the estrogens appear to be diluted immediately so that no single organ except for the

vagina receives a particularly high dose. Within four hours of applying the cream, the blood levels of estradiol and estrone reach their maximum levels.[75] Since standing or moving about may cause the cream to leak out of the vagina, the cream is applied at bedtime to counteract the force of gravity (which is why most women prefer other methods of hormone delivery). When one is lying down, the hormone can be absorbed through the vaginal walls most completely. Be aware, however, that sexual intercourse is to be avoided immediately after the application of vaginal estrogens. If the estrogen has not yet been absorbed into the vaginal skin, it will rub off on the penis and might be absorbed into the man's body through his skin. But the amount absorbed is transiently circulated.

Placing the micronized* estrogen (Estrace) under the tongue works like the patch and creams do when absorption is maximal. The hormone is absorbed through the skin, enters into the blood stream rapidly, is diluted by the blood as it circulates through the body, and then reaches the liver.

STARTING HORMONE THERAPY

Women begin losing mass from their bones as early as their late thirties and early forties. Cholesterol levels start to rise at that time. Hot flashes and other menopausal symptoms often begin well before menopause. Patterns of menstrual bleeding change for many who are in their early forties. Unfortunately, hysterectomy is frequently recommended as a "cure" for the bleeding, and surgery is often performed when appropriate hormone therapy could be used instead to control the menstrual bleeding, prevent bone loss, promote cardiovascular health, and alleviate the symptoms associated with the perimenopause. But just as there is controversy about the safety of HRT for menopausal women, so is there controversy about HRT for women who have not yet reached menopause.

Between 1986 and 1988, six studies[44, 53, 55, 85, 89, 101] were published that described the effects of HRT on women in their late thirties and early forties who were still spontaneously menstruating. Women con-

*The word *micronized* means "broken into minute particles, which permits more rapid absorption into the body."

sidered at special risk for hormone use were excluded from participation. The smallest study[53] included 13 women; the largest[55] included 434 women and evaluated 7,600 menstrual cycles. In these studies, no pregnancies occurred in women using HRT. (Nonetheless, despite these studies, pregnancies have occurred; HRT is not an effective contraceptive.) Menstrual bleeding became more regular. It also became lighter for everyone, heavy bleeding was eliminated, and painful menstruation disappeared. HRT had no significant effect on blood pressure, liver function, or white-cell count.

At the 1987 meeting of the International Menopause Society, several sessions were devoted to hormone therapy for premenopausal women over thirty-five. The conclusion of those scientists and physicians at the conference was that, given the benefits of hormonal contraception after the age of thirty-five, only patients seriously "at risk" should be deterred from hormone therapy. This conclusion is reinforced by the results of the studies noted above. For women in their late thirties and early forties, oral contraceptives offer hormone therapy that can be beneficial. Provided a woman is a nonsmoker and has none of the at-risk conditions listed on page 128, low-dose oral contraceptives can probably be safely used for contraception, the control of uncomfortable menstrual bleeding, and the alleviation of symptoms associated with the perimenopause. Oral contraceptives are available in a variety of doses. In general, lower doses have fewer associated adverse side effects than higher doses do. So women using oral contraceptives should take the lowest dose that can provide them with symptom relief.

Estrogen is the generic term for a class of steroid hormones that have a number of physiological effects in common. There are two classes of commercially available estrogens. A *natural estrogen* is one whose molecular configuration is identical to a form found in nature and includes 17β estradiol, micronized estradiol, estrone, and estriol. *Conjugated equine estrogens* (for example, Premarin) refer to a mixture of estrogens and other substances derived from the urine of pregnant mares and are considered natural estrogens. A *synthetic estrogen*'s molecular configuration is not the same as a comparable estrogen that occurs in nature; its actions, however, are similar to those of natural estrogens. Common synthetic estrogens include ethinyl estradiol, and mestranol. All estrogen-containing oral contraceptives available today contain one or the other of these two synthetic estrogens.

WHAT IS A BENEFICIAL DOSAGE?

If you decide to take HRT, you should review with your doctor the reasons for using natural estrogens. You should also realize that every woman has a unique metabolic pattern. A tall, slim woman will need more hormonal support than a short, slim one. A heavy woman will probably need less hormones than a thin woman because the fat cells of a woman serve as miniature "conversion factories," changing the androgen hormones contributed by the adrenal glands and the ovaries into the estrogen she needs. When you know what taking too much or too little hormone feels like, you will be able to work with your physician to find the type and dose of hormonal support that is best for you.

When estrogen levels are adequate, hot flashes usually stop. The Kupperman index on page 78 can show you what your level of menopausal distress is. The higher your score, the more estrogen your doctor will need to prescribe for you to get relief. If you take your estrogen pill by pill, 1 mg. of micronized estradiol or .625 mg. of conjugated equine estrogen is probably a good starting measure.[79] Then, if you find you are taking too much of the hormone (for example, your breasts have become swollen and heavy), you can discuss with your doctor decreasing the dose. Persistent swelling of your ankles should be brought to your doctor's attention so that your blood pressure and kidney function can be tested. If you find you are taking too little of the hormone (hot flashes are continuing), increasing the dose will help. Within this dose range, most women find relief from distress and protection for both their bones and their cardiovascular system. (However, if you have started using hormone therapy late—after vaginal atrophy has already begun—an initially higher dose of estrogen will be needed to achieve relief.) If you take estrogens in cream form—that is, placed via an applicator directly into the vagina—lower doses will solve the vaginal problems than if you take the hormone by mouth.[60] Estrogen creams placed in the vagina will also reverse atrophic (deteriorating) urogenital tissue.[11]

Since Premarin is the most widely sold hormone therapy in the United States, this is the hormone cream that published studies have most thoroughly evaluated. Moreover, we have had over fifty years' experience with its use. Recent problems with some generics that have different batch potencies make Premarin the most reliable option. The dose of 1.25 mg. in cream form seems to be fully effective. Lower doses may be safer and can be achieved by using the cream on alternate nights or by administering only a fraction of an applicator quantity each night. Estrace, in vaginal-cream or tablet form, has also been well studied and shown to be effective. But just about every hormone regimen tested has been shown to be effective in relieving menopausal distress, provided the dose is correct. The decision that you and your physician reach, should you opt for hormones, requires a careful consideration of which route (the pill, the patch, or the cream) to select.

PROGESTERONE

While estrogen appears to produce a variety of feminizing effects— from breast development to skin suppleness—progesterone functions differently. Progesterone is an important part of a safe HRT regimen. It protects the endometrium from estrogen stimulation that might lead to hyperplasia. Chapter 6 provides details. Progesterone also seems important to the emotional life of a woman. Previously, in the discussion on the role of progesterone in beta-endorphin secretion and the sense of well-being, we described our developing understanding of the connection between these two substances. Progesterone also appears to play a role in weight control. In the progesterone phase of a normal menstrual cycle, a woman burns about 9 percent more calories per day. We do not know whether progesterone therapy has the same effect, but it is likely that, as you take progesterone therapy, your metabolism speeds up.

The word *progesterone* refers to natural hormones. The words *progestagen* and *progestin* are applied to synthetic progesterones that can be taken as part of an HRT regimen. Natural progesterone for HRT is currently available in pill and cream form throughout Europe and may soon become available in North America.[5, 38]

Synthetic progestins, as you can see in Table 5, are composed of two basic types: the 17α progestagens (for example, medroxyprogesterone acetate) and the 19-nortestosterones such as norethisterone acetate. The 17α progestagens appear to be better tolerated, even at high doses, than the 19-nortestosterones; but in either case, when the doses are sufficiently low, the 19-nortestosterones seem to have no negative side effects.

TABLE 5   Oral Progestins: High versus Low Doses with Respect to Lipid Changes

HORMONE USED*	HIGH DOSES	LOW DOSES	REFERENCES
19-NORTESTOSTERONES			
Medrogestone	5.0 mg.		94
Norethisterone ac-	5.0–10.0 mg.	1.0 mg.	43, 100
etate	2.0 mg.		44, 87
17α PROGESTAGENS			
Medroxyproges-	5.0 or 10.0 mg.	2.5 mg.	43, 67, 87
teroneacetate	twice/day	twice/day	
(MPA—Provera)		5.0 mg.	83, 85
		once/day	
PURE NATURAL PROGESTERONE			
		100.0 mg. twice/day	66, 67
		300.0 mg. once/day	26

*Usually 10 to 13 days per month.

Table 5 lists the three classes of progestins according to high and low doses. These doses have been determined by studies that analyzed the plasma cholesterol level before and after hormone therapy. This research has shown that when the doses are high, the plasma levels are altered in ways that place a woman at risk for cardiovascular disease. When the doses are low, any of these progestins appears to be equally good in preventing that risk. For details of cardiovascular health reactions to different hormones, see Chapter 10. For now, if you want to know what constitutes a safe, low dose of any of the currently marketed progestins, refer to Table 5. Safe dose levels of natural progesterone for preventing endometrial hyperplasia await further rigorous research.

If you experience sore breasts (transient mastalgia) while on progestin, this could be a reaction to too much of the hormone.[21, 99] Likewise, the synthetic progestins, either the 19-nortestosterones or the 17α progestagens, may produce mild breast irritation, but this usually stops within the third month of the therapy.[21] Thus, you will want to take enough progestin to protect the endometrium and breast (as is described in greater detail in the next chapter) but not too much or your blood lipids will be at risk.

THE BLEEDING DAY TEST

Fortunately, in 1986, a group of investigators in Great Britain presented "a simple method for determining the optimal dosage of progestin in post menopausal women receiving estrogens."[68] We call this the *Bleeding Day Test* because you can use information from your own cyclic bleeding to tell you whether you are getting enough progesterone or not. The study, which evaluated 100 postmenopausal women, searched for a way to protect the endometrium without requiring an endometrial biopsy (see the next chapter) because biopsies are uncomfortable and costly. The researchers, investigating different hormonal regimens that used synthetic and natural estrogens and progesterones, came to some helpful conclusions.

The estrogen treatment (whether oral, skin cream, patch, or implant) was taken every day of the month; the progestin, at first, was taken 12 to 14 days of the month. Counting the first day of progestin therapy as day 1, if bleeding did not begin before taking the eleventh tablet, the woman was *not* at risk for endometrial disease.[68] If she began bleeding *before* day 11, indicating that she was not taking enough progesterone and was thus at risk for endometrial disease, she could delay the bleeding by increasing either the dose or the duration of the progestin. Because these investigators are highly esteemed professionals with respect to their studies of endometrial health and HRT, their results are particularly comforting and trustworthy. Although no HRT regimen can guarantee against endometrial disease, this method is clearly able to lower the incidence dramatically. For more detail about HRT and cancer, see Chapter 6.

ANDROGENS

One 1985 study provided data indicating that women who had taken estrogen for several months showed a reduction of about 30 percent of normal levels in circulating free testosterone.[68] Although this was the only report that studied this subject, if you do take HRT without androgen and later begin to experience a decline in libido, this may be the reason and you may want to discuss with your physician the possibility of low-dose testosterone treatment.

Investigators of HRT regimens have begun to consider the role that androgens play in the therapy.[36, 86] Using anecdotal reports that he had obtained, Dr. R. B. Greenblatt, an eminent pioneer in HRT for menopausal women, concluded that androgens are psychotropic drugs (that is, drugs that affect the emotions) that influence the way women feel.[36] When doses are kept sufficiently low (to prevent virilization), they complement the estrogens, to the benefit of the women who are on this regimen. A study conducted by Dr. B. B. Sherwin on the role of androgens in restoring lost libido[86] supports this theory. Even though we have no systematic body of published research on these benefits of androgens on which to draw, we must remain alert for future studies on this important, possibly useful, therapy.

We should mention, though, several studies reported in 1988 and 1990. These studies have begun to evaluate relationships between androgens (such as testosterone) and cardiovascular health factors. The findings suggest the following:

- Women with cardiovascular disease are likely to have been hirsute when they were in their fertile years.[99a]
- Thus, women who are hirsute should rigorously monitor those cardiovascular risk factors that they can control (that is, diet, exercise, stress reduction)[63a] and should consider taking hormone replacement therapies balanced with estrogen.
- Testosterone therapy can produce hirsutism. The higher the testosterone dose, the greater the odds that this side effect will occur; by cutting the dose, the problem diminishes.
- When testosterone therapy is added to HRT regimens to overcome libidinal and energy deficits after surgically induced menopause, lipids are not adversely affected provided that (1) the dose is in the moderate range (see Table 5) and (2) estrogen is given with the testosterone.

Although the two-year duration of the studies so far reported[84a, 94a] will need to be extended, the results look promising. But since the reports of lipid responses have been published as symposia in private meetings sponsored by hormone manufacturers rather than in peer-reviewed biomedical journals,[84a, 94a] we believe that caution is advisable in the early 1990s.

The data suggest, however, that *low doses* of testosterone taken orally are generally safe for the cardiovascular system. Until more studies have been completed, women who want to consider such therapy should work with their physician to keep a close watch on their plasma levels of cholesterol and other risk-determining lipids. Also, newer progestagens are being developed (and some are presently used in Europe) that do not have these unfavorable effects on the lipids. But caution is advised by Dr. A. Z. Teran and Dr. R. D. Gambrell, who point out that progestin must be added to the estrogen and testosterone to protect the uterus.[94a]

PILLS, PELLETS, PATCHES, AND CREAMS

The most common way to take estrogen is by swallowing a pill or tablet. When the first edition of this book appeared, there was concern that taking estrogen orally might adversely affect the liver. This issue has now been studied, and it appears that taking hormones orally does not compromise liver health.[29, 63] Regardless of whether estrogens were administered by pill or by injection, the metabolism in the blood was shown to be similar.[49]

Estrogen can also be taken by placing a pill of micronized estradiol under the tongue; estrogen is then absorbed from there into the blood stream.[12]

Hormones can be delivered by surgically implanting pellets under the skin. This procedure, which involves injecting a solid pellet of hormone under the skin after the region is numbed with a local anesthetic, can be uncomfortable.[30, 59] We do not recommend it because the dose of hormone cannot be easily adjusted.

Other ways in which hormones can be taken have been well studied. The patch is an estrogen-filled Band-Aid that is placed on the skin (usually the buttocks). It should not be placed on the breasts because breast tissue is hypersensitive to estrogen and should not risk receiving the initial undiluted dose. The hormone is absorbed through the skin into the blood stream. Each patch lasts several days and will leave a series of harmless stains on the skin that take a few days to fade. The only other apparent drawback to this method of taking estrogen is that hormones delivered in this way do not seem to have the same beneficial effect on blood lipids as estrogen delivered by other means. Studies on this are summarized in Chapter 10.

In Europe, estrogens have been taken two other ways not yet available in North America. Estrogen-impregnated vaginal "rings," designed to be carried comfortably in the vagina, have been used to deliver low doses of estradiol directly to the vagina.[45] The method has proved effective in reversing urogenital atrophy in elderly menopausal women: women noted a reduction in vaginal dryness, and pain on urination and frequent urination (a manifestation of urethral irritation) were also reduced.[43] In Sweden, both estrogen and progestin are available as vaginal suppositories,[17] which appear to deliver effective amounts of hormone to the vagina and blood stream. We look forward to a time when North American pharmaceutical companies will be able to offer these methods of hormone delivery.

Progesterone, applied as a vaginal cream, can successfully affect the blood levels of progesterone. (In the case of the Myers *et al.* study, the university pharmacy had to compound the substance because it was not yet available from a pharmaceutical company.)[64]

Long-term hormone therapy (in this case, unopposed estrogen in the form of mestranol—a synthetic hormone) was reviewed in a 1989 study.[4] The investigators showed that even after 15 years of hormone use, former, earlier reports of a risk for venous thrombosis were not confirmed. The hormones appear to be safe.

One other method of hormone delivery that is widely used in Europe is hormone creams—both estrogen and progesterone—that are spread on the arms. The two come in natural form and are well received. Pharmaceutical companies in the United States have applied for FDA approval to market these creams, and we look forward to their availability here.

AVOIDING SYNTHETIC ERT

By 1990, the route of HRT administration had become less important than an awareness of the appropriate use of natural estrogens and low-dose progestins. Provided that you balance the dosages correctly, the particular issues to watch for remain as follows:

1. Monitor your blood pressure regularly. Your blood pressure may increase, although this is unlikely. Only oral hormone therapy (pills) has caused this problem in the rare cases where it did happen. Here is how. The liver responds rapidly to the oral ingestion of hor-

mones. Large increases of certain blood molecules that sometimes increase the risk of hypertension (high blood pressure) have been clearly noted.[34] One liver hormone, renin substrate, increases when oral estrogens are ingested.[69] Renin substrate does not increase in women who take their estrogen by means of vaginal cream, and this is one reason why the cream is sometimes considered a safer route of hormone administration. In young women who take oral contraceptives, these renin-substrate increases have been associated with hypertension. In menopausal women, the increases in renin substrate have not caused hypertension. Nonetheless, the very rapid response to oral hormones by the liver is cause for caution.

If you are one of those rare people whose blood pressure increases upon orally ingesting hormones, you need to address this condition. You should consider reducing the salt in your diet and taking other measures that your internist may prescribe, including possibly stopping your hormonal regimen until your blood-pressure problem is assessed by your doctor. If your blood pressure remains elevated, then you may choose to switch from oral administration of hormones to another route or, if this isn't helpful, to give up hormone therapy entirely. Your doctor should be able to help you make this decision.

2. You should be knowledgeable about your endometrial health. (See Chapter 6.) All routes of estrogen administration appear equally safe for endometrial (the cancer-prone) tissue, provided the doses you use are not excessively high. If you take hormones in cream form to reverse vaginal atrophy, you can use less hormone to get the same relief because the sensitive tissues are getting the needed dose before the hormones are diluted.

3. You should be informed about your cardiovascular health by having your cholesterol and other lipid levels checked at least annually. (See Chapter 10.)

CONSTANT AND CYCLICAL THERAPIES

Cyclical hormone therapy regimens involve going off hormones for a few days per week or month. Other regimens involve constant use of estrogen therapy coupled with either constant low-dose progesterone or cyclical use of progesterone (taking progesterone 12 to 15 days each month). The use of the term *constant* in HRT prescriptions is often confusing because it is applied differently by people who use it. *Constant HRT* usually means that a similar dose of hormones is taken every day, no exceptions. We do not yet have a universally accepted term that describes the taking of a constant dose in a cyclic fashion. Nor is there a term that would show which regimen has days off and which does not.

Provided the dosage is adequate and you are not having symptoms on the days when you are not taking hormones, all regimens seem effective.[2, 47] If symptoms occur, you should consider another regimen. The critical differences among the hormonal preparations have to do with their safety.[1] And, fortunately, the natural estrogens and low-dose progestins used in North America have all passed rigorous tests.

However, there are some differences in bleeding response. Monthly bleeding in women who continuously take hormones tends to stop within 4 to 12 months (or sooner) of beginning this regimen. [52, 90] Women who have a cyclic component to their hormone regimen (either some days without any hormone or some days without progestin) tend to continue having withdrawal bleeding for a longer period of time and to an older age. But all women who use cyclic HRT eventually do stop their monthly withdrawal bleeding regardless of the hormone regimen that they take. For those who use a cyclic regimen, the menstrual-like flow often continues for variable intervals even beyond the age of sixty. And in one investigator's research, 60 percent of the women seventy years or older continued to show monthly bleeding.[31] The option of constant HRT that averts the bleeding is always available.

Some women prefer the predictable levelness of a constant regimen. Others prefer the cyclical variation characteristic of feminine cycles. Biomedical investigations have not yet published data indicating which therapy is better.

SUMMARY

Hormone replacement therapy relieves the symptoms of menopausal distress, promotes a sense of well-being, may facilitate cardiovascular health, prevents or halts bone degeneration, and may even positively affect one's natural immune responses. How often you take the hormones depends on the route of administration, the strength of the dosage, the symptom relief, the presence of side effects, and the other factors discussed in this chapter. There are many different regimens that are being used successfully. An individual plan can best be worked out by means of cooperation between you and your health-care professional.

In 1983, the *Journal of the American Medical Association* published a study of estrogen use and all-cause mortality. Two thousand two hundred sixty-nine white women had been followed for six years. The results were that estrogen users had a lower incidence of any kind of death than nonusers. Oophorectomized women who took hormones had only 12 percent the incidence of death than oophorectomized women who took no hormones; hysterectomized women who took hormones had only 34 percent the incidence of death as hysterectomized women who took no hormones; and intact women who took hormones had half the risk of intact women who took no hormones.[14]

More recent developments in the area of breast cancer and hormone therapy indicate that progestin opposition to estrogen replacement therapy programs may offer protection against the disease.

HRT is rapidly developing into a wonderful, viable option for many women. It is critically important, before embarking on a hormone replacement regimen, to consider the one set of risks against which women need to protect themselves: the cancers. (This is discussed in the next chapter.) And for women who cannot take HRT, Chapter 14 will suggest alternatives.

6

HORMONE REPLACEMENT THERAPY II:
The Cancer Risk

Cancer is scary. If left unchecked, it can kill you. So can walking across the street. We don't stay inside to avoid being killed by a passing car, but we do not take walks along the freeway either. We ought not to avoid hormones before evaluating how low the risks are when proper hormone doses are taken. And make no mistake about it. With new regimens whose doses are lower than regimens that were common 10 years ago, the risks, too, are low and must be balanced against the benefits to bone and cardiovascular health that hormones provide. When the first reports came out in 1975 showing an association between cancer of the endometrium and estrogen replacement therapy, the signs were ominous. But the publicity tended to obscure the facts, and in certain crucial ways the public was left uninformed and was thus misled. Such events continue to recur whenever a published report suggests cancer.[3] Recent studies have shown that while high doses of estrogen do, over time, tend to affect endometrial health adversely, there are alternative courses of treatment available: (1) lower doses of estrogen and (2) adding the correct doses of appropriate progesterone to counterbalance the negative effects that too much estrogen sometimes causes. Both approaches radically alter the risks of developing endometrial cancer.

Ovarian cancer is not a problem for those receiving hormone therapy, and the risk of contracting the disease does not appear to increase either during or after therapy. Naturally produced hormonal activity is not considered a risk factor in this disease,[36] but recent studies suggest that some infertility patients may experience a higher incidence of this form of cancer.[51] Furthermore, although ovarian-cancer patients show increased blood levels of androstenedione and estrone,[58] HRTs do not seem to have an adverse influence on development of cancer of the ovary. And the same holds true for oral contraceptives: the Centers for Disease Control have provided data supporting the finding that taking oral contraceptives protects against developing ovarian cancer. Unfortunately, since the development and causes of ovarian cancer are not well understood, it is difficult to take preventative action against this rare but very serious disease.

Breast cancer and fibrocystic breast disease also represent an important issue for menopausal women and are addressed later in this chapter.

Cancer can be understood as an aberrant cellular growth that reproduces in your body, replacing healthy cells with malignant ones and destroying tissues as it voraciously spreads and forms tumors. Surgery can often remove tumors. The greater danger lies in the tendency of malignant cells to migrate. Little pieces of the tumor break off and travel throughout the body much like the seeds of a dandelion are dispersed across a great field with the help of the wind. In the case of the tumor, the blood stream acts like the wind, spreading malignant cells to other parts of the body.

ENDOMETRIAL CANCER

Since the endometrium responds to HRT and the appropriate dosage is critical, we begin the chapter with a discussion of endometrial cancer.

Your endometrium is a gland that lines the central cavity of the uterus. It is illustrated in Figure 7, page 92. The endometrium grows and thickens with each menstrual cycle, finally sloughing off during the menstrual flow. This tissue sometimes develops an overgrowth (a condition called endometrial hyperplasia) or, rarely, evolves into the more diseased state—the cancer.

HOW COMMON AND SERIOUS IS IT?

On average, 1 woman in 1,000 per year is diagnosed as having endometrial cancer.[86] Other diseases hit menopausal women more frequently: 14 per 1,000 die each year of cardiovascular attacks;[85] more also die each year after osteoporosis-induced hip fracture. The average age of detection for endometrial cancer is about sixty. Seventy percent of the cases occur between fifty and seventy years of age,[62] although endometrial cancer does strike women from twenty-one on.

It appears to be a slow-growing cancer. The earlier it is detected, the better the cure rate; and close to 90 percent of the earliest cases are cured. In contrast, the more developed cases have a poor prognosis: only 32 percent of these cancer patients survive the next five years. While advanced stages of endometrial cancer are life-threatening, the early stages are much less so. Moreover, it is reasonable to assume from our current knowledge of reproductive physiology that before such an early-stage cancer occurs, there is a long—more than a 12-month—progression of hyperplasias. Furthermore, these hyperplasias appear in response to high doses of unopposed estrogen (that is, estrogen taken without progesterone). You can take progesterone (which opposes the influence of estrogen on endometrial tissue) to reduce the risk of endometrial cancer.

DEVELOPMENT OF THE DISEASE

Before the cells of the endometrium reach a state that can be called cancerous, they appear to pass through three abnormal but noncancerous stages. These stages of endometrial hyperplasia[7, 13, 21] seem to be progressive in that the earlier, less severe stage *always* precedes the development of the later, more severe ones. The first stage is called *cystic hyperplasia,* the second *adenomatous hyperplasia,* and the third *atypical hyperplasia.* Pathologists can, with a microscope, look at slides on which smears of endometrial tissue have been placed to distinguish one stage of hyperplasia from the next. These scientists employ seven criteria:

1. appearance of the reproductive glands. The glands become progressively more swollen and enlarged and begin to show overcrowding.

2. number of cells per slide. Cystic hyperplasia shows counts of about 100 cells per slide while the more severe atypical hyperplasia shows about double this number.
3. number of clumps of cells per slide. Milder conditions show, on average, fewer cell groups, per slide.
4. average cell size. Individual cells get larger with increasing hyperplastic severity.
5. average size of the cell nuclei. With increasing severity, the area gets larger.[66]
6. increased number of mitotic figures. This indicates increased cell multiplication.
7. variations in the size and the staining properties of the cell nuclei. The nuclei may look darker (or lighter) than usual under the microscope.

If the hyperplasia increases in severity, it may develop into endometrial cancer.[30, 66] From a superficial cancer, it can spread into the uterus or into another part of the body by means of the circulatory or lymphatic system. Once malignant cells are in another part of the body, a lump or discrete tumor can form.

How likely is it that cystic glandular hyperplasia will develop into endometrial cancer? It appears to be very unlikely. In one study of 544 premenopausal women with cystic glandular hyperplasia (who were traced and followed for up to 24 years), less than 1 percent of the women developed endometrial cancer.[62] Other studies give higher figures for untreated hyperplasia.[87] Fortunately, hyperplasia can be treated with progestins.[68] Adenomatous and atypical hyperplasia are much more dangerous.[30, 68]

When endometrial cancer develops, it is diagnosed according to grade and to stage—from the lowest of I to the highest of IV. The more clearly defined the tumor(s) is (are), the lower the grade that is assigned. Staging of the tumor from a low of I to a high of IV is also assigned. The higher number denotes a greater size and degree of involvement that the body is experiencing with respect to the malignancies. Cancer cells, unlike benign tumor cells, invade your tissue and metastasize (spread). The dangerous highest grade (grade IV) indicates that the cancer is no longer neatly isolated in clumps but rather has changed into an undifferentiated state much like pepper sprinkled on eggs. A low-grade cancerous tumor can be identified and removed—usually without trouble. A high-grade, less differentiated tumor spreads easier, metastasizing to other parts of the body, where new tumors can form. This is where the greatest danger lies—when a cancer spreads to another part of the body via blood or lymph circulation.

Once a diagnosis of cancer of the uterus has been made, the stage and grade it is assigned helps predict how curable it is. Low-grade and early-stage endometrial cancers are almost always curable.[60, 61, 62]

SYMPTOMS

The most common symptom for endometrial cancer is abnormal (that is, unexpected) vaginal bleeding.[60] Not all abnormal vaginal bleeding indicates a cancerous condition. But if you are bleeding abnormally, it is important for you to see your physician.[24, 76] Both endometrial hyperplasia and endometrial cancer can exist without any telltale bleeding to signal their presence.[5, 7] However, this is rare. [5, 76] You may have apparent symptoms and most likely not have a disease, or (much less often) you may even have a disease but not have symptoms. Speedy diagnosis and treatment can save life and health.

EXAMINATION OF THE ENDOMETRIUM

To define the state of the endometrium, one must remove cells from it. One cannot use vaginal cells as a way of estimating the state of endometrial cells.[6, 50, 52] One must examine those cells that line the uterus. Once the cells are retrieved, they are smeared onto glass slides and studied under a microscope by pathologists.

Several methods are available for retrieving endometrial cells. The older, conventional method is a D & C—dilatation (expanding the opening of the cervix) and curettage (using a spoonlike instrument to scrape a bit of tissue from the lining of the uterus). "Cell samplers," an alternative method to D & C for obtaining endometrial cells, are simpler, faster, and make the utilization of anesthesia unnecessary. One of several cell samplers available is used: the Garcia Endometrial Curette (developed by Celso-Ramón García),[66] the Isaacs Endometrial Cell Sampler,[43] or the Endopap. Each is pictured in Figures 17, 18, and 19. Another, comfortable suction sampler is the Pillpelle Endometrial Sampler. The Vabra Endometrial Biopsy Suction de-

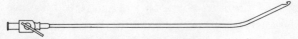

FIGURE 17   The Garcia Endometrial Curette

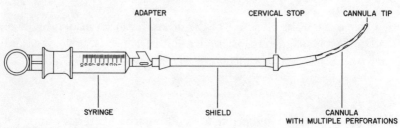

FIGURE 18   The Isaacs Endometrial Cell Sampler

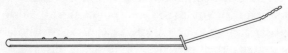

FIGURE 19   The Endopap

vice, however, while frequently used, causes more pain; thus, the other samplers are preferable.

The cell sampler is introduced into the vagina, narrow end first, passes through the opening of the cervix, and reaches the walls of the endometrium. The cervical stop prevents any other part of the instrument from gaining entry into the uterus. If you have a narrow cervix, the Isaacs Endometrial Cell Sampler will stretch the area as it penetrates through the narrow opening (os) to the womb. This stretching open of the narrow cervical canal can be uncomfortable. The Endopap, because it is thinner, does not cause this discomfort. Likewise, the Garcia Endometrial Curette is gentler. Once the cell sampler has entered the uterus, some of the endometrial cells are removed—either by gently scraping the endometrium (using the Endopap or the Garcia Endometrial Curette) or by using a syringe attached to the hollow end of the shield (Isaacs Endometrial Cell Sampler or Garcia Endometrial Curette). The syringe, illustrated on the Isaacs Endometrial Cell Sampler (Figure 18), would be attached in the same way to the Garcia Endometrial Curette. The head of the syringe is manipulated to create a vacuum. This vacuum causes some of the cells from the endometrium to be sucked into the sampler. Very few women find this alternative to D & C more than "slightly uncomfortable."[43] The Endopap does not provide as much tissue and, therefore, is more limited to screening (rather than diagnostic) techniques. Studies comparing the accuracy of diagnosis between conventional D & C and the diagnostic endometrial suction curettage support that both produce adequate tissue for accurate diagnoses.[12] More recent studies suggest that vacuum curettage has increased the accuracy of diagnosis over the D & C.[79]

Lately, two new diagnostic tools have been increasingly utilized. Due to improvements in ultrasonography and the addition of a wand that is inserted into the vagina to perform the evaluation, significant changes in the endometrium often can be detected and used to identify those women who might be at risk for endometrial cancer.[64a] And MRI (magnetic resonance imaging), while very effective, is extremely expensive. These methods are not yet readily available in gynecologists' offices, but they should be. Eventually, we expect ultrasound to be as widely used as Pap-smear screening is now.

WHO IS AT RISK?

Women with endometrial cancer are more likely to be obese, nulliparous (have never had a baby), hypertensive (have high blood pressure), and to have taken high doses of unopposed estrogen for a long duration.[24] The least critical factor turns out to be the high doses of estrogen, even though it has received the most publicity.

The greatest risk for endometrial cancer appears to be obesity. Usually this is defined as being more than 30 percent overweight.[31] One research group compared those with endometrial cancer to age-matched healthy women for a 30-year period. Obesity turned out to be the best predictor of endometrial cancer. Obesity accounted for much more cancer than did nulliparity (never having given birth), and nulliparity accounted for much more cancer than did estrogen use. Another 30-year study of 1,590 cases of uterine cancer found that a startling 51 percent of the cancer victims were obese.[63] If you are very overweight, you should monitor your endometrial health carefully. Have either regular (annual) endometrial checkups (endometrial biopsy), or take the Progestin Challenge Test, described later in this chapter. Readers who want information on nutrition, dieting, and exercise can find three separate chapters on these subjects (see Chapters 11, 12, and 13).

If you are short (5 feet 1 inch or less) and obese, the risks have been shown to be less since these risks apply predominantly to taller women. And women over 5 feet 6 inches are taking the biggest cancer risk of all if they become obese.[57, 93] We do not know why. With regard to your weight, one other point is worth noting: slender women who take estrogen may be at a higher risk than other women who take estrogen for a different reason. As described earlier, your fat cells actively convert androstenedione (an abundant menopausal hormone secreted by the adrenals and the aging ovaries) into estrone. The more fat you have, the higher your estrone level is likely to be. Thin women have, on average, lower levels of estrogen and, consequently, may suffer greater menopausal distress than heavier women. They may overcompensate with dosages of estrogen that are disproportionately high for their small body size. Currently, consideration of a woman's size is not taken into account when hormone therapy is prescribed, but it should be.

Being nulliparous also places women in the higher-risk category for endometrial cancer.[57, 63] It was shown that having had even one child sharply reduces the risk for endometrial cancer.[57] Apparently, the endometrium changes in some unknown way after having supported a growing fetus and placenta to make the development of a uterine cancer less likely.

Hypertension is the third most critical risk factor.[63] Almost half of the endometrial cancer patients have diastolic blood pressures of more than 100 mm. Hg. (normal values should be around 60 to 80).

HORMONES AND ENDOMETRIAL CANCER

Estrogen is a critical hormone that controls the growth of the endometrium during each cycle. Estrogen therapy at menopause likewise influences the growth of the lining. Too much estrogen can lead to overgrowth. High doses of estrogen have, not surprisingly, been shown to be associated with endometrial overgrowth (hyperplasia).[7, 13, 27, 42, 46, 48, 79, 94] This overgrowth often looks like the beginning growth of cancer. The biomedical research community is not agreed on whether hyperplasia and cancer are directly connected or separate entities. In any case, there is evidence that high doses of unopposed estrogen predispose some women to endometrial cancer. Unfortunately, when the first reports appeared and caused such a scare, they failed to point out that it was high, not low, doses that were largely responsible. Even though very few (7 per 1,000) women who take this risk will have a problem, there is no reason for you to gamble, because low doses fully relieve the distressing symptoms of menopause, prevent the devastation of osteoporosis, and do not appear to place you at risk for endometrial cancer.[56] In fact, in one 30-year study that monitored the women of a county in Minnesota, those with endometrial cancer were no more likely to have used low levels of estrogen (less than 1.25 mg. of conjugated oral estrogen) than those without cancer.[56] In that study, just as in the others described, high doses of unopposed estrogen did increase the risk, as was expected. Moreover, by adding progesterone in the proper way, you can actively reduce your risk of endometrial cancer to levels below that of women who take no hormones.[27] (More about this later.) Moreover, for women in their forties, HRT may be able to protect against the hormonal imbalances that cause the hyperplasia. The Bleeding Day Test on page 142 describes the method.

ESTROGEN AND ENDOMETRIAL CANCER

Each drug company packages its estrogen in several doses of increasing strength. See Tables 3 and 4 (pages 132 and 134, respectively). Your doctor can show you the guidebook he or she uses and go over with you the range of doses of the particular brand he or she selects for you. The *Physicians' Desk Reference,* published yearly, is one such text. You might even find it in your local library or at the book store. While it is not a complete compendium of drugs, it does reflect the information that is found in drug-package inserts. These are required by the Food and Drug Administration. For example, as of 1989 for Premarin (which has fifty years of clinical and scientific use), the pill form comes in doses as low as .3 mg. and ranges upward to 2.5 mg. For vaginal cream, the low dose begins with .3 mg. per day when one-eighth of the applicator capacity is used. The total cream applied each day to yield this low dose of estrogen is one-half a gram's worth. Clearly, the lower your dose of estrogen, the less stimulated your endometrium will be. The choice of estrogen dose must reflect a consideration of endometrial safety that is balanced against the benefits that were described in the previous chapter: relief from menopausal symptoms and improved general health of the skeletal and cardiovascular systems. The more unopposed estrogen you take each day, the greater the risk that you will overstimulate your endometrium.

PROGESTERONE AND ENDOMETRIAL CANCER

Progesterone helps prevent or oppose endometrial disease. In fact, the old term, *ERT* (estrogen replacement therapy), has finally given way to a newer term, *HRT* (hormone replacement therapy), reflecting the developing perception that proper therapy should include more than just estrogen. Investigators en masse now realize that since the normal-cycling woman has a repeating sequence of estrogen plus progesterone, it makes sense to mimic these ingredients in menopausal replacement programs.

Beginning with the work of Dr. Robert Kristner,[49a] investigators have found that progestagens in adequate dosages could reverse hyperplasias that had been induced by estrogen therapies.[75, 90] In 1978, a review of 8,170 women, evaluated by Dr. R. D. Gambrell of the Medical College of Georgia, showed that women who took estrogen in combination with progestagens had less incidence of endometrial cancer than women who took no hormones. (The terms *progestin* and *progestagen* are the names given to any substance with progesteronelike activity.) Women who took estrogens (at a time when high doses were common) without progestin had three times the incidence of this cancer than nonhormone users.[81] In 1986, Dr. Gambrell published updates of his original data. The results were similar to those of 1978 (see Table 6): estrogen-progesterone therapy, when combined, produces a lower incidence of endometrial cancer than when no HRT is taken.[20]

In another study, long-term estrogen users (5 or more years) were compared with nonusers to show that while estrogen alone did increase the risk of endometrial cancer, progesterone protected against developing this cancer. No cancer appeared in any of the patients treated with progestagen supplements.[33] Other studies have supported these findings.[7, 24, 26] Nonetheless, endometrial cancer does occur (though rarely) in women who take judiciously balanced HRT. Apparently, there are other nonhormonal factors that can also affect this disease.

The influence of progesterone on endometrial tissue has been studied by molecular biologists, who have shown that progesterone acts

TABLE 6   Incidence of Endometrial Cancer at Wilford Hall USAF
Medical Center, 1975–1983

THERAPY GROUP (5,563)	PATIENT YEARS OF OBSERVATION*	PATIENTS WITH CANCER	INCIDENCE PER 1,000
Oestrogen†-progestogen users	16,327	8	.49
Unopposed-oestrogen† users	2,560	10	3.90
Oestrogen† vaginal-cream users	2,716	2	.74
Progestogen or androgen users	1,160	0	—
Nonhormone users	4,480	9	2.50
Total	27,243	31	1.10

Source: From reference 20, courtesy of Dr. R. D. Gambrell.

*Patient years are calculated by adding up the number of years that all the patients are followed.

†Although *estrogen* is the usual American spelling, *oestrogen* is used in certain European communities; we use the same spelling that the investigators have used.

on endometrial tissue in such a way that the endometrium loses its usual ability to grow in response to estrogen.[12, 29, 49, 77] The literature on this issue is consistent. Unopposed high doses of estrogens may be dangerous; low doses of estrogens (e.g., .625 mg. per day of Premarin) are usually not harmful; and the influence of progesterone on endometrial health is good, even reverting hyperplastic tissue back to normal.[23]

Studies published in the last eight years have continued to show the unequivocal benefit of prescribing progestin in opposition to estrogen in order to protect the endometrium. A particularly noteworthy study, published by Dr. W. B. Wentz in 1974 (with an update in 1985), shows that one progestin (megestrol acetate), when given for 8 weeks in 4 daily doses of 20 mg. each, completely reversed adenomatous hyperplasia in 80 patients and atypical hyperplasia in 30 patients. In the five-year follow-up of that study, no person had a recurrence of the disease. In another study, reported by the same author, a higher dose 4 times a day was tried; the results were not as good: at double the dose, 3 percent of the patients had a recurrence of disease.[87, 88] These results are similar to the progestin results described in Chapter 5: lower doses of progestin may be more effective than higher doses in preventing endometrial cancer. In *all* cases, Dr. Wentz noticed that when HRT did not prevent the occurrence of the cancer, the women involved were obese.

By contrast, the newer, natural progesterone therapies being used in Europe have not been studied as thoroughly for endometrial response. One investigator, in a study that involved 32 women, found that natural progesterone delivered in daily oral doses of 200 mg. or 300 mg. sometimes did not adequately protect the endometrium.[34a] Another study—but of only 11 women—showed good protection at these doses. During Dr. C.-R. García's efforts in the early development of the oral contraceptive—in 1956 and later—he used natural progesterone orally (oral crystalline progesterone) at doses of 450 mg. to 1,000 mg. a day to oppose the natural secretion of a young woman's estrogens in order to protect the endometrium. Because all data have not yet been collected, we suspect it will take some years before the appropriate dosage of progesterone will be defined for women who still have a uterus and want to protect it as they take HRT. More important is to discover that point in the increasing dosages of natural progesterone at which the plasma-lipid changes become adverse to cardiovascular health.

ADMINISTERING PROGESTERONE

Once it was appreciated that progesterone is an important part of a conservative hormone replacement program, doctors asked: How much progesterone should be taken and for how many days each month?

The earliest report, in 1937, was that of Dr. Fuller Albright of the Massachusetts General Hospital. The next significant report, in 1966, was by Dr. Georgeanna Seegar Jones, a pioneer in female endocrinology, who went on record saying, "The most effective hormonal support can be given by the administration of a progestogen in combination with estrogen for 20 days each month. If hysterectomy has been carried out, continuous estrogen therapy is quite satisfactory."[45] Dr. Robert Greenblatt of the Medical College of Georgia was another early pioneer in progestin therapy.

The researchers who compared the reduction in cancer risk as a function of progesterone use did not have available to them women taking progesterone for as many days as Dr. Jones had recommended. Those few physicians who were prescribing progesterone tended to limit its use to 5 or 6 days out of each month. Even when used for 5 or 6 days, the beneficial results were unambiguous and startling.[76] More recently, a series of studies makes it clear that it is not how much progesterone you take that matters, but for how many consecutive days you take it. It is far better to take a little bit each day for 10 to 13 days than to flood your system with a high dose over a 5- or 6-day period.[7, 26, 76, 80] In fact, when doses were too high, the side effects tended to cause women to stop participating in hormone regimens.[22] And the higher the dose of progestin, the higher the dropout rate because of adverse effects. Fortunately, in order to be adequate, the dose does not have to be so high that it produces these side effects.

There are now two viable ways for planning an individual hormone regimen with respect to endometrium safety. The first, the Progestin Challenge Test, has proved effective in releasing built-up tissue from the endometrium and in indicating that no more bleeding will be necessary for safety (because the endometrium has now turned atrophic). The Progestin Challenge Test, pioneered by Dr. R. D. Gambrell,[24, 26] is so named because a dose of progesterone "challenges" the endometrium to produce a withdrawal bleeding 10 to 15 days after starting the hormones. The estrogen therapy causes endometrial tissue to build up; the progestin induces a withdrawal-like menstruation. If you use this method, you may menstruate each month until you reach your late sixties. In effect, you are mimicking nature's hormone cycle, and a menstrual-like flow often occurs when hormones (estrogen and progesterone) are cyclically taken. According to Dr. Gambrell, if a woman takes 10 mg. of medroxyprogesterone acetate per day for 12 days and, after 3 months on this routine, no menstrual-like flow ensues, eliminating (for 3 months) the progestogen appears to be safe for the endometrium.[24, 26] In other words, the endometrium has been challenged with progestin and has not responded with a menstrual flow. Thus, if no menstrual period follows the Progestin Challenge Test, you can assume that your endometrium is not simply overstimulated due to the unopposed estrogen you had been taking.[26] It could be atrophic. If it is, this is all right. By stopping the progestational agent, you may allow the endometrium to build up once again and to benefit from the estrogen you are taking. The balance that the Progestin Challenge Test produces is one of neither depriving nor overstimulating the tissue of the endometrium. Every 3 months, the woman without a flow once again takes progestin to see if the buildup has been large enough to induce a flow.

The bleeding after the challenge is good for you. It represents a sloughing off of the endometrial tissue that had been building up in response to the estrogen therapy. This Progestin Challenge Test is a useful way of monitoring your endometrium without endometrial examination and has been shown to be remarkably effective at preventing endometrial cancers.[26] For women who are obese and are not taking hormones, this test provides a useful way of reducing the risk of undetected cancer. If you are heavy, you would be wise to discuss the test with your physician, even if you are not taking HRT.

The second, more recent, Bleeding Day Test has also emerged as a safe way of protecting the endometrium when hormone therapy is taken. See page 142 for a complete description.

Several forms of progestins are available in pill form, with variations in the package doses occurring from one country to another. Appropriately taken, each seems to prevent the development of a hyperplastic endometrium.[34] The recommended procedure is to take progestin for at least 10 days during each cycle.[34] Four chemical forms of progestin are commonly in use today: norethindrone, norethindrone acetate, medroxyprogesterone acetate, and norgestrel. The effective doses are now believed to be 2.5 to 10 mg. of norethindrone, 1 mg. of norethindrone acetate, 2.5 mg. of medroxyprogesterone acetate, or .15 mg. of d/l* norgestrel per day during each of the last 10 to 13 days that you take the estrogens.[89, 90, 91] These dosages are about one-fifth the dosages first tried, and the newest studies suggest that these low doses protect the endometrium fully. Moreover, your lipid levels will respond well to these low doses. Either the Progestin Challenge Test or the Bleeding Day Test should inform you as to whether your endometrium is safe at these low doses. If it is, it makes sense to stay at the lower dose but to take the progestin for a longer period of time—at least 13 days and up to 16 days or more (which research now confirms).[54, 65, 11]

Women taking higher doses of progestin sometimes report discomfort the first few months—premenstrual tension, a bloated feeling, or some menstrual cramping. These symptoms usually vanish by the fourth month. The lower doses may turn out to have no side effects at all, but the question is still being studied.

---

*All compounds have mirror images (i.e., two forms)—the "d" and the "l." The term *d/l* means that the substance in question contains both.

BREAST CANCER AND FIBROCYSTIC BREAST DISEASE

Perhaps no disease has had more frightening publicity than breast cancer. The specter of disfigurement and potential metastasis is terrifying, and the media continually seem to feed on this terror with front-page stories overexposing and extending the signficance of the results of research publications.

Benign breast change (fibrocystic breast change) also creates problems. The condition is common, occurring in 1 out of 3 women, and women naturally wonder whether these benign lumps predispose them to breast cancer.[11]

The terminology surrounding fibrocystic breast disease, benign breast disease, and fibrocystic change has caused a great deal of confusion and lack of consistency in the medical community. In 1989, the textbook *Benign Disorders and Diseases of the Breast: Concepts in Clinical Management* presented a series of chapters, suggesting to physicians both the conditions and a more appropriate terminology that could be universally agreed upon. Table 7 shows the variety of diseases that have all been grouped under the heading "benign breast disease." The relationship between benign breast disorders and breast cancer are also indicated in this table.

HOW COMMON AND SERIOUS ARE THEY?

Fibrocystic breast changes are very common, occurring in 1 out of 3 women. Breast cancer is much less common, with statistics showing variable incidence rates. Although the textbooks that physicians read often tell them that 10 percent of women will experience breast cancer, the actual data are different.[74] We know that by the time women are seventy-five years old, 6 percent to 10 percent of them will have breast cancer. Consider this. After menopause, the lifetime risk of dying of coronary heart disease is 31 percent; breast cancer, 2.8 percent; and endometrial cancer, less than 1 percent.[10] This is very different than the more general statement that 6 percent to 10 percent of all women will develop breast cancer. Studies of women who died have shown that about 6 percent had breast cancer but never knew it; and it didn't seem to interfere with the quality of their lives.[74]

Another way to get a more accurate picture of this problem is to realize that the age-adjusted deaths due to ischemic heart disease

TABLE 7 Relative Risk for Invasive Breast Carcinoma Based on Pathological Examination of Benign Breast Tissue

NO INCREASED RISK
Adenosis, sclerosing or florid
Apocrine metaplasia
Cysts, macro and/or micro
Duct ectasia
Fibroadenoma
Fibrosis
Hyperplasia (mild: 2 to 4 epithelial cells in depth)
Mastitis (inflammation)
Squamous metaplasia

SLIGHTLY INCREASED RISK (1.5 TO 2.0 TIMES)
Hyperplasia, moderate or florid, solid or papillary
Papilloma with fibrovascular core

MODERATELY INCREASED RISK (5 TIMES)
Atypical hyperplasia
Ductal
Lobular

INSUFFICIENT DATA TO ASSIGN A RISK
Solitary papilloma of lactiferous sinus
Radial scar lesion

Source: American College of Pathologists Consensus Statement.

(heart attacks) in white women are 4 times higher than the deaths due to endometrial and breast cancer added together.[68] Other studies that publish data continue to show a lower incidence rate than the textbook reports that doctors study. For example, one report published in 1984 described 10 years of evaluations (office exams) of close to 9,000 patients.[60, 63] Using manual palpation (by hand), mammograms, and fine-needle aspiration biopsy whenever a suspected tumor appeared, only 25 cancers among all 9,000 patients over those 10 years occurred.[64] Statistics for female death rates confirm this less frightening pattern. The annual incidence of death from all cardiovascular diseases in women in the United States is 485,000; the annual incidence of death from breast cancer in the United States is less than one-tenth this figure—38,400.[11] The risk of an asymptomatic forty-year-old woman having breast cancer within the next year is now shown to be 1.1 per 1,000 women.[15] Although the disease appears to be less common than the media would have us believe, it still occurs, and it should be understood and prevented where possible.

DEVELOPMENT OF FIBROCYSTIC BREAST DISEASE

Fibrocystic breast changes are sometimes viewed in relation to hormonal imbalance.[59, 72] It has been suggested that women whose breasts become cystic while taking HRT may be at a slightly increased risk of developing breast cancer. But according to several studies, this incidence is only found in users of higher doses of unopposed estrogen (more than .625 mg. of conjugated estrogen).[38, 68]

The slightly increased rate of breast cancer in this subgroup of women with cystic breasts could be due to the difficulty of detecting early-stage cancers in cystic breasts. Why? Because cystic changes can obscure premalignant changes.

Fibrocystic breast changes tend to increase with age until the men-

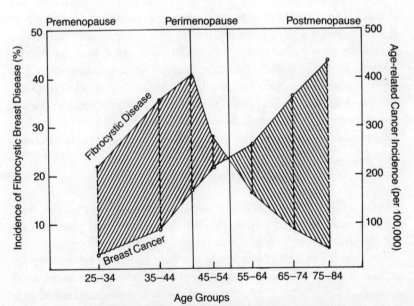

Figure 20   Incidence of Fibrocystic Breast Changes and Cancer

opausal transition, when these changes sharply decline.[28, 83] Figure 20 shows this age dependency in fibrocystic breast changes.

Progesterone deficiencies have recently been targeted as a cause of these changes. Studies of the progesterone level in the blood have shown that women with fibrocystic breast changes tend to have much lower progesterone levels during the luteal phase of their menstrual cycle than women without the disease[56, 72] and that progesterone therapy, administered in the appropriate dosages, helps raise those levels.[83, 84] The conclusion of some researchers who have been working directly with the development and care of fibrocystic breast changes is that benign breast changes may be partial indicators of future breast cancer; but this pathway to disease can be overcome with progesterone.[59] The value of progestational agents is further illustrated by studying oral-contraceptive use: the lowest incidence of fibrocystic changes occur in women who take oral contraceptives. Progesterone has been shown in laboratory studies to lower the estrogen receptor levels and to inhibit the conversion of androstenedione into estrogen. These two actions serve to reduce the mitosis, cell division and cell proliferation, in women who have been studied in the laboratory.[83]

Breast cancer has a different life-history pattern. As Figure 20 also shows, breast cancer increases during the menopausal years.[21, 84] Breast cancer is a slow-growing disease whose appearance may make itself known only after many years of development.[39] So long a developmental process could entail nine years of silent growth before the cancer becomes apparent as a tiny lump. Breast cancer, like the other cancers described earlier, poses the greatest danger when the disease metastasizes—that is, spreads—through the blood or lymph. The longer its silent presence, the greater the potential for metastasizing.

SYMPTOMS AND DETECTION

Fibrocystic breast changes are often painful.[44] As the cysts grow, they press against adjacent tissue, producing pressure and pain. Breast cancer, in contrast, may produce no symptoms for many years.

Because of the threat of silently growing cancer of the breast, detection methods of the disease are actively sought by the biomedical research community. Ultrasonography is now being developed as a method of breast-cancer detection and, as of 1988, seems to be able to differentiate accurately among breast changes,[47] especially among cystic and solid breast masses. It is less reliable, however, in making the distinction between benign and malignant masses.[8]

Breast self-examination has also proved very valuable in discovering tumors when they are small and relatively less developed.[78,*]

For the present, however, no other examination approaches the accuracy of mammography. Perhaps the largest study of breast-cancer detection was reported in 1982: the Breast Cancer Detection Demonstration Project.[1] In that study, 29 health centers in 27 widely distributed U.S. locations had enrolled more than 280,000 women. The original intent was to give each woman a mammogram every five years. Most of the mammography was confined to women over the age of fifty. This study also included *high-risk women* (women who had a mother or sister with breast cancer or an abnormal physical exam) under the age of fifty. Since the younger subjects were at high risk for breast cancer to begin with and were the only ones in their forties to be followed, the discovery of breast cancer in a number of these women is not surprising. What is unfortunate is the widespread conclusion that low-risk women should be X-rayed. The failure to cite that only high-risk women in their forties were followed has misled the public, resulting in a current misappropriate citation of this study as evidence for why low-risk women in their forties should undergo routine mammograms. It is important not to go too far in the other direction. However, for women in their forties who are *not* low risk, routine mammograms can be helpful—they often effectively identify the first sign of a developing tumor.

Should you have regular mammograms? According to the American Cancer Society, a baseline mammogram between the ages of thirty-five and forty should be followed by annual or biannual screenings until age fifty and annually thereafter. The preponderance of opinion favors this, and this opinion represents current conclusions from the American Cancer Society, the American Radiology Society, and other groups in the medical establishment. However, even though groups express this view, it does not change the low rate of mammograms that are currently being performed and the disagreement among reasonable people as to the appropriateness of the procedure. In terms of absolute safety, mammograms help. In terms of

*See Appendix 3.

absolute necessity, the data have not yet been fully gathered. What can we conclude? At age thirty-five, at least a baseline mammogram is sensible. How often you should be X-rayed after that depends on whose advice you choose to follow. The data clearly show an increased survival time after an X ray detects a malignant tumor.[82] Other data show that close to 90 percent of breast cancers detected by mammography emerge in the *baseline* reading.[4] So, after your baseline reading, although subsequent mammograms are less likely to find tumors, they will serve as a point of comparison for marginal or other changes. But the question of the appropriateness of mammograms before age fifty has not yet been resolved because the necessary studies of low-risk patients have not been completed. Nonetheless, women with mothers, aunts, and siblings who develop breast cancer should probably undergo annual mammograms throughout their adult lives in order to insure their own well-being and to allow for early treatment, should cancer develop.

The news may not be so good for women with breast implants since the implants tend to obscure the view. One recent report questioned the reliability of mammographic screening for these women.[35] Greater expertise or possibly some other method will need to be devised to provide these women with a viable means of cancer detection, but as of this writing, no confirmed screening method has yet been developed and tested.

WHO IS AT RISK?

For women who have benign breast changes, the risk of developing cancer is greatest in the 25 percent who have hyperactive breast tissue.[41] These women would likely profit from new research that suggests that hormone therapy be considered. Hormone therapy (the regimen that includes progesterone to mimic fertile-type luteal-phase levels of progesterone) in the appropriate dosages appears to be effective in reducing the incidence and experience of benign breast disease.[59, 72] Some investigators prefer to use the stronger progestins for benign-breast-disease hormone regimens.[72] If you follow that approach, it will be very important to monitor your blood lipids because these progestins, when given in high doses, can adversely affect plasma lipids.

The risk pattern for breast cancer is different. Not only does family history of breast cancer play a role in the risk of contracting the disease, but a particular kind of benign breast disease also increases the risk: *proliferative disease*—that is, the proliferation of breast cells. Fortunately, in one study of more than 10,000 such lesions, proliferative disease was shown to be absent in 70 percent of women with benign breast disease.[14] Unfortunately, when proliferative disease was present, the risk of breast cancer was increased. Therefore, if you have proliferative disease, you will need careful medical monitoring and expert medical management.

Smoking also substantially increases the risk of breast cancer. Although the reasons have not yet been proved, it is known that smoking suppresses the immune system, which may play a role. Chapter 12 discusses helpful hints for breaking the smoking addiction.

Although obesity or just being overweight has been suggested as a risk factor for breast cancer, the actual data are less convincing. Two recent studies (conducted in 1989 and 1990, respectively)[53, 69] that systematically addressed the question concluded that gross obesity or very large weight gain (more than 40 pounds) in the postmenopause is associated with a small increase in the incidence of breast cancer. When they compared 216 breast-cancer patients with age-matched controls, researchers showed that the breast-cancer population tended to have a higher weight, more body fat, and a thicker waist-to-hip ratio than the control group. However, there was so much overlap between those with cancer and the controls that strong assertions could not be made.[69]

More to the point was a prospective study of over 120,000 women nurses, age thirty to fifty-five when the research began in 1976.[53] These nurses were contacted every 2 years and followed for 10 years. By the time the study was published in 1989, more than 115,000 women had been followed; a little over 1,000 of these women developed breast cancer—that is, about 1 percent of the study's population within the 10 years. This research shows that in the premenopause—before age fifty—the heavier the woman, the more protected she was against breast cancer; and in the postmenopause, no such relationship emerged either way. However, one obesity relationship did appear in this study: postmenopausal women who had gained more than 40 pounds since the age of eighteen showed about a 40-percent higher risk of developing breast cancer than their contemporaries. We can compare this 40-percent increase, which amounts to slightly less than half of the cases of breast cancer, to a fivefold or 500-percent increased risk of heart attacks in smokers.[69] In other words, although major weight gain in the postmenopausal years is something to avoid, its relative influence on breast cancer is moderate compared to the effects of other behaviorally induced actions (such as smoking) on the body.[2]

The studies of the role of alcohol in the development of breast cancer are discussed in Chapter 11 (pages 275–276).

MASTECTOMY OR LUMPECTOMY?

Once breast cancer is detected, does mastectomy or lumpectomy best reduce the risk for subsequent cancers? Fortunately, the news is good. In 1989, the conclusion of a study of 2,200 cancer patients was published.[16] This study, an 8-year extension of a study reported several years earlier, again showed that lumpectomy followed by radiation therapy is just as effective as mastectomy (removal of the breast) in patients whose breast cancers are in the stages before metastasis— that is, where the tumors are still small (less than 4 cm). This study also provided clear data indicating the importance of early detection of breast cancer to the prolongation of life. Eight years after lumpectomy, the same percentage of women were still alive (over 90 percent) and free of disease (over 60 percent) as those who had undergone the more severe procedure involving the removal of the entire breast.

HRT AND BREAST DISEASE

An overwhelming amount of evidence indicates that in almost all cases of breast disease, accepted hormone therapies play no causative role.[92] Studies of women taking oral contraceptives or HRT have shown the benefits of the appropriate dosages of hormones in reducing the incidence of cancer of the breast for women who were not already at high risk for this disease before they began taking the hormones.[22, 83] Although some investigators have concluded, after studying several thousand menopausal women, that postmenopausal estrogen use can neither be indicted as causing nor be considered to prevent breast cancer,[83] in a 1982 report of a large sample of menopausal women, when breast cancer did develop, HRT users fared better. In this study, women who were taking hormones had a 50-

percent better chance of not dying than women who were not taking hormones.[84] However, there have been two reports at variance with the many studies supporting hormone therapy. Table 8 shows a summary of oral-contraceptive and breast-cancer publications through 1986.[84]

One 1986 study evaluated the use of conjugated equine estrogen in the presence of fibrocystic breast changes.[44] In that study, a higher rate of fibrocystic breast changes was found in users of estrogen replacement therapy than in nonusers. But the author discussed and then concluded that it could not be discerned from these data whether the higher rate of fibrocystic breast changes was due to the hormone use or to the improved detection of breast changes in women who were coming for their therapy and, at the same time, having their breasts examined.[44]

More recently—in 1989—a large epidemiologic study of over 23,000 women over the age of thirty-five in Uppsala, Sweden, was published[3] in which two populations were evaluated. The first consisted of 23,000 women who had prescriptions for HRT. Over a

TABLE 8   Oral Contraceptives and Breast-Cancer Risk*

AUTHOR	DURATION	RELATIVE RISK†	COMMENT
Centers for Disease Control (1983)	Ever-use	0.9	Neither duration of use nor time since first use alters risk of breast cancer.
Centers for Disease Control (1984)	≥ 11 years 4–6 years	0.8 0.8	No association between high use of progestin pills and breast cancer.
Pike et al. (1983)	> 6 years 4–6 years (use before age 25)	0.9 2.0	High use of progestin pill for 2 to 4 years and 4 to 6 years increases breast-cancer risk by 2.4-fold and 4.1-fold, respectively.

Vessey et al. (1983)	> 6 years
	Ever-use age 16–35
	Interval since last use:
	  1–4 years
	  4–8 years
		4.9
		0.9
		
		0.9
		1.2
			No patterns of breast-cancer risk emerge in younger women.

Hennekens et al. (1984)	> 8 years Ever-use	0.5 1.0	More-than-10-year users are slightly lower breast-cancer risks than never-users.
Rosenberg et al. (1984)	Ever-use ≥ 5 years	1.0 1.0	Use of oral contraceptives for 5 or more years was not associated with breast cancer.

*Reference 83.

†A relative risk of 1.0 means no risk. When the relative risk is less than 1.0, the data suggest a reduction in risk.

6-year period, the incidence of breast cancer for these women was compared to the rest of the women in that city who did not have prescriptions for HRT. The investigators suggested that their data showed an increased incidence of breast disease (in this case, cancer) among those women who were having HRT prescriptions filled. The overall increased "risk" was 1.1. Based on this information, the *New York Times* published a front-page story about how HRT users were at risk for breast cancer.

A close look at the Swedish study, however, leads to serious questions about whether the data do indicate indeed an increased risk of breast cancer due to hormone therapy. Here's why. The incidence of breast cancer among the 23,000 women using HRT was 1.1 percent (253 cancer cases divided by 23,000 HRT users) in 6 years; this percentage was higher—but only slightly—than the percentage of the nonhormone users who developed breast cancer during the same period. But a detection bias may be at work in this study. The report did not provide any evidence that the women who were not getting hormone therapy were having their breasts examined. In contrast, before a woman could get a prescription for HRT, she had to see her doctor. Presumably, HRT prescriptions followed breast exams. Since—as stated earlier—close to 90 percent of breast cancers are discovered when the first mammogram is taken, a greater search for and consequent "detection" of existing disease may occur in women who go to their doctors for medical care. And since early detection may have been what emerged rather than the incidence of cancer, we don't know what was actually discovered: early detection of the disease or an increased incidence in the population of HRT users.

When the investigators looked more closely at their data, they concluded that there was no increased risk for those who used conjugated equine estrogens or the estriol form of estrogen. The increased incidence of breast cancer emerged in the users of estradiol (the strongest of the estrogens). By letter (to Dr. Cutler), the researchers explained that the synthetic estrogen estradiol valerate (not available as an oral preparation in North America) tends to be the estradiol prescribed in Sweden. The investigators also evaluated progestin in opposition to estrogen and said that the number of cancer cases were too few to allow the researchers to evaluate specific progestins. In general, however, progestin use emerged as a risk factor after 6 years of combined hormone use. Because women with benign breast disease are often being treated with progestin opposition to estrogen, and because one benign-breast-disease subtype, proliferative disease (see page 169) (1) occurs in 30 percent of the women with benign breast disease, (2) increases the risk of breast cancer, and (3) often leads to progestin treatment, the discovery of a higher incidence of breast cancer in estrogen and progestin users is not surprising.

But these results cannot logically lead to a conclusion that HRT increases the risk of breast cancer. The study did not present any data on the incidence of benign breast disease in the hormone users. Moreover, this epidemiologic study confounds rather than clarifies the risk factors of breast cancer. This epidemiologic report is not a study with an appropriate control group, capable of proving cause and effect. Under ordinary circumstances, a good epidemiologic report points the way toward a plan for rigorous double-blind, controlled studies, which this report does not do. We mention these details because the study has drawn a great deal of publicity and because the publicity has not helped the public to get to the truth.

But other properly controlled studies have already shown a decreased incidence of breast cancer in the populations of not-at-risk women using estrogen with progestin.[22] In Dr. R. D. Gambrell's study, reproduced in Table 9, women using combined estrogen and progestagen showed the lowest rate of breast cancer. However, this study also must be evaluated with reservations because women at increased risk for breast cancer were not included in hormone-therapy groups.

What can we conclude from these seemingly varied results? For women who are not at an increased risk for breast cancer (they do not smoke or have sisters or mothers with breast cancer), the evidence seems to weigh in favor of the benefits of HRT (specifically a combination of estrogen and progestin), which may lower the risk. For women at risk for breast cancer, no proper data have yet been collected.[92] Thus, each woman must make the decision on whether or not to take HRT on the basis of her knowledge of the situation and her interaction with her physician. We wish we could offer more clear-cut advice, and we look forward to the time when the data will have been collected and published on this important question. All we can say is that there is nothing substantive to show that hormones cause cancer when the hormones are prescribed in the estrogen-progestin combination referred to throughout this book.

TABLE 9   Incidence of Breast Cancer at Wilford Hall USAF Medical Center, 1975–1983

THERAPY GROUP	PATIENT YEARS OF OBSERVATION*	PATIENTS WITH CANCER	INCIDENCE PER 100,000
Estrogen-progestagen users	16,466	11†	66.8
Unopposed-estrogen users	19,676	28†	142.3
Estrogen vaginal-cream users	4,298	5†	116.3
Progestagen or androgen users	1,825	3†	164.4
Nonhormone users	6,404	22	343.5
Total	48,669	69	141.8

Source: From reference 22, courtesy of Dr. R. D. Gambrell; adapted from *Hysterectomy: Before and After,* p. 135, Table 4.

*Patient years are calculated by adding up the number of years that all the patients are followed.

†Includes individuals who were not using hormones at the time the cancer was discovered.

CONCLUSION

Concerns continue to erupt whenever the news reports that long-term estrogen use has just been linked to an increased disease risk. The sophisticated consumer should realize that, because of the time constraints on publication, long-term results may cover a span from two years ago to perhaps twenty years ago. Thus, a 1991 announcement could reflect data gathered from 1969 onward.

Any study of long-term estrogen use probably covers women who were using very high doses of unopposed estrogens since it is only from about 1985 that progestin opposition and low estrogen have been appropriately balanced by most prescribing physicians.

Ultimately, it is you who reaps the benefits that hormone therapy provides. It is you, not your doctor, who must make an "informed" choice about what benefits and risks you will accept. Specific conditions that can allow for hormones but that require careful consideration and frequent checkups include a past history of any hormone-dependent cancer or pelvic disease (like fibroids or endometriosis). Gall-bladder disease also requires a careful medical monitoring. If you decide to take hormones with such a history, then any symptoms of pain or uncontrolled bleeding will probably cause your physician to take you off hormone therapy. Likewise, if you have high blood pressure, diabetes, varicose veins, or smoke heavily, or are more than 30 percent over your proper weight, you may decide to forgo hormone therapy, although many women who have these conditions safely enjoy the therapy with careful medical monitoring.

You should not take hormones if you have any of the following: undiagnosed vaginal bleeding, acute vascular thrombosis (sudden onset blockage of blood vessels), or neuro-ophthalmologic vascular disease (disease of the blood vessels in the visual system).

In any case, you should know that there is a risk whenever you take a medication. No one knows for sure what the effects will be for a specific person. Every experience in life carries with it some risk. Walking across a busy street, exerting oneself in a strenuous game of tennis, driving or riding in a car, and so forth carry risks of death from internal or external accident. From the abundance of rigorously designed studies, the increased risks of properly dosed hormones appear to be low, provided that you are not in the "should not take hormones" category. And for those of you who are in the "careful consideration" category, you must weigh the risks (low though they may be) against the benefits (which are many and significant) and choose the alternative best suited to you.

With a clear understanding of the benefits of HRT, you now have the knowledge to make an intelligent choice. The medical community has accepted the responsibility for health care of society, but the individual has the final responsibility for her own health care. To do this effectively requires motivation, the willingness to take that responsibility, and knowledge. Although it is up to you to gather the information that you need (and that this book provides) and to initiate and maintain the motivation to establish your best possible health, this does not mean that you do not need the help that your physician can provide. Rather, you should use the information in this book to help you work *with* a health-care professional in order to maximize your own proper care.

SUMMARY

Taking too much estrogen can lead to overgrowth of the endometrium and may increase the risk of developing endometrial cancer. But, according to the best studies available, relatively low doses of estrogen relieve menopausal symptoms and prevent the development of osteoporosis without causing a woman to risk endometrial cancer. Moreover, taking progestagen in combination with estrogen—in effect, mimicking the body's natural hormone cycle—appears to reduce the risk of getting endometrial cancer or suffering from benign breast changes when compared with taking no hormones at all. According to the extensive studies of Gambrell, the lowest incidence of breast cancer occurs in those women who have been on long-term HRT. And for those women who do develop breast cancer, the prognosis is better for HRT users. In any decision about taking ovarian hormones, endometrial safety should be a major consideration. Your doctor can help you decide what kind of a program is right for you. Although there are women who, for a variety of reasons, should not take hormones, if you are like most pre- and postmenopausal women, you can have the benefits of HRT without compromising endometrial safety.

7

HORMONE REPLACEMENT THERAPY AND COEXISTING DISEASE

B y 1990, although a large proportion of physicians and patients in North America were aware of the benefits of HRT, there was still concern about whether HRT can affect coexisting diseases. Now, we can all take comfort from the results of studies that deal with hormone therapy and its benefits and risks to women who both have disease and are also suffering from menopausal signs.

While there remains a need for more prospective studies (and this research will be forthcoming), we must not lose sight of the enormous body of data that have already been collected clinically on the oral contraceptive as well as on HRT. For the history of HRT, we can go back about fifty years; for the history of oral contraceptive, the data are more extensive but cover a shorter time span—about forty years. Because it is now well documented that the menopausal conditions of bone loss, cardiovascular disease, and vaginal atrophy will respond beneficially to HRT in the appropriate dosages, what is of critical concern is whether the disease that exists is going to be adversely affected by the hormone treatment.

In rare circumstances, the use of HRT in a woman who has a coexisting cardiovascular problem could exacerbate the condition. For example, fluid retention might overload the heart (the mechanism by which this happens is complex). What matters here is that despite the disease, HRT can be overwhelmingly beneficial as long as the patient is monitored in order to avoid swelling from fluid retention.

The use of HRT with coexisting osteoporosis is generally beneficial, can often halt the continuation of bone loss, and may even produce a slight accumulation of additional bone mass. (For details, see Chapter 4.)

Sexual dysfunctions due to hormone deficiencies can occur and are discussed in Chapter 8. In general, each dysfunction (loss of libido, anorgasmia, lack of arousal) improves after the appropriate sex hormone is taken.

Finally, for a review of HRT and cancers of the reproductive system, see Chapter 6.

Let us look next at how HRT relates to some common problems:

* uterine fibroid tumors
* endometriosis
* urinary incontinence
* polycystic ovary disease
* prolapsed uterus
* ovarian cancer

UTERINE FIBROID TUMORS

Fibroid tumors, also known as leiomyomas or uterine myomas, plague many women. Probably 1 in 4 women past the age of thirty has these benign tumors lodged in the muscular wall of her uterus. Most of the time, fibroids cause no problems. Even when they do grow and become troublesome, more than 99 percent of the time there is no cancer.[16] For extensive details on the nature of this disease and current treatment available for it, see *Hysterectomy: Before and After,* written by Dr. Cutler and available in paperback (New York: Harper & Row, Perennial Library, 1990). Meanwhile, as to the question of whether HRT leads to changes in these fibroid tissues, the data are not all in yet. Moreover, other factors besides estrogens and progestagens seem to be involved.

In 1989, scientists in Japan published a study evaluating over 100 fibroid tumors that had been removed during hysterectomies. The researchers were trying to learn whether estrogen, progesterone, or a combination of the two was responsible for changing growth rates in these tumors. Results were mixed. The tumors were about 8 times more active (that is, cells from the tumor multiplied 8 times the normal rate) during the luteal phase of the menstrual cycle, when both estrogen and progesterone are normally being produced.[10] From those data, it seemed as if progesterone added to estrogen stimulated the growth of these tumors. However, another part of the study seemed to indicate the opposite effect. As women were approaching menopause and losing both their luteal phase and its progesterone production, the incidence of fibroid tumors was increasing dramatically. Once menopause was achieved, a sharp drop in the incidence of the tumors occurred. The relatively unopposed estrogen characteristic of the premenopausal years may have been responsible for the increasing incidence of fibroid tumors as women neared their menopause; thus, it seemed that the drop in progesterone increased the incidence of fibroid tumors in women as menopause approached. One of the confusing factors is that not all patients showed this pattern: fibroid tumors did not in every case increase in size as menopause approached. And for postmenopausal women, when the tumors do increase rapidly, there are serious grounds for concern because these tumors have the greatest potential of becoming cancerous. Moreover, HRT at the dosages now used do not usually affect one way or the other these postmenopausal tumors.

One hormone treatment seems to be effective in shrinking fibroid tumors, producing on average a 20-percent reduction in tumor volume; but it only works for as long as the hormones are taken continuously. This treatment, using *GnRH* (or gonadotropin-releasing hormone) *analogs,* causes a shutting down of the pituitary secretions of the gonadotropins* and triggers a sharp reduction in the ovarian secretion of sex hormones (estrogen and progesterone). As hormone secretion diminishes, the size of the fibroid tumors shrinks.[12] In late 1989, some studies showed the effects of different doses, brands, and routes of administration (nasal spray and injection) on the shrinkage of these tumors and on coexisting side effects.[4, 7, 8] Other studies evaluated the prospects of giving progestagens with the GnRH ana-

---

*For the technically interested reader, GnRH analogs are hormones that are analogous to—i.e., that mimic—the brain hormone GnRH (gonadotropin-releasing hormone).

logs because it is known that while analogs are successful in reducing tumors, they also produce menopause-like symptoms such as hot flashes.[2, 6] Thus, while GnRH treatments may reduce the size of fibroid tumors, they must not be taken for more than 3 to 6 months unless they are combined with HRT because of the effects of these treatments on the metabolism, which are the same as those of sudden onset of menopause: hot flashes, rapid skin aging, loss of a sense of emotional well-being, adverse blood-lipid changes, sexual dysfunctions, and bone loss. Fibroids grow back promptly on cessation of treatment.

The perceived value of GnRH analogs lies in their limited ability to shrink fibroid tumors, thereby permitting the tumors' surgical removal with minimal blood loss and the patient's rapid postoperative recovery.[11, 14] The ability to minimize blood loss and promote rapid healing is critical. For example, in surgically competent myomectomies,* average blood loss should be less than 200 cc. This is about two-fifths of the amount that a woman typically donates per session at a blood bank and generally will not hinder her recovery from surgery or her well-being. But GnRH analogs will not make surgeons better than they are. And, ultimately, it is the surgery that is critical in the complete removal of these tumors.

If you have fibroid tumors and are experiencing hot flashes, vaginal dryness, or other menopause signs, this should not deter you from using HRT. However, you will need to work closely with your physician, watching for growth of these tumors. But even if there is growth, it may have nothing to do with the simultaneous use of HRT. The growth of these tumors in a postmenopausal woman may be a reflection of cancerous changes, particularly if there was a solitary tumor. Your objective should be to find a regimen that maximizes your health without leading to tumor growth. Because both the uterus and (probably) fibroid tumors tend to shrink with advancing menopause, the benefits of HRT in promoting good bones health, a sense of well-being, and sexual function will need to be weighed against the distress associated with benign tumors. For further details on this disease and its treatment, the more extensive discussion in *Hysterectomy: Before and After* may be of help (see page 89).

Myomectomy (from *myoma*, a benign muscle tumor, and *ectomy*, "removal") is the surgical removal of one or more uterine fibroid tumors while preserving the uterus.

ENDOMETRIOSIS

While endometriosis principally affects women in their premenopausal years and tends to diminish with age, there are those who wonder about HRT and either previously or coexisting endometriosis.

About 15 percent of women suffer from endometriosis, a disease in which tissues formed in the uterine lining (the endometrium) and intended for discharge from the body during menstruation make their way into the pelvis instead. There, an autoimmune reaction may occur in which the body "sees" this tissue as a disease.[13] This endometrial tissue can then affix itself to the ovaries, to the bowel, to the outer wall of the uterus, and sometimes within the vagina, growing and shrinking in response to the changing estrogen/progesterone pattern of the woman. For women who have this disease, menstruation days can be very painful as internal bleeding occurs simultaneously with the vaginal bleeding.

When the level of hormones that HRT provides is very low, these hormones do not seem to cause adverse effects on women with this disease. According to Dr. Felicia Stewart, a practicing physician in a large health-care group and co-author of *Understanding Your Body,* postmenopausal HRT use does not aggravate existing endometriosis.[16] (This has been our experience as well.) Also, GnRH analogs have been effective in reducing endometriotic lesions in some women. And GnRH analogs, unlike another widely used drug, Danazol, were shown not to have an adverse effect on plasma lipids.[3] However, they may affect bone. Review with your physician the prospects for trying these treatments.[3, 11]

Great strides are being made in the study and treatment of endometriosis, and the 10,000 physician-members of the American Fertility Society are particularly focused on the disease and its treatment. To obtain the name of a local physician-member of this society, write to the American Fertility Society, 2140 Eleventh Avenue South, Suite 3200, Birmingham, AL 35205.

URINARY INCONTINENCE

The causes of urinary incontinence and their relationship to aging (and the decline of female sex hormones) were discussed in Chapter

3. Unless the urinary incontinence is due to either a neurogenic bladder problem or a mechanical problem such as a fibroid tumor pressing against the urinary structure, HRT will usually help.

But HRT can only partially address the problems that may produce the incontinence; it cannot address others. The sex hormones play a vital role in maintaining the structural integrity of the body's muscles, cellular tissue, and certain support structures. Thus, replacement hormones serve this system. Since the urinary tract and the vagina have similar tissue structure (mucous membranes, connective tissue, blood vessels, and muscles), both undergo atrophy during periods of estrogen deficiency. Incontinence follows urinary-tissue atrophy. Moreover, urinary-tract atrophy and tissue infections will combine to increase urinary-incontinence problems. For all of these problems, the hormone component of an HRT regimen is helpful in restoring and maintaining the structural integrity of the tissue.

Optimal dosage will depend on the degree of the deficit as well as on how much of the estrogen gets to the tissue that needs it. If estrogen is applied as a vaginal cream and spread over the vaginal/urethral area, most of the estrogen will be absorbed directly at the target site before spilling into the blood stream. Many forms of vaginal estrogen—from the strongest estradiols to the weakest estriols—if given in the appropriate dose, will help to restore deficits. If you have had an ovariectomy, are younger than fifty, and suffer from incontinence caused by severe estrogen loss, you have a good chance of completely reversing the pathology if you combine the estrogen treatment with an exercise program to restore muscle strength.

Hormone therapy, particularly its estrogen component, should be combined with pelvic-muscle exercises (see page 90) and healthy fluid intake. If you suffer from urinary incontinence, be sure to drink plenty of water—a minimum of 8 to 10 glasses a day. By restricting water, a woman produces a more acid urine, which irritates a weak urethral structure. By drinking a great deal of water, she will dilute the acidity, thereby treating her urethral tissues more gently.

In 1989, gynecologic surgeons were just beginning to publish studies on the benefits of estrogen for urinary incontinence. One group, formerly studying surgical techniques for treating urinary incontinence, reported on how estrogen replacement therapy could be used instead of surgery.[1,9]

POLYCYSTIC OVARY DISEASE

When women develop polycystic ovary disease (PCOD) or syndrome, it reflects that their ovaries produce excess estrogens and androgens. Recently, the first set of comparative data was published to show how the plasma lipids of polycystic-ovary-syndrome patients compared to those of age-matched healthy women. The results were clear: PCOD patients suffered from increased levels of triglycerides and (harmful) LDL cholesterol, and their (beneficial) HDL-cholesterol levels were lower than normal.[17]

Although studies have not yet been published to show the reactions of such patients to HRT, it is more than likely that estrogen replacement therapy may be helpful in reversing these adverse lipid effects (see Chapter 10). It is possible that PCOD patients will need only estrogen if the increased androgens are having an effect similar to what progestin opposition would normally provide. Your physician should be able to assess this.

PROLAPSED UTERUS

Under normal circumstances, the uterus is supported well above the bladder, as shown in Figure 21. Ligaments from above and muscles from below hold the uterus in place. The pelvic floor, a sheet of muscles that supports the pelvic organs, connects the coccyx (labeled as lower spinal bone in Figure 21) to the pubic bone. Sometimes, because of childbirth and the advancement of age as well as decline in hormonal support to the muscles, these supportive muscular sheets become weak, sag, and permit the stretched ligaments to drop the uterus into the vagina or even beyond, the uterus now emerging between the legs.

A prolapsed uterus must be corrected in order to avoid what is otherwise an inevitable progression of the problem and, with it, associated pain and distress to the rest of the pelvic organs. The condition is uncomfortable and gets worse unless treated. Moreover, a prolapsed uterus can also add to urinary-incontinence problems by weakening the bladder.

HRT combined with the Kegel muscle exercises described in Chap-

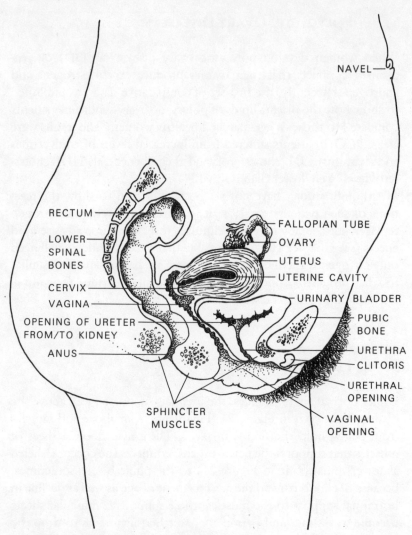

NAVEL

RECTUM

FALLOPIAN TUBE

LOWER
SPINAL
BONES

OVARY

UTERUS

UTERINE CAVITY

CERVIX

VAGINA

URINARY BLADDER

OPENING OF URETER
FROM/TO KIDNEY

PUBIC
BONE

ANUS

URETHRA

CLITORIS

URETHRAL
OPENING

SPHINCTER
MUSCLES

VAGINAL
OPENING

FIGURE 21   Sagittal Section of the Female Pelvis

ter 3 could be the simplest remedy for the early stages of the problem.
HRT will help rebuild the tissue structures that are inclined toward
atrophy when sex hormones become deficient. All of the sex steroids
estrogen, progesterone, and testosterone serve to strengthen muscle
tone. Thus, HRT in any combination should be helpful for the muscular structure. In any event, you will want to balance hormones
appropriately, as described in Chapter 5.

If this simple approach does not rapidly improve the condition, surgical correction will probably be necessary. This takes the form of "surgical suspension," where the stretched-out ligaments are surgically shortened and attached to the internal pelvic structures, pulling the uterus up into the pelvic cavity where it belongs. Unfortunately, if you seek medical help for a prolapsed uterus, a hysterectomy may be prescribed—not because this is the only way to solve the prolapse, but for other reasons. Current medical attitudes focus on cancer prevention and the concern that a recurrence of the prolapse might occur if surgical suspension is undertaken. We believe that it is no more valid to remove a uterus to prevent cancer (when no cancer is present) than it is to remove any other body part as a preventive. As informed health consumers agree with our perspective, the current medical attitude may then change (as it has with other medical procedures that have become less invasive as knowledge has grown). If a prolapsed uterus is your problem, seek out a gynecologic surgeon who specializes in surgical suspension procedures. Dr. Harold A. Kaminetsky, Director of Practice, Activities Division, American College of Obstetricians and Gynecologists, 600 Maryland Avenue SW, Washington, D.C. 20024, or Dr. Raymond Lee, Secretary, Society of Gynecologic Surgeons, Mayo Clinic, Rochester, MN 55905, should be able to help you.

OVARIAN CANCER

The benefits and risks of HRT for women with reproductive-system cancers have not been resolved. One example may help to show the nature of the problem. In 1989, the first report appeared in which the effect of estrogen in promoting cell growth was studied.[15] The scientists compared two different ovarian-cancer types, each of which had been isolated and could be put into "growth dishes" in a laboratory setting. When estrogen, in a dose range that was proportionally normal for the human body, was added to the dishes along with other "growth factors," one of the cell lines began to multiply rapidly, and the other did not. Even though the cell line that did not multiply had been known to have estrogen receptors on it, the addition of estrogen to the media did not promote any cancerous growth. This study was highly detailed and very significant for cancer researchers. What we can learn from this study is the following:

- In a cancerous condition, estrogen may increase the growth of the tumor cells but will not necessarily increase them.
- When estrogen receptors are found on the cancer cells, the subsequent addition of estrogen will not necessarily have any effect on the growth of the cancer.
- There is, therefore, a variable response in different cancer cell lines to hormone treatments.

Women who have developed reproductive-system cancers have already experienced great physiological distress, both with respect to the disease process and to the loss of premenopausal hormone levels. Compared to other women, most women who have recovered from cancer of the breast, uterus, or ovaries are suffering from more severe menopausal effects: their hot flashes may be worse, their vaginal dryness may be extreme, their sense of well-being may be drastically reduced, their bones may be losing mass.

The critical questions of efficacy and safety of HRT for these women have yet to be established by the scientific community. In the meantime, actions must be taken as the days of our lives are lived. Whatever you choose contains risks and benefits—but, ultimately, the choice is yours. We hope that the information we have been able to provide will be of service to you, and we look forward to apprising you of new information as it becomes available.

8

SEXUALITY IN THE MENOPAUSAL YEARS

I personally have had a satisfying relationship with my husband. He is very much in love with me and requires a lot of sexual attention. Almost every other night. I think, because of all this affection, I am a very contented female. His appetite hasn't changed at all, but he has become more tolerant of my disinterest many nights. I enjoy sex, find it more of an effort to reach orgasm, but can if I put my mind to it. I don't crave it. I have many activities and work every day, and constant worries about my 2 grown daughters (one who has been very ill) that drain my efforts to concentrate more on bedtime romance. . . . I am 51.

I obtain less satisfaction from sex and find myself making more excuses as to not have sex. I am 51 years old.

The complexity of human sexuality and the diversity of human sexual experience is clearly evident in the comments of different menopausal women.

If you are fortunate enough to have a partner you value, sex can be one of the most pleasurable experiences that life has to offer. There is comfort in being held and caressed. Erotic pleasure takes many forms unique to each individual. At every age, it can be wonderful. But since our society tends to be youth-oriented, it is easy to get the idea that sex is only for the young. Then, too, many people equate sex with reproduction and believe that the end of a woman's reproductive years brings a decline of sexual desire and pleasure. While these notions are by no means universally true, it is natural enough for you to wonder about your own sexuality during menopause. Is there a difference in sexual appetite? How does the change of life affect your capacity for sexual pleasure?

These are not easy questions to answer because a person's sexual feelings are related to many different things. A sense of health, well-being, and vigor can make you feel sexy. You will probably feel less so if you are flushing, tired, or depressed. What is your attitude toward sex—generally positive or more negative? Have your past sexual experiences been good ones or bad ones? Sexual feelings can be intensified by the presence of an interesting partner and by your partner's interest in you. Each couple forms its own world, and these deeply personal and private experiences cannot be fully studied in the same way that hormones or bone mass can. Masters and Johnson, pioneers in the study of the physiology of sexual response, and others have contributed enormously to our understanding of sexuality. They have shown how the nervous system activates muscular response as well as other physiological responses during sex. But no one has been able to examine adequately the range of individual experience that occurs within the private domain of a man-woman relationship. In physics, the problem is defined by "the Heisenberg Uncertainty Principle," which states, in simplified form, that the tools one must use to measure a dynamic process inevitably disturb and distort the very process one is trying to measure. For this reason, investigators are bound to produce "uncertain" results. Although this chapter reviews the best information available on the subject, it should be understood that studies of human sexuality have only just begun to explore seriously this most complex area of human experience. And they will, undoubtedly, continue to produce "uncertain" findings.

CHANGES IN FREQUENCY OF SEXUAL ACTIVITY

A number of studies have shown that women tend to be less sexually active with the passage of years.[1, 20, 21, 26, 32, 34] This may be due to changes in either partner. Consider the following comment from a fifty-five-year-old woman:

Sex drives and desire for me doesn't change much except that our husbands don't have the same sex drive as before. They perform, but it's not the same—more like a feeling of obligation than an actual drive. It's no wonder so many middle age men leave their wives for younger women—they have to prove to themselves they are still the "macho guy."

A fifty-year-old woman simply said:

My sex drive has diminished slightly.

In the Stanford Menopause Study, 49 percent of the women said that sexual activity had declined since their menstrual cycles had begun to change; 38 percent reported no change; and 14 percent told of an increase in activity. A variety of reasons were given for the decrease in sex. Some women told of being less interested in sex. Others found it more difficult to locate a suitable male partner. Some found new living arrangements that offered them less privacy. Privacy problems tended to diminish the pleasure in sexual encounters and, therefore, to make their occurrence less likely. But some women found a new love, and these women tended to report an increase in sexual activity—as we would expect.

Recently, the first study of very old people—80 to 102 year olds—documented this trend. The older the people got, the less often they were likely to have intercourse, even if they were married or had a partner. But while intercourse frequency declined, the caressing did not.[7]

Whatever your situation, knowing about the physiology of sexual response can help you to understand your own sexuality during the menopause years.

CHANGES IN SEXUAL PHYSIOLOGY

In women of reproductive age, one of the first signs of sexual arousal is when the walls of the vagina produce droplets of fluid that quickly form a slippery coating throughout the vaginal barrel. The same moistening reaction occurs in response to any vaginal irritation, including infection. This response is nature's mechanism for diluting and washing out the contents of the vaginal tract. With the characteristic diminution of estrogen at menopause, the vagina is much less moist. In addition, the walls of the vagina become tissue-paper thin and lose some of their ability to lubricate quickly and efficiently in response to sexual arousal. So even if you feel yourself becoming aroused, it may take several minutes before your vagina catches up and begins to lubricate.

Not surprisingly, estrogen therapy improves vaginal lubrication in menopausal women.[8, 33] One of the mechanisms responsible for this lubrication appears to be increased blood flow brought about in response to the hormones, which results in vaginal transudate ("sweating of the vaginal wall"). This "sweating" acts as a lubricant.[6, 38, 39]

The sensitivity of the vagina changes both with age and with alterations in hormone levels.[44] There is an ongoing controversy over the existence of a sensitive area known as the "G spot." One 1989 study of vaginal sensitivity to electric stimuli[37] supported much older knowledge: the existence and physiological location of the G spot.[37] An unusual series of studies by Dr. Heli Alzate, culminating with a 1990 publication, supports that women vary in the specific vaginal region most sensitive to stimulation and argues against one universal G spot location.[3a–i] The G spot (named after Dr. Ernst Gräfenberg, who discovered it) is a sexually sensitive region of the vagina that, for a woman lying on her back, is located at the "12-o'clock high" position about 1½ inches from the entrance to the vagina. What does this suggest for heterosexual behavior? When stimulated by rhythmic thrusting of an erect penis, as experiments have shown with stimulation by hand, the area forms a mound of tissue somewhat like the tensing of the abdominal region during a sneeze. Since these new studies of electrical sensitivity were conducted on hormonally rich young women, we do not yet know about the potential change in sensitivity at menopause. In 1990, in a survey of over 1,000 professional women,[11] 82 percent acknowledged the existence in themselves of that sensitive vaginal region as described by Gräfenberg and, later, by Perry and Whipple.[33a]

The hormone declines of menopause also cause the vagina to become smaller (shorter and narrower) and to lose some of its elasticity. Vaginal dryness and a decrease in elasticity can make intercourse painful—a condition known as *dyspareunia*.

Thick vaginal walls serve as kind of a cushion during intercourse, protecting the bladder and the urethra from the pressure produced by the thrusting of an erect penis. With the loss of this cushion, it is common for intercourse to be followed by a strong urge to urinate. Some menopausal women also complain of a burning sensation during urination that persists for several days after a long session of intercourse.[11, 29, 30]

In women of all ages, orgasm is often accompanied by strong contractions of the uterus. Lacking sufficient estrogen, the uterus of a menopausal woman shrinks, and for some women the uterine contractions during and after orgasm can be painful. One woman over sixty described the contractions as being "almost like labor pains except that they occur more rapidly."[30] We do not know the reason for this pain but suspect that it is related to hormone deficiencies because of the timing of its appearance.

Some menopausal women taking estrogen report a significant improvement in sexual interest, activity, satisfaction, experience of pleasure, sexual fantasy, and capacity for orgasm.[13, 18] But other studies do not find this to be true.[16] According to Masters and Johnson, HRT with both estrogen and progesterone is necessary in order to eliminate the discomfort that some women experience from orgasmic uterine contractions. Neither hormone used by itself will relieve complaints of this kind.[29, 30] So if you are having this problem, you may want to discuss with your doctor the possibility of using this combination therapy. But he or she may not have a ready answer for you because the issue has not yet been rigorously researched.

Not every woman is affected in the same way by the change of life; not every woman needs HRT. In some menopausal women, the ovaries and/or adrenal glands continue to produce sufficient estrogen so that there are few, if any, menopausal symptoms. In such women, the vagina retains much of its tone and natural appearance, and continues to lubricate during sexual arousal in a pattern characteristic of a younger woman.[29]

Although vaginal dryness is a frequent complaint of menopausal women, Masters and Johnson[29, 30] note an interesting exception. They found that three women in their study—each over sixty years old—lubricated rapidly when aroused. These women had continued to have sex on a regular basis (once or twice a week) throughout their adult lives. The facility with which these women lubricated is particularly remarkable because, in each case, their vaginal skin had atrophied to the tissue-paper thinness characteristic of other menopausal women. Why were they exceptions? Note what one fifty-year-old woman in Philadelphia had to say:

My friends complain about how dry they have become and resort to lubricants. I never had any such problem. I attribute it to the fact that through my husband's efforts and insistence, I am still sexually active.

Regular sexual activity may promote the capacity for rapid vaginal lubrication and, in this respect, counteract at least one of the effects of a paucity of estrogen. Using an appropriate vaginal moisturizer (such as Replens®, from Columbia Laboratories in Miami) may help to provide the lubrication that will serve as a background against which regular sexual activity will keep the system going.

Regular sexual activity may have other beneficial effects. Data from the Stanford study show that women approaching menopause who have regular weekly sexual intercourse tend to be either entirely free of hot flashes or to experience milder ones than women who either abstain from sexual activity or who are only sporadically sexually active.[9, 28] The data also show that these women have higher levels of estrogen and a tendency to maintain these levels as the months pass. In contrast, the sporadically active and celibate women had lower levels of estrogen and, 3 months later, had lost an additional 10 percent of their estrogen concentration.

Other studies, by Dr. Sandra Leiblum and her colleagues, showed that regular masturbation also reduced the incidence of vaginal atrophy.[27]

As difficult as the above-mentioned natural hormone-related changes are, the problems of women who have had pelvic or genital cancer are even more severe. Recent research has shown that a variety of sexual dysfunctions are almost inevitable after cancer surgery and recovery.[36] Women report declines in sexual frequency, satisfaction, and capacity. Studies show that hysterectomy (regardless of the cause) and cancer surgeries both signal these declines. See Chapter 9 for details on hysterectomy-induced changes as well as reference 9, this chapter.

Hormones and Sexual Desire

If the walls of your vagina have thinned and you have trouble lubricating, intercourse can be uncomfortable, even painful. Are you flashing, itching, and depressed? All of these common signs of menopause may lessen your interest in sex. These signs are relieved by estrogen, and this may be one reason why some menopausal women report an improvement in sexual desire after starting HRT.[13] The capacity for reaching a comfortable orgasm and for achieving a feeling of sexual satisfaction are also improved among menopausal women taking hormones.[13, 18]

Relatively recent studies show that hormones and sexual interest are linked.[6, 25, 27] The precise mechanisms elude us because, as human beings, we can intellectually overcome the messages that our hormones are sending us. Thus, research in this field is difficult. However, there are data that cannot be ignored. For example, in one study of 590 fertile-aged women, those who had regular menstrual cycles showed the highest incidence of "autosexual" activities during the middle of their cycle.[3] These autosexual activities included masturbation, sexually arousing fantasies, and dreams. For these women, sexual desire seemed to peak around the middle of the menstrual cycle, when they were also more likely to initiate lovemaking with their partner. The middle of the cycle, which is when a woman ovulates, is the time when intercourse is most likely to initiate pregnancy. So, from a purely reproductive point of view, it makes evolutionary sense that an ovulating woman should be most interested in having sex at this time.

At the middle of the cycle, just before ovulation, the ovary secretes high levels of estrogen. Testosterone and androstenedione levels are also maximal at that time because the ovaries secrete a large amount of these androgens, too. Since sexual desire in women who are still having menstrual cycles seems to fluctuate with changing levels of ovarian hormones, it is likely that these hormones play an important role in desire.

Results of a study by Dr. B. B. Sherwin begin to address this point. She studied 43 women scheduled to have a hysterectomy along with surgical removal of the ovaries.[40, 41] Each woman rated the intensity of her sexual desire before and after surgery. After surgery, women were randomly assigned to different groups: some women received estrogen, some received testosterone, some received estrogen and testosterone in combination, and a control group received a placebo. Sherwin reported that sexual desire, arousal, and sexual fantasies all declined after surgery for the women receiving a placebo; the same was true for women receiving estrogen. In contrast, women taking either the testosterone or the testosterone-estrogen combination had relatively high levels of desire, arousal, and fantasies, and in this respect were little different from women in an additional control group who underwent a hysterectomy without having their ovaries removed. Conclusions? The ovaries apparently make an important contribution to a woman's sexual health. Certainly their effect on sexual feelings is supported by Sherwin's observation. The effectiveness of testosterone replacement therapy in restoring sexual interest after ovariectomy shows that androgens may stimulate sexual interest in women in much the same way they do in men.

Even after menopause, the ovaries continue to secrete androgens into the blood stream; the adrenal glands are also an important source of these hormones. However, hormone output varies widely from woman to woman. In some women, blood levels of androgens actually increase after menopause; in others, androgens decrease by 50 percent or more (but are still higher than in women without ovaries). Furthermore, estrogen replacement therapy may reduce the amount of free testosterone in the blood stream.[31] So if you are menopausal and are currently taking estrogens, your testosterone level could be 30 percent lower as a consequence.

What does this mean? We don't yet know. The data that deal with the reduction of testosterone indicate that the women taking estrogen replacement therapy still had circulating in their body adequate levels of the hormone. Until studies are made that look at exact amounts of testosterone and how they relate to sexual desire, we cannot offer complete advice. Nonetheless, if you have noticed a decrease in sexual desire that seems to be related to your menopause, it could be due to the decreased presence of androgens, and testosterone replacement therapy could be a beneficial adjunct to estrogen replacement therapy.

No studies have yet been published in peer-reviewed journals to evaluate the lipid (cholesterol) response to oral testosterone therapy. We know that men, with their much higher levels of testosterone, show much higher levels of cholesterol; and we also know that estrogen therapy reduces cholesterol in women. In Chapter 10, we discuss the relationship between lipids and hormones as far as we currently understand them.

But you should know that in women, when testosterone exceeds the appropriate level, the result may be an increase in facial hair and a deeper voice.[2] Since there are only a few studies published on women who are taking testosterone replacement therapy, there is little information about what constitutes a suitable dose of testosterone and what side effects can be expected. A pioneer in this field, Dr. R. B. Greenblatt of the Medical College of Georgia, promoted the cause of testosterone replacement therapy for women whose hormonal changes with age included a loss of testosterone.[19] He defined the appropriate dosage of one of the widely available testosterones. Table 10 shows Greenblatt's recommendations for androgen treatment. Note that he outlined a variety of androgens and routes, representing those hormones with which he had had positive clinical experiences over his long career.

If you suspect that changes in your sexual feelings may be related to a decrease in testosterone, discuss this with your doctor. You may need to have your blood tested to determine your level of testosterone. The "ideal" level of testosterone for women has not yet been determined, but the results of this assay (blood test) will show how it compares with what is normal for your age. This information is essential in deciding whether or not you would benefit from androgen replacement therapy. And even if you and your physician conclude that you would benefit sexually from testosterone, the selection of a therapy will be fraught with uncertainty. (See pages 142 ff.)

But remember that not everyone is the same. Some women notice an increase in sexual desire around the time of menopause. Since androgens are still being produced by the ovaries and adrenal glands and for some women blood levels of androgens rise around menopause, an increase in sexual interest could be one result.

A word of caution. If you still have irregular cycles, you are probably ovulating some of the time and thus can become pregnant from unprotected intercourse. Therefore, if you are sexually active and do not want to become pregnant, use some form of contraception until you stop menstruating altogether.

Desire is clearly related to factors other than one's underlying level

TABLE 10   R. B. Greenblatt's Recommendations for Androgen Treatment

THERAPY	DOSAGE
Oral Androgens	
Methyltestosterone	5–25 mg.
Fluoxymesterone (Halotestin—Upjohn)	5–10 mg.
Danazol (Danocrine—Winthrop)	50–200 mg.
Injectables	
Testosterone cypionate	
(Depo-Testosterone—Upjohn)	50 mg./ml.
Testosterone enanthate	50 mg./ml.
Testosterone propionate	25 mg./ml.
Testosterone-estrogen combinations for parenteral use	
Depo-Testadiol (Upjohn)	2 mg. testosterone cypionate and 2 mg. estradiol cypionate
Pellets	
Testopel (Bartor)	75 mg.
Oreton (Shering)	75 mg.
Estrogen-androgen combinations for oral use	
Premarin with Methyltestosterone (Ayerst)	.625 + 5 mg.; 1.25 + 10 mg.
Estrone sulfate and methyltestosterone	
Estratest (Reid-Rowell)	1.25 + 2.5 mg.
Estratest H.S. (Reid-Rowell)	.625 + 1.25 mg.
Estrogen-androgen combinations for topical use	
1% testosterone ointment (can be made up by the pharmacist)	—*

Source: see reference 19.

*Dosage depends on how much is applied to the skin to attain the desired effect.

of sexual interest. The availability of an interesting and interested sexual partner is obviously relevant; the influence of hormones on desire may be relatively modest in comparison with these and other social influences. As one forty-seven-year-old sexually interested woman from California put it when describing her recent sexual history:

One romance 2 years ago—but there are no men available! Sad—sad!

Masturbation

For people of any age, finding a suitable sexual partner isn't easy. If you are alone, masturbation may be a good way to experience pleasure and discharge sexual tensions. Such activity is common, harmless, and may be health-promoting.

The Hite Report devotes thirty-four pages to detailing the different ways women masturbate. Although there has been controversy about the book, it does contain valuable information. When women were asked to describe the importance of masturbation in their lives, there was a wide range of answers: masturbation was used as a substitute for successful coitus; it helped prevent one from going "nuts"; it provided health (by dissipating stress) during the times when a partner was not available; it increased one's understanding of one's own body, thereby promoting better sex with another person; it produced a calming effect; and it was an important part of one's sensuality.[24] Also, regular massage of the genital area will slow the atrophying of the tissues.[27]

The Power of Touching

In 1989, an extraordinary study was published that showed the importance and interrelationship among beta-endorphins, social isolation, and subsequent social contact for pairs of primate animals.[25] The research is intriguing because it carries with it a metaphor for humans. Scientists conducted four experiments that involved different combinations of social isolation, social contact, chemical inhibition of the beta-endorphin system, and its stimulation with morphine injections.

To understand how this experiment might apply to the human condition, it helps to know a little "monkey language." Adult monkeys show a characteristic "grooming behavior" and a "grooming invitation." The "invitation" involves one monkey approaching another and either (1) spreading its arms wide and offering its chest while it turns its head to the side or (2) bending over and, in a similarly undefended manner, offering its rear end. This grooming invitation clearly represents an offer for interaction. Sometimes the

response is positive: the invited animal responds by petting and strok-
ing the body part offered. Other times the response is negative: the
invited animal walks away. These experimenters showed that when
animals had been isolated and then allowed to have social contact,
the quantity of grooming behavior increased dramatically (lonely animals try to make up for lost time). As the grooming behavior increased, the beta-endorphin levels in their blood also increased.
When animals were socially isolated, their beta-endorphin levels
dropped. When animals were given injections of morphine (imitat-
ing high endorphin levels), they lost all interest in grooming behavior or interactions (that is, once the endorphin levels got high
enough, the animal appeared to be satisfied with itself).

We know from other research that the power of touch and its
importance to people never loses its luster. Even in very old age (80
to 102 years), the power of physical intimacy is reported to be very
important.[7] Being hugged and petted may be critical to the physical
and mental well-being of humans. And this may be mediated through
the beta-endorphin system.

AGING AND MALE SEXUAL PHYSIOLOGY

The gamut of interpersonal attitudes affects sexual experience. How
two people relate to each other is probably more important than the
mechanics of sexual physiology, but it helps to understand the latter.
If you have a male partner over fifty, you may notice that his sexual
physiology is changing, too.

For many men, erections occur quickly. For men over fifty, it may
take longer, and direct stimulation of the penis can become more
important. Even with direct stimulation, it can take several minutes
before an older man's penis becomes really firm. While young men
often ejaculate prematurely, older men seldom have this problem.
One of the usual things about getting older is that the drive to ejaculate becomes less urgent so that intercourse can last longer. Or the
older man may be unable to maintain his erection.

On average, as a man ages, the volume of his ejaculate decreases
and the force with which it is expelled diminishes. After a man ejacu-
lates, his erection softens, and there is a waiting period before he will
be ready to have—or will even be capable of having—another erection of sufficient firmness for intercourse. In a young man, this re-

fractory period is usually measured in minutes; for a man over fifty, the detumescence can occur much faster, and it may take several hours or more before the capacity for a full erection returns.

Difficulties in erection appear to be increasingly common as men approach their fifties. This may account for the result of a 1987 study of married men that showed that as they pass through their sixties, coitus decreases while masturbation increases.[46] Regardless of the true cause of the difficulty, most of the men who are willing to seek professional help believe that their problem is physical in origin.[47] And this often turns out to be the case. In one recent investigation of a group of men willing to be studied for erectile dysfunction, the most common problem was vascular impairment. However, at least half of the men had problems that were not physical in nature, but rather psychogenic. And these problems could be effectively treated through psychotherapy.[47]

Some drugs can also cause erectile difficulties. In 1988, the first prospective double-blind carefully controlled study to investigate the effects of different, commonly used beta blockers on sexual function was published.[35] In this study, several kinds of information were analyzed: the hormone levels; the physiologic response of the penis; the subjective impression of each man. The authors found that some drugs were more likely to produce erectile difficulties than other drugs. Beta blockers are commonly prescribed to treat hypertension. If your partner is taking a beta blocker and is having erectile difficulties, discuss this (or have your partner discuss this) with the prescribing physician, suggesting the possibility of switching to a different beta blocker. Other drugs can also influence sexual desire. If you are concerned about a loss of sexual desire in someone who is taking any drug, it is appropriate to consider whether the drug itself is responsible.

Sometimes a man does not ejaculate during sexual intercourse. This does not mean that he cannot continue to ejaculate each time, but only that he may come to accept that ejaculation is not as important to his sexual satisfaction as it used to be. Putting it another way, a man in his sixties may continue to have sex eagerly and frequently and to express satisfaction even though he may not ejaculate each time. Each man is different and follows his own timetable: some may be in their forties or fifties when these changes occur; others may be well into their eighties.[7]

Why do these changes occur? This is a very complex question.

They may be the result of a gradually declining level of testosterone or simply one of the many consequences of the aging processes or of some other factors that have not yet been quantified. Systematic study of testosterone replacement therapy and sexual functioning in aging males could answer this question, but so far no such studies have been reported. We do know that, for the vast majority, the decline in testosterone levels parallels the declining frequency of erection.[12] And *very* low levels of androgen have been related to declining sexual function.[5, 19] But testosterone therapy may not be of any value. When investigators in one study restored the low levels of testosterone to moderate levels, sexual function did not change regardless of how high the testosterone level got.[18] Men need a minimum of testosterone. If they already have this minimum, testosterone therapy will not help. However, a decline in a man's level of testosterone with age is not inevitable.[22]

Even in this age of relative sexual enlightenment, it is a popular fallacy that the aging process robs a man of his capacity for sexual pleasure. Few men are immune to fears of losing their sexuality and may view with alarm as a sign of impending sexual failure age-related changes in their sexual activity.[23] Anticipating difficulty with achieving an erection, a man may avoid the expected humiliation of impotence by withdrawing from opportunities for sexual contact. If he has been monogamously attached, he may blame his partner for his difficulty and perhaps seek rejuvenation by having sex with another woman. In the short run, the sexual power of a new relationship may do wonders for his self-esteem and perhaps ease his fears. But a man who fears impotence might also fail to perform with a new partner. In any case, the likelihood is that these changes in a man's sexual capabilities are as natural and as inevitable as the other physical changes of aging. If a man is in good health, however, he could retain the capacity for erection and sexual pleasure into his eighties and perhaps beyond.[7]

Age, then, can affect the sexual abilities of your partner. If you view these changes with alarm, it is likely that he will do the same. As a man ages, the fact that he may take longer to achieve an erection may not mean that he finds you less attractive as a sexual partner. It may only mean that in some instances, in order to get a full erection, it may be necessary for his penis to receive more direct stimulation than when he was younger. Many women feel that they have not satisfied their partner unless intercourse results in his orgasm (ejaculation). You should understand that as your partner gets older, he may be satisfied with sex even though he does not ejaculate.

Parenthetically, certain interpretations of the *Tao* have long held that if a man wants to live a long and healthy life, he should not ejaculate with every sexual encounter. However, no studies have been published on restraint in ejaculation that allow us to confirm its value.

Good sex has a lot to do with how well two people communicate. Men and women often find it difficult to talk about what is bothering them, particularly when it comes to physical intimacy. Men in particular sometimes feel that any expression of fear or insecurity on their part will be seen as unmasculine, and they will go to extraordinary lengths to preserve an illusion of confidence and control. The man who acts the most secure may be the one who feels the most insecure. This is unfortunate because talking about one's fears often helps to relieve them. If a relationship is a good one in other respects, sexual problems can probably be resolved; but some effort at communication is required. If communication cannot be achieved without help, counseling may be effective.

SUMMARY

Menopause need not herald the end of your sexual life. Although some people may happily choose that route, many do not. If sex has been important to you as a younger woman, it is likely to be important to you as you approach and pass through your menopause. You will probably notice some changes in your sexual physiology that parallel other changes you are experiencing. This is natural since all of these effects can be traced to the continuing changes in ovarian hormone output, which represents the menopausal stage of life. Just as HRT alleviates the other signs of menopause, the appropriate HRT can prevent (or reverse) the vaginal and uterine atrophy of menopause and help you to continue to have a healthy and satisfying sex life throughout your postmenopausal years. In fact, with the knowledge that comes from experience, your capacity for sensuality can mature as your body does; you may find that sexual pleasure can become better than it was before. If you come to experience sex as an expression of love, as a means of building a close relationship, as a way of communicating sharing and caring, as a source of erotic pleasure, as a time for feeling, a time when problems cease and pleasure is meaningful, a time of acceptance and being accepted, then aging can be a period of growth. In fact, to the mature person, as the body ages, the sexual responses slow and the spirit can grow. Shall you embrace the wisdom of your body? If you slow down and focus on those areas of sexual activity that provide pleasure, full sexual enjoyment can become better than it was. After periods of sexual abstinence, you should expect some degree of narrowing and thinning of the vagina as well as a loss of lubrication response. But these problems will disappear if sexual activity is resumed with gentle and limited coital thrusting and perhaps the use of a lubricant.

9

HYSTERECTOMY

By 1988, the startling fact had emerged that the medical establishment would prescribe a hysterectomy for 1 out of 2 North American women sometime during her life.[18] With such a high incidence of hysterectomies being performed here, it behooves every woman to learn as much as possible about this operation—to prevent it if it is unnecessary and to make her aware that if she has had this surgery, her menopausal life will be different than if she had not had it. In the United States, hysterectomies are performed five times more frequently than they are in western Europe: by the age of forty-two, 21 percent of American women have had a hysterectomy; by the age of forty-two, 4 percent of European women have had a hysterectomy.[18]

The removal of a uterus—hysterectomy—requires major surgery. The removal of the ovaries—ovariectomy or oophorectomy—is commonly performed at the same time. Why? Why are women in record numbers having these vital organs removed? Should the organs be removed? Apparently not always. A physician speaking about the uterus stated:

I am unaware of any other important organ that is effectively removed without first assessing its degree of malfunction.[31]

Such highly critical views are being expressed more often. By contrast, twenty-one years ago a very different view was expressed by another gynecologist:

The uterus has but one function: reproduction. After the last planned pregnancy, the uterus becomes a useless, bleeding, symptom-producing, potentially cancer-bearing organ and therefore should be removed.[84]

In a sense, this doctor is right. The uterus does cause problems for many women: approximately 1 in 3 develops a fibroid tumor; probably 1 in 2 experiences some degree of unexpected, apparently abnormal, bleeding. If you think of the uterus in the same way you think of your teeth—valuable but in need of maintenance and repair—a more rational way to approach problems than surgical removal can be perceived.

Increasing evidence indicates that the uterus is anything but useless. It is a muscular glandular organ, a living, functioning tissue that responds to ovarian hormones. Besides its well-known role of housing a growing fetus, it appears to have other functions. It responds to certain important hormones.

In 1989, three research studies were published that provide new facts about the anatomy and physiology of the reproductive organs of women. These facts show that the reproductive organs are important to the health of the rest of the body. The first research studied cadavers. The veins of the pelvic region were injected with barium sulfate (a contrast medium used for X-ray visualization) in order to define anatomical relationships.[68] The study showed that the valves (in veins) transmit blood in one direction only—from the rectal area toward the uterine region. Investigators from Egypt suggested that this new knowledge would be useful in treating pelvic cancers by allowing toxic doses of drugs to be injected appropriately in the pelvic region, thus bypassing the general circulation, thereby reducing the drugs' toxic effect on other organs.

The second study evaluated ovaries after the women had had these organs surgically removed.[53] These investigators proved that postmenopausal ovaries contain specific areas (binding sites) for pituitary hormones to activate them. The researchers further showed that the outer regions of postmenopausal ovaries are actively manufacturing hormones, even at advanced ages.

The third study was the result of a collaboration among investigators in Japan, Canada, and the United States.[52] This investigation demonstrated that the smooth muscle of the uterus responds to the nervous system in the promotion of uterine contractions. Through both electron microscopy and electrical stimulation of pieces of muscle tissue, the investigators showed that the uterus is a highly active organ with a physical capacity for both sensation (sensory input from the organ into the nervous system) and muscular contraction that occurs at orgasm.

Taken together, these three studies have added important information to a growing arsenal of data, all published within the last ten years, showing how richly alive and variably functioning the reproductive organs of a woman's pelvis are.[18] These organs are no more "used up" and "useless" than are the testes or prostate of a man who ages.

While not life-threatening, hysterectomy may lead to—or even directly produce—certain sexual deficits in some women. This is more likely to occur when the surgery has had complications such as infection, scarring, or adhesions. If sex is important to you and you are considering having this operation, you should also consider the possible effects of the operation on your sex life, which may improve or get worse.[54] A chapter devoted to sexual changes after hysterectomy and what can be done about them is available in Dr. Cutler's book *Hysterectomy: Before and After* (New York: Harper & Row, 1988, 1990).

Your ovaries also serve very vital functions throughout your life. Remember that in a modified way your ovaries continue to secrete important hormones even though you might have passed your reproductive years. Even when you must lose your uterus, your ovaries can continue to serve you well.

HOW MANY WOMEN HAVE HYSTERECTOMIES?

Since the early 1960s, the incidence of hysterectomy has been rising in the United States. In 1962, about 31 percent of the menopausal women had had their uterus surgically removed.[73] Four years later, this figure was up to 35 percent.[46] By 1974, it rose even more—to 40 percent.[73] In 1975, hysterectomy had been performed on a startling

59 percent of the 369 menopausally distressed patients of one medical group.[14] More compelling is the study of 763 women whose menstrual history had been followed for forty-five years. These women were all healthy when they started recording their menstrual history; 31 percent had been hysterectomized before their menstrual cycles had stopped.[78] Figures are not yet available for that group to define how many will have had a hysterectomy throughout the full span of their lives. But by 1978, the lifetime chance for having a hysterectomy in the United States was estimated to be greater than 50 percent.[60] The incidence seemed to have stabilized at this level by 1983. According to the best estimate, about 650,000 hysterectomies are performed annually in the United States.[27] Hysterectomy is second only to D & C or laparoscopy (examination of the interior of the abdomen) as the most common operation performed on women.[45] While this surgery may be justified, the reason for its increase has only begun to be apparent.

REMOVING THE UTERUS

Different reasons are given for the removal of the uterus. This is not surprising since different doctors have different attitudes about the importance of the uterus. Clearly, it should be removed when it is diseased and threatens your well-being.

Many gynecologists spoke out in 1976 at a medical meeting that was evaluating hysterectomy. One respected woman in particular listed reasons that are "appropriate indications for hysterectomy," given the current state of knowledge. Modifying them in light of knowledge fourteen years more advanced, we list below the indications that we consider "appropriate":

- premalignant states of localized invasive cancers of the cervix, endometrium, ovaries, or Fallopian tubes
- symptomatic nonmalignant conditions of the uterus such as leiomyomas (nonmalignant tumors of the uterine smooth muscle—also called fibroids) compressing adjacent pelvic structures, thus giving rise to uterine bleeding—and only if the bleeding or the removal of the tumor is unresponsive to other, less drastic treatments

- uterine bleeding that endangers a woman's energy/health and is not responsive to progestagen hormone therapy[67a,*]
- in rare circumstances, diseased Fallopian tubes—when infection is life-threatening
- prolapse of the uterus due to loss of the supporting structure's health (that is, if the uterus was prolapsed, it would drop down into the vagina), providing it is not amenable to surgical sacro-spinus suspension
- cancer of adjacent structures
- uterine rupture

Although some diseases warrant hysterectomy, few studies have assessed the "indications" (reasons) that physicians give for prescribing surgery. But in 1989, a group of physicians did analyze 584 hysterectomies to learn what indication the physician or the surgeon had listed before undertaking the hysterectomy. See Table 11 for the data.[27] The Naval Hospital in this table may represent an institution where the surgeon has great autonomy. Thus, one can appreciate a medical facility that has a control so that the autonomy of the surgeon can be balanced by peer reviews.

Some of the reasons listed for surgery in Table 11 are appropriate for hysterectomy, but others are not. For ways in which a woman can avoid undergoing a hysterectomy while curing the condition, see Dr. Cutler's *Hysterectomy: Before and After,* which devotes several chapters to satisfactory and less dramatic alternative treatments that often eliminate fibroid tumors (leiomyomas), recurrent uterine bleeding, pelvic relaxation, and stress incontinence.

But there may be other, valid reasons for the surgery such as endometriosis. The important thing is to find unbiased, compassionate, expert advice. Before a diseased organ is removed, it is sensible to try to heal it first. Initially, the reason for excessive bleeding should be determined; depending on the cause, perhaps the bleeding could be better treated with hormones or endometrial ablation.[10a, 10b, 28]

In 1989 and 1990, published studies began to appear on the new use of an old technique: resectoscopic removal of tissue, now of intrauterine lesions. Called *endometrial ablation* or *laser ablation,* the

*However, hysteroscopic endometrial ablation (see pages 207–208 and 210) may prevent the need for hysterectomy.

TABLE 11 Indications for Hysterectomy at the San Diego Naval Hospital

INDICATION FOR SURGERY	NUMBER OF WOMEN	PERCENT OF WOMEN
Acute condition	18	3
A-1: Pregnancy catastrophe	12	3
A-2: Severe infection	6	1
A-3: Operative complication	0	0
Benign disease	338	58
B-1: Leiomyomas	179	31
symptomatic	(170)	
asymptomatic	(9)	
B-2: Recurrent uterine bleeding	47	8
B-3: Endometriosis	13	1
B-4: Adenomyosis	29	5
B-5: Chronic infection	8	2
B-6: Adnexal mass	62	11
B-7: Other	0	0
Cancer or premalignant disease	87	15
C-1: Invasive cancer	62	11
C-2: Premalignant disease	25	4
C-3: Adjacent or distant cancer	0	0
Discomfort	133	23
D-1: Chronic pelvic pain	33	6
D-2: Pelvic relaxation	57	10
D-3: Stress incontinence	43	7
D-4: Other	0	0
Extenuating circumstances	8	1
E-1: Sterilization	3	0.5
E-2: Cancer prophylaxis	5	0.8
E-3: Elective	0	0
Total	584	100

Source: see reference 27.

method involves destroying by means of cautery or laser the endometrial lining of the uterus. For almost all patients, this procedure usually stops the bleeding permanently, can render the patients sterile, and preserves the uterus, thus preventing hysterectomy. Unfortunately, the technique is very new. Our particular concern is the lack of long-term follow-up.

While this technique can be used on patients with a small submucous fibroid, the best results are achieved in those women with a normal uterine cavity. In other words, if fibroid tumors are changing the shape of the cavity, the entire fibroid must be removed (not just its surface) to prevent subsequent bleeding. Moreover, fibroid lumps can render this technique more difficult. A smooth endometrial shape allows for the best use of the technique.

Two principle problems must be understood in relation to this technique: (1) a high level of specialized surgical skill is required to complete accurately the ablation while preventing the accidental perforation of the uterus; (2) the method could "bury a cancer" if one were present and delay its detection.

Specialists who believe the technique to be useful point out that the time in a woman's life (the late thirties and forties) when heavy bleeding may be a predisposing factor for a hysterectomy is the same time when cancer is rarely the cause of the bleeding. In other words, during these years, heavy bleeding is more likely to represent the presence of benign fibroid tumors or hormonal imbalances than of cancer.

We will be alert to future studies of the technique because of its three benefits to women: compared to a hysterectomy, this procedure is 75 percent less expensive, 75 percent less painful, and 75 percent less time-consuming. And so far the results look good when highly skilled surgeons do it.[10a, 10b]

How many of the hysterectomies being performed in the United States today are being done for one or more of the uncorrectable reasons listed above? We do not know.[11] There is no systematic and retrievable reporting system among medical communities, except for the hospital record room and tissue committees, that would allow such information to be retrieved. Hospital tissue committees are formed of medical professionals who accept the responsibility of reviewing the results of recent hospital activities, including the outcome of individual surgical operations. The information that the tissue committees evaluate is privileged in a legal sense and, therefore, not readily available.

From statements reported by gynecologists at medical meetings and in several published studies, it appears that many hysterectomies were done for purposes of birth control (permanent sterilization), to prevent cancers, or "to improve the quality of life."[11, 23, 37] Hysterectomy is major surgery and has its risks, both in pain and potential complications. Most now believe that the removal of a healthy organ for reasons of birth control or cancer prevention is not in the best interest of the patient. For instance, there are, obviously, alternative methods of birth control that avoid hysterectomy. Before you undergo surgery, be sure that you have explored these alternatives first. A complete review of alternatives to hysterectomy for birth control is available.[29]

It is not wise for you to undergo major surgery unless you must. But if you must, it is important to know what to expect.

HYSTEROSCOPY

Hysteroscopy, perhaps the most thorough form of uterine examination involving no invasive surgery, has been used since 1869. But because of its diagnostic capabilities and its potential to reduce the number of hysterectomies performed, its use has recently increased.[43, 71] Two studies published within the last year have confirmed hysteroscopy's tremendous diagnostic value, particularly if it is compared to D & C when, in a case of abnormal bleeding, the site to be biopsied has been identified.[43] If you have abnormal bleeding or other undiagnosed uterine diseases, before considering a hysterectomy, discuss with your surgeon or physician enhancing the diagnosis to identify the problem. By doing this, you may obviate the need for surgery.

Hysteroscopy "scopes," or views the lining of the "hyster" (uterus) by distending the organ with gas or another substance (in most cases) while the patient is under anesthesia and then inserting the hysteroscope through the vagina and cervical opening into the uterus. Since the hysteroscope is equipped with lights and lenses, the uterus can be clearly seen. And since surgical tools can be passed through the scope, a biopsy can then be done.

The results of this kind of evaluation have prevented unnecessary surgery in 60 percent to 85 percent of cases because hysteroscopy revealed that, in spite of abnormalities in bleeding, the uterus was normal and had no disease worthy of the organ's surgical removal.[43] For these reasons, if you are having problems with your uterus, we strongly urge you to learn about this procedure and then discuss it with your health-care provider. (For more details on hysteroscopy, the reader is referred to reference 18.)

TYPES OF HYSTERECTOMIES AND THEIR AFTEREFFECTS

There is confusion in regard to terminology. For most people, a *hysterectomy* means the removal of the uterus, tubes, and ovaries, and is often—and incorrectly—said to be a "total hysterectomy." The correct names for the removal of uterus, tubes and ovaries is *total hysterectomy and bilateral salpingo ovariectomy.* If only the uterus and cervix are removed, this is correctly called a *total hysterectomy,* although some call it a *partial hysterectomy* because the tubes and ovaries remain. A *subtotal hysterectomy* or *supracervical hysterectomy,* sometimes confused with a partial hysterectomy but actually quite different, means that the cervix is left behind. Figures 22, 23, and 24 depict the different kinds of hysterectomies.

The uterus can be removed in either of two ways: through the vagina or through a surgical opening in the abdominal wall. A good physician will be able to select the best approach for each case.

Vaginal hysterectomy is advisable, first, when the anatomy allows for the easy removal of the uterus from below. For instance, in a woman who has borne many children, the vaginal opening is generally more relaxed and permits this easy access. Second, vaginal hysterectomy may be performed when the woman's health shows no disturbances in either blood circulation or skeletal structure that might be aggravated by the prolonged operative position in stirrups that the body must assume. Finally, the surgeon should be proficient in this approach or be supervised by a skilled and experienced pelvic surgeon who is guiding and assisting him or her.

Both forms of the operation, vaginal and abdominal, produce about the same amount of sickness although the particular kinds of discomfort may vary.[24] Vaginal-hysterectomy patients may show a much higher incidence of postoperative fever and higher numbers of localized infections of the vagina. They also experience a greater postoperative vaginal blood loss.[83]

With both approaches, the intestine may be inadvertently wounded. This is more likely to occur in patients who have had prior abdominal surgery. Depending on your medical history, you may have a greater or lesser risk of these operative complications. For example, those who have had a cesarean delivery or pelvic inflamma-

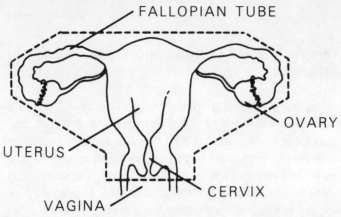

FIGURE 22 Total Hysterectomy and Bilateral Salpingo Ovariectomy

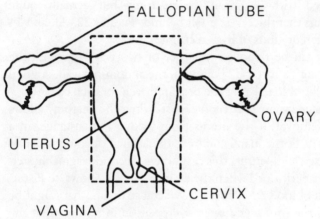

FIGURE 23 Total Hysterectomy

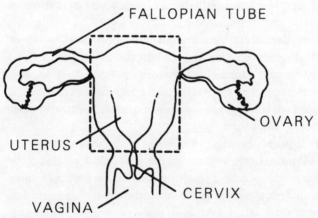

FIGURE 24 Subtotal or Supracervical Hysterectomy

tory disease before the hysterectomy have a greater chance of having their intestines stuck to the uterus or tubes or ovaries before the operation has begun. If this were your situation, your surgeon would first have to separate these tissues before removing the uterus. In the process of detaching the tissues, there is a chance that a wound to the intestine (caused by the separation itself) could lead to postoperative complaints. And if this happens, the small bowel can become paralyzed; until it heals, there will be many digestive problems to contend with, principally vomiting and pain.[83]

Although the aftereffects of abdominal and vaginal hysterectomies are different, with either approach you might be sick afterward. Different studies give different results, but between 25 percent to 80 percent of women are sick after the surgery.[26, 27, 41] In other words, the aftereffects of a hysterectomy can be unpleasant.

Some studies support the theory that blood flow to the ovaries is temporarily altered when the uterus is removed.[35] As a result of this reduction in blood flow, estrogen secretion (of young ovaries) or other hormone secretions (of older ovaries) have been reported to be temporarily suspended.[75] There is an immediate hormone drop that is quite large and has been observed to occur more often on the second day after surgery.[34] This reduction of ovarian blood flow may account for the hot flashes that women frequently report right after hysterectomy. Commonly, the flashes reach their maximum by about the fourth or fifth day after surgery.[2] When full blood flow is eventually restored, the flashes stop.

However, not all patients get flashes. One group of doctors reported that 69 percent of their patients experienced postoperative flashing;[62] another group rarely found flashing in women they interviewed after surgery.[16] What might explain this? Different surgical techniques may be the answer. Perhaps some techniques do not disrupt the flow of blood from the ovary.

Other internal tissue traumas occur including injury to the blood vessels of the operated pelvic area, the rectum, the bladder, and the ureters.[24, 40]

Bladder trouble is sometimes a postoperative problem.[26] You may experience difficulty in voiding, for instance. This is related to alterations in the sensation, which occurs when the bladder is surgically separated from the uterus; in order to remove the uterus, the surgeon must separate these two organs, which are normally attached to each other. These urinary problems are always temporary, and most women do not experience them at all.

Sexual discomforts are also common. The temporary ones, such as pain on first attempting intercourse after surgery, indicate that coitus has been resumed too early. Abstain from sexual intercourse until the healing is complete—that is, when you are no longer sore. After surgery the abdomen feels sore and is easily bruised. It usually takes three to four months before coital pressure can be enjoyed rather than merely tolerated.[1] There is often a temporary narrowing and shrinking of the vagina. These difficulties can combine to make sexual intercourse unpleasant at first. However, with a considerate and understanding partner, one who is willing to be gentle, resumption of coital activity can promote the return of pleasurable sex. Most women who previously were sexually active become sexually active again between two and four months after hysterectomy.[17]

There are also the complications that can occur after any surgery. Such a list is not included here. But most of the immediate problems of hysterectomy surgery are annoying and not life-threatening. They are, however, sufficiently discomforting for you to seek a hysterectomy only if it is really necessary. Choose your surgeon carefully because these problems are less likely to happen with a highly skilled gynecological surgeon. Since there is wide variation in the quality of surgeons, finding a good one should be an important priority.

There may be occasions where differences of opinion are expressed concerning the need for hysterectomy. For example, a woman that wants to bear children in the future and has extensive fibroids of the uterus might better benefit from removal of these fibroid tumors (*multiple myomectomy*) than from a hysterectomy since hysterectomy would preclude future childbearing. Saving such a uterus may necessitate the seeking out of an experienced and able gynecological surgeon adept at such conservational surgery. The myomectomy may take much longer than a hysterectomy to perform because it can be technically more difficult and time-consuming for the surgeon to remove individual tumors and then repair the uterine areas from which these tumors have been removed than to remove the entire uterus. And the surgery will be significantly more expensive because of the greater skill and time needed for this type of reconstructive surgery. Moreover, most insurance companies will not adequately reimburse the patient for this procedure perhaps because they do not yet appreciate the greater skill and time involved. For example, at the Hospital of the University of Pennsylvania, the 1990 surgeon's fee for a myomectomy is $4,000, for a hysterectomy $2,500. Even though Blue Shield of Pennsylvania allows only $960 for myomectomy and $1,350 for hysterectomy, the federal government is guided by the standards of Blue Shield in setting Medicare and Medicaid reimbursement levels. Other insurance carriers cover up to 80 percent of the fees and are, therefore, more realistic.*

If you are well informed, you should insist that your special needs be reflected in the approach that your physician outlines for you. There is a delicate balance between the needs of the woman and the propriety of what the physician can and should do. There are no simple answers. Getting the proper opinion depends upon how you approach the specific physician and how you weigh the importance of what he or she and others offer to provide you with. The more knowledgeable you are, the better you are able to ask the right questions. (See Dr. Cutler's *Hysterectomy: Before and After* for details.)

In order to get two independent opinions about the possibility of having surgery to solve your problem, you may want to find two surgeons who are not professionally connected with each other. To do this, each physician should form and render an opinion on the basis of personal judgment, unbiased by the knowledge of where and what judgment was rendered elsewhere. You will optimize objectivity if you require the same rigor of judgment about your case that researchers require of their studies. It is like the double-blind requirement, discussed earlier. If you lack tact, however, you could be misunderstood and might insult the person you are going to for help. While it is perfectly reasonable to seek two unbiased opinions, it is unreasonable to behave as though you do not trust the ability of your physician. You must maintain a delicate balance when you seek two truly objective opinions. If from the start you are tactfully able to communicate the truth—that you are seeking two independent and unbiased judgments—you should be able to secure competent medical help. Yes, it will cost you an extra fee since some insurance companies may not reimburse for a second opinion. When you need the operation, it can enhance your well-being to have the surgery. In any

---

*But insurance companies have guidelines, too. Therefore, it would be wise to find out from your insurance carrier the ceiling for a procedure, should surgery be necessary.

event, it makes sense to consider carefully the reason for surgery before you decide to have your uterus removed.

KEEPING YOUR OVARIES

Some doctors routinely remove the ovaries when they remove the uterus. Fortunately, this practice has become less routine since the first edition of *Menopause* was published. In part, this change is attributed to a paper that Drs. García and Cutler published in 1984 in the medical journal *Fertility and Sterility*. That paper, "Preservation of the Ovary—a Reevaluation," resulted from the authors' discovery that the then-common practice of routine ovariectomy performed during hysterectomy was based on an error—a statistical misstatement—that had been perpetuated in the literature. The current textbooks at that time were advising surgeons—*incorrectly*—that if an ovary were not removed when a hysterectomy was being performed, there was a 5-percent chance that it would become cancerous. This was inaccurate: the true rate is about one-tenth this figure. When the authors checked the references for this statement, they found that not only had an error been made, but the literature was quoting the error instead of uncovering and correcting it. Unfortunately, not everyone has either read the above-mentioned paper or has been convinced by the authors' logic. The American College of Obstetrics and Gynecology now recommends that for each patient having a hysterectomy for benign disease, the removal of the ovaries be decided on a case-by-case basis.

In 1982, statistics indicated that for women over forty, half of those who underwent hysterectomy also had their ovaries removed.[23] Too commonly, one would hear comments like "As long as I'm cleaning out your uterus, I might as well clean out your ovaries, too." With the development of modern science, reproductive researchers have provided clear evidence that shows how important your ovaries are, regardless of your age![18] Thus, the ovaries should not be removed unless they are diseased. Some gynecological surgeons—particularly gynecologic oncologists—are beclouded by the great many ovarian cancers they see and tend to extrapolate the risk of cancer to retained ovaries. This occurs precisely because they are experts in that field and, therefore, see a preponderance of malignant cases. Hence, such specialists may feel the need to remove ovaries in women routinely after age forty-five to fifty. We do not agree. We think that each case must be considered on its own merits. The studies suggest that ovarian-cancer risk is no higher in those hysterecto-mized women who keep their ovaries than in those women who have never had a hysterectomy. Moreover, removal does not assure absolute prevention of ovarian-tissue cancer.[77] These facts strongly support the view that ovariectomy of healthy ovaries is unnecessary.[3, 77]

Ultrasound equipment has become more available and more refined in its resolution. The use of the new vaginal wand for ultrasound has permitted ovaries to be monitored unobtrusively and noninvasively. Early published results are very promising for ultrasound's ability to evaluate ovarian health.[66] Ultrasound permits an internal view of the body (like X-rays do) but does not bombard the body with gamma radiation. Rather, it uses the echo characteristics of sound waves. These sound waves do not appear to be harmful.

Since postmenopausal ovaries are active hormone producers (see Chapter 1 to review the facts), one can expect benefits from retaining the ovaries. The removal of the ovaries will induce a profound shock and an immediate menopause. As described in Chapters 3 and 4, when the ovaries are removed from a premenopausal woman, one expects rapid skin aging,[32, 56] bone deterioration, and other hormone-related changes that would not occur if these hormone-producing glands (the ovaries) were retained. Even after age fifty, removal of the ovaries will cause physiological changes, and simply replacing estrogen and progestagen will not bring the hormonal environment back to its presurgical state.[72]

Since, as described in Chapter 1, a woman's ovaries probably continue to function throughout her life, it is not surprising that ovariectomy leads to loss of bone mass. Four years after ovariectomy and no HRT, most young women show beginning signs of osteoporosis.[33] The largest loss of bone mass occurs within the first three years after ovariectomy, and even women who have had only a hysterectomy are more subject to bone loss.[18] Even in the aging ovary, ovariectomy will influence the speed with which osteoporosis develops.

If you lose your ovaries before age fifty to fifty-five and don't take estrogens, your skin will begin aging rapidly. It will wrinkle, dry out, and sag much the way a plum turns into a prune. This condition will get worse as time goes by.[56] But there is hope. Hormone therapy seems to prevent this unfortunate condition.

Young women who are hysterectomized and retain their ovaries often continue to show a normal cycle of ovarian hormone secretion; and though menstruation has stopped, the other cyclic changes (like mood swings, breast swelling, etc.) often go on until the age of natural menopause.[5, 13, 21, 25, 58, 59] The postmenopausal ovary continues to produce hormones; women in their sixties have been shown to have active ovaries when tested during surgical procedures.[44]

Unfortunately, recent studies have shown that hysterectomy tends to hasten the onset of the ovarian menopause.[18] Nevertheless, when surgery is mandated, it is a good idea to remove as little body tissue as is prudent.

During the menopause years, it makes sense to retain the ovaries, if possible. Hysterectomy, both with and without ovariectomy, was evaluated in one study of 122,000 women. The women whose ovaries were retained enjoyed a reduced risk of heart attack (myocardial infarction) when compared with those women whose ovaries had been removed.[67] The younger the woman, the greater the benefit in keeping the ovaries intact; but at every age, the ovaries provided a reduced risk of heart attack. Such a finding makes sense if you understand that, due to the estrogen (and possibly progesterone) secreted by the ovaries, women enjoy a lower heart-attack rate than men do. On the other hand, it has recently been suggested that the "liberation" of women has produced a new breed of hard-driving woman who, like her male counterparts, is going to be subject to an increased risk of heart disease because of coronary-prone behavior patterns.[81, 82] While such a suggestion may turn out to be true, it still seems likely that ovarian secretions will offer additional protection against heart disease, a protection that men do not enjoy. More on this hormonal influence is found in Chapter 10.

Remember that even when an older ovary stops producing estrogen, it continues to manufacture the androgens androstenedione[48, 49] and testosterone.[49] If you are menopausal, losing your ovaries will result in a 50-percent fall of androstenedione and testosterone in your blood. These hormones, along with estrogens, can be important to your health and sense of well-being.[75a] The ovaries continue to be vital even during menopause.[44, 47, 48, 49, 72, 76] Keep them if you can. Should your ovaries be routinely removed at hysterectomy? No! Is it safe to keep them in? Yes, it appears to be safe[57] unless uterine cancer is found or the ovaries are diseased—in which case your doctor will probably recommend that the organs be removed. But even the issue of cancer prevention by ovariectomy is controversial. Recent evidence has shown that ovariectomy of normal ovaries does not prevent cancer.[77] This makes routine ovariectomy less defensible.

RECOVERY AFTER HYSTERECTOMY

What is the recovery period like? One California woman put it pretty clearly:

After my hysterectomy, I had the usual post operation discomfort. About one week after the surgery I became very depressed and cried all the time. My feelings reminded me of how I felt after I had child birth. I really had no reason for feeling so blue. My family and friends had been very supportive and loving. I had my tubes tied 7 years ago so it wasn't that I was upset about not being able to have children. I remember when I was taking a shower one day, I was crying so hard I thought I was drowning in my emotions. I talked to my doctor and he said it would pass. That probably there was a shock to my ovaries and that they had stopped producing estrogen and that it was a change in my chemistry that was causing my depression. He was right. In about a week later I felt much better. I have felt better all the time and the fact that I don't need to worry about heavy periods draining me every month is such a relief.

Things probably do settle down, but recovery from the operation can be—and often is—difficult. Although some women seem to bounce right back after surgery, the vast majority find recovery slow and painful. One study compared 56 hysterectomized women with age-matched control women undergoing other surgical operations. Since hysterectomy is a more complicated abdominal surgery than most other operations, it is not surprising that it produces the slowest convalescence of all: on average, it took about 13 months for a woman to feel as if she were her old self again, and this compared to an average of 4.2 months for recovery from other operations (for example, removal of the appendix, thyroid, breast, gall bladder).[62]

More recently, researchers have shown that recovery time after pelvic surgery is longer the longer a woman has spent on the operating table, the shorter the operating time, the faster the subsequent recovery time.[4] For the postoperative patient, intravenously administered Premarin (a conjugated estrogen) may be used until oral estrogens can be taken. This will prevent the estrogen deprivation that often occurs postoperatively.

Postoperative adhesions are common after any form of pelvic surgery. These adhesions are the result of scar tissue developing internally at the site of the wounds that are healing after surgery. Because adhesion formation is frequently seen even after excellent and careful surgical performances,[9] investigators are continually seeking new methods to prevent them.[9, 10, 74] In all of these investigations, the necessity of meticulous surgical techniques is stressed in addition to the new prevention methods.

LONG-TERM PROBLEMS AND REMEDIES

SEXUAL FUNCTION DEFICITS

The following are the most frequent difficulties that women encounter when they resume sexual activity after having undergone a hysterectomy:

• a shortened vagina and, more rarely, narrowing of the vaginal vault
• dryness of the vagina and failure to lubricate during intercourse
• dyspareunia (painful intercourse)
• bleeding during intercourse
• loss of libido

Vaginal wetness in response to sexual arousal can occur with or without the uterus. But the cervix—the lower tip of the uterus—is responsible for a fluid that contributes moisture. In fact, for cycling women, as their mid-cycle ovulatory stage approaches each month, this fluid becomes copious—more so than at any other time during the cycle. While physiologists may show that vaginal lubrication resulting from sexual arousal is unimpaired by hysterectomy and mainly originates in the vaginal walls, the total amount of fluid may be diminished by the loss of that produced by the cervix, particularly in younger women. For women past fifty-five, substantiation of a cervical contribution to vaginal moisture is not yet available. Fortunately, ERT, whether applied locally in the form of a cream or by another route of administration, should help restore this lubrication by increasing vaginal transudate (the "sweating" reaction that produces vaginal lubrication).

LOSS OF LIBIDO

The loss of sexual desire after hysterectomy is common. This is true even when ovaries are retained.[18, 22, 51, 79, 80] Between 25 percent and 45 percent of women lose their sexual appetite after losing their womb. And taking estrogens doesn't help.[80] In fact, one double-blind study showed that although estrogen eliminated the dyspareunia, it did not influence the libido.[22] These libido effects have been studied in hysterectomized women at different times after surgery and were found to occur at all times studied: immediately;[51] up to two years after surgery;[80] even five years after the operation.[22]

Why would a decrease in sexual desire follow the loss of a uterus? First, the uterus itself could be a sexual center whose pleasure helps promote appetite. Studies conducted at the University of Pennsylvania of young women and at Stanford University of women in menopausal transition support such an idea.[19] Other studies have also considered it.[51] Here is what one woman had to say:

The greatest change since the surgery is this. Before, each time the penis is pushed hard against the cervix, I would feel intense excitement deep inside me, huge waves of pleasure going from the area of the cervix all through my torso. This was by far the most exciting part of sex for me, the real climax. I've tried to be satisfied with the orgasms I get from stimulation of the clitoris, that is mildly pleasurable contractions in the muscles in the front part of the vagina. Maybe I'll get used to it in time, but it isn't nearly as good, and I feel sad.[86]

Scientific data from Scandinavia were published that support the fact of the sexual role of the cervix after hysterectomy. Investigators compared the postoperative effects on women who had had a complete hysterectomy versus those who had had a subtotal hysterectomy (that is, the cervix was retained, and only the uterus was removed).* The researchers found that among married women, sexual activity was greater and the incidence of painful intercourse lower in the women who had retained their cervix than in those who had had a complete hysterectomy.[38]

---

*Three conditions had to be met to qualify for this study: (1) normal Pap smears; (2) normal cervical tissue determined by colposcopy; (3) willingness to have endocervical cauterization.

In their second report, the investigators evaluated the same women for the effects that the complete hysterectomy and the subtotal hysterectomy had on libido and orgasm. They found there was no difference between the two surgeries with respect to libido. But for the women who had had the complete hysterectomy, there was a significant and large loss in capacity for orgasm (from 30 percent preoperatively who had experienced orgasm at intercourse less than 1 time in 4 versus 47 percent of the group one year after hysterectomy who now experienced orgasm at intercourse at that same low rate). The women who had kept their cervix did better. There was no increase in the number of women postoperatively who had difficulty experiencing orgasm.[39] Maintaining the cervix appears to play some role in the postoperative experience of sexuality, but libido itself does not seem to be related to the presence of the cervix.

Second, removal of the uterus and ovaries accounts for an apparent loss of a significant quantity of the natural secretion of the androgens. Evidence for this lies in the return of the libido in women who take testosterone therapy after hysterectomy with ovariectomy.[69, 70] Although we know that testosterone affects libido—that is, testosterone increases interest in and the drive for sex among women—what remains to be determined is whether there is an appropriate dose that can be administered to achieve this effect without creating plasma levels of testosterone that are higher than that which is normally found in a woman's body. Studies have begun to be published that resolve this problem. High blood levels of testosterone have the potential to promote cardiovascular disease through alterations in lipids and through other, as yet undefined mechanisms. Lower doses—at least in the two-year-long studies—appear to be safe.

Third, there may be psychological reasons for a decrease in sexual appetite after hysterectomy. Many women integrally link sexual pleasure with childbearing. Knowing that their childbearing days are over may decrease sexual appetite for such women. Still others may be involved in deteriorating relationships and find it convenient to use the operation as the "reason" for loss of libido.

DEPRESSION

The word *hysterectomy* has an interesting history. It is derived from the Greek and the Latin. The Greeks called the womb *hystera*. The

Latin *hystericus,* suggesting disturbances of the womb, became associated with the English word *hysteria,* an emotional disorder. The thinking at that time implied that the uterus has a controlling influence on the female brain.

Depression hits in different ways and at different times in life. There are occasions when being depressed is normal. To react to a serious loss with depression is to be expected. Hysterectomy produces a loss of something very important. Not surprisingly, younger women—those in their childbearing years—are more prone to depression after hysterectomy than are older women.[50, 61] If you lose your ability to have children before you have had a chance to start or complete your family, you have reason to be depressed; and 55 percent of women under forty who have this surgery do go through a period of real and, by established medical standards, severe depression afterward.[61]

But sometimes depression is not to be "expected." A menopausal woman whose family is complete has no obvious reason to bemoan the childbearing loss associated with the loss of her womb. And, therefore, more troubling is a series of studies that have suggested a menopausal posthysterectomy depression syndrome. In 1957, a paper reported on a group of women who had been hysterectomized and followed for ten years by one physician. The author suggested that most postoperative troubles begin after the last routine follow-up that a surgeon performs and showed how physicians could be under the false impression that women recover nicely from hysterectomies because, usually, the doctors have stopped seeing their patients by the time the troubles begin.[20] Here are the facts: in the first year after the operation, 83 percent of the women were satisfied with the results of their surgery; between one and five years after the operation, 41 percent were satisfied; between six and ten years postoperatively, this figure dropped down to 33 percent. Another investigator, eleven years later, found that there was a two-year delay after surgery before the postoperative depression was most likely to happen.[7]

By 1989, the possibility of a biochemical link for this depression had been raised.[18] Pelvic surgery causes beta-endorphins to fall, and the decrease in the beta-endorphin level might be responsible for the psychological distress. Clearly, this is not the only cause for the depression that women experience; there are probably several biochemical changes that can provoke depression after hysterectomy.[18]

Hysterectomy is more likely to produce depression than other operations. When hysterectomized women were compared with age-matched women undergoing other surgical procedures, the hysterectomized women fared badly: 70 percent of the women who had had their uterus removed were severely depressed, which was more than double the rate of other postoperative depressions.[61] Two other published studies have confirmed this finding.[7, 50]

In 1990, a report of Dr. B. Sherwin's presentation to scientists at the 1989 inaugural meeting of the North American Menopause Society presented some startling results: evidence for surgically induced deficits in cognitive function. Although the measured deficits were statistically significant, the degree of impairment was small. Still, it gave support to what many women had been saying—that after hysterectomy and removal of both ovaries, they had noticed a reduced ability to concentrate.[70a] And it reaffirmed Sherwin's study published in 1988.[68a] In both studies, a series of psychological tests had been given to women before surgery and then at intervals of several months. Some women had taken ERT after their hysterectomy with ovariectomy; others had taken a placebo. The good news was that ERT produced a recovery from the cognitive impairments.* Whether there is a link between these particular cognitive-function changes and general depression has not yet been studied. Moreover, a person's values can affect her perceptions.

Why is hysterectomy so much more traumatic an operation than other surgical procedures? Or is it? Is it possible that women who are depressed are more likely to have their uterus taken out than women who are not depressed? Unfortunately, this seems to be true.[30, 55]

One investigator demonstrated that in large population samples, the highest incidence of depressive illness occurs in women who are going through the change of life. In that age span, 40 percent of the women show scores indicative of clinical depression.[6] This 40-percent figure compares with a lower (25 percent) figure for all other age groups in that study. Women in the forty-five- to forty-nine-year-old age group (the menopausal-transition years) are most likely to develop depression.[6] Preoperative depression was measured in age-matched women before hysterectomy and before other surgical operations. And preoperative depression was twice as common in the

---

*These studies also showed that estrogen plus testosterone did, too.

women about to undergo hysterectomy.[62] Hysterectomy was most difficult when it occurred during the change of life and best tolerated in women over the age of fifty-five.[20]

Depressed patients frequently have perceptions that their symptoms are worse than they would have judged them to be if these patients were in a nondepressed state.[31] Since many women slated for hysterectomy appear to be scheduled on the basis of a self-report of heavy bleeding,[37] it is possible that the uterus is sometimes being removed because the patient is depressed. In fact, one study showed that women who were depressed preoperatively were much more likely to have a normal uterus (discovered after the surgery) than women who were not depressed preoperatively.[7] Patients often do not appreciate that a hysterectomy may not correct the symptoms that produced a depression. What a terrible thought! Obviously, it doesn't happen in every case, but any case in which it does occur is unfortunate.

Time and the care of a loving person are probably the most reliable emollients for the depression that women feel after a hysterectomy.[42] Whether or not the hormones are available to you, we should not lose sight of the truth that a loving person in your life will greatly enhance your sense of wellness. Love is always available in the form of service to others in one context or another. If you suffer from depression, try helping someone less fortunate than you are. Maintain contact with other people. But if you find you are unable to overcome a debilitating depression, seek medical help. There are remedies available in the form of psychotherapies in combination with HRT. HRT, if the estrogen and progesterone are appropriately balanced, should replenish the diminished beta-endorphins, thus reducing the depression (see pages 125–126).

HEART DISEASE

Hysterectomy increases the risk for heart disease, according to one investigator who reviewed many small studies. The risk of coronary heart disease increases three- to fivefold over what is expected in similar-aged women who have their uterus intact.[15] A closer look at the individual studies indicates that while hysterectomy alone often shows negative heart health effects, ovariectomy plus hysterectomy may be even worse when no hormone therapy is taken. By 1990, this picture continues to elude concensus. For more detail, see the review in reference 18. If you must give up your uterus, the retention of your ovaries may help limit the risk.

In one large-scale evaluation, compared to other women of the same age who had had no surgery, ovariectomy was associated with three times the risk of heart disease (nonfatal myocardial infarction). The younger the woman, the greater the risk for having a heart attack. For example, a thirty-five-year-old woman who had had an ovariectomy was more than seven times likely to have a heart attack than a thirty-five-year-old woman who had not had the surgery. Hysterectomy by itself, with the ovaries left intact, did not seem to be a risk factor in this study.[67] Apparently, the risk of heart attack increased in that sample only when the ovaries were also removed at the time the hysterectomy was performed. While a heart attack proves the presence of heart disease, the process that precedes the attack is often silent but insidious. Several studies have explored the question of whether hysterectomy increases the risk of developing heart disease. The evidence suggests that it may.[18]

ATHEROSCLEROSIS

Atherosclerosis, a condition in which the lining of the blood vessels becomes so clogged with cholesterol droplets that circulation is sometimes blocked, is a serious problem for many older people. Atherosclerosis leads to heart disease. Ovariectomy significantly increases the incidence of the problem when no ERT is offered.[64, 85] In one study of several hundred hysterectomized women, those whose ovaries and uterus were removed before the age of forty-five showed four times the incidence of atherosclerosis than those whose ovaries were retained.[65] But a different team of investigators, asking similar questions, concluded that any hysterectomy (with or without ovariectomy) significantly increases the risks of atherosclerosis in both younger and older women.[63] In this study, there was, however, a difference in cholesterol levels that appeared to relate to the presence or absence of ovaries in the body. Cholesterol levels were consistently higher among those hysterectomized women whose ovaries were removed than among those whose ovaries were retained. Levels increased with age; they increased even more for any given age when hysterectomy was performed; and they increased even further if ovari-

ectomy was performed along with the hysterectomy.[63] *One could conclude that hysterectomy increases the rate of precipitators of heart disease and
that ovariectomy compounds the problem.*

Why the removal of the uterus, with the retention of the ovaries,
should influence heart-disease rate is not known. Some investigators
have suggested that the presence of the uterus may contribute something that keeps the ovaries more active.[18, 63] Estrogens, in some as
yet undiscovered way, appear to prevent the development of heart
disease. For those who smoke, the risks of these surgeries may be
worse since smoking greatly increases the chance for atherosclerotic
disease. Reports have not yet been published that directly address this
combination of factors to see if the risks are compounded when these
factors occur simultaneously.

HRT AFTER HYSTERECTOMY

In 1989, we were able to confirm what we had hypothesized in 1982.
We were able to say in 1982 that the evidence strongly indicated that
HRT was beneficial. Then we were able to discuss two reports in
which more than 1,000 women were studied for up to two years after
their hysterectomies.[12, 13] All of these women were taking ERT. If the
ovaries were intact, the therapy was initiated when menopausal symptoms (hot flashes, night sweats, etc.) began. If the ovaries were
removed, estrogen therapy began immediately after the operation.
The hormone doses were prescribed at the lowest level needed to
maintain comfort. Results clearly showed a marked drop in deaths
from all causes. At every age, the death and disease rates were much
lower among estrogen users than in age-matched comparison populations who were not taking estrogens. The hormones improved the
health outlook. The main improvement in longevity was the result of
reduced heart-attack rates and reduced cancer deaths. Both of these
diseases, as described earlier, are connected to hormone levels. Non-
hormone-related deaths (car accidents, for example) were equivalent
in both the patient population and the population norms. Our research for *Hysterectomy: Before and After* (1988, 1990) continued to
support the benefits of HRT after hysterectomy.

Taking hormones, especially when there is no uterus to stimulate
into a hyperplasia, appears to maximize one's health, longevity, and

well-being. But to undergo hysterectomy in order to take hormones without risk doesn't make sense even though premature death after hysterectomy is unlikely.

One more point should be made. You might hear about the often-cited, very impressive Boston Collaborative Drug Surveillance Program, which followed the cardiac health of a large population of men and women for many years. In this study, 14 of the postmenopausal women developed heart disease, and the authors noted that half of them used estrogen therapy and half did not. Although at first glance it seems as if the taking of hormones may be associated with heart disease,[36] a closer look does not support that conclusion. Nor do results of an earlier study that compared estrogen use to no estrogen use among 600 hysterectomized and oophorectomized women to test directly whether hormones are bad for hysterectomized women.[63] Hormone use did not increase the risk of heart disease in hysterectomized women, although the operation did increase the risk of heart disease over age-matched women who did not undergo hysterectomy. In the Boston Collaborative Study, of the 14 postmenopausal women who developed heart disease, 12 had been hysterectomized at an age younger than their natural menopause. Information was not available that could tell how many of these 12 had also been ovariectomized. Since we know that hysterectomy and ovariectomy increase the risk of coronary heart disease, it may be that the precipitating factor in these cases of heart disease was related to the premenopausal hysterectomy, not to the hormone use. Unfortunately, we cannot test the question properly with the facts available. The data that were published in the Boston study did not break down the facts that would be needed to analyze cause-and-effect relationships properly. One would need to know what dosages and durations of hormones had been taken, how much time had passed without any hormone therapy in these hysterectomized women, how many hysterectomized women were taking estrogen compared to a population of similar-aged nonhysterectomized women, and so forth.

One well-known epidemiologist, Dr. E. Barrett-Connor, published her study with colleagues in 1989. Comparing hormone users and nonusers aged fifty to seventy-nine in an upper-middle-class California community, her study showed that when ERT was used alone as compared to using estrogen with progesterone in combination, equal results on blood pressure, plasma glucose levels (relevant for those with diabetes), and lipoprotein levels were obtained. She noted that the cardiac risk profile of current users was not more favorable than that of nonusers, but current users were more likely to have had a surgically produced menopause.[8] In fact, twice as many of the hormone users (24 percent) had had surgically induced menopause as had the nonusers (12 percent).

In correspondence with us, Barrett-Connor agreed that the following is, by 1990, becoming apparent: surgically induced menopause* appears to increase the risk of cardiovascular disease. Once women have had a hysterectomy and go on HRT, their risk is no higher than nonhysterectomized women. This reduction of risk to presurgical levels is a powerful benefit of hormone therapy in surgically induced menopause. We can now say, therefore, that, as indicated in the large-scale studies of hysterectomized women taking ERT as well as in the large-scale studies of hormone-therapy users who have had and have not had a hysterectomy, HRT is beneficial to heart health in mature women (that is, over the age of fifty).

Should progesterone be taken in opposition to estrogen after hysterectomy? When we wrote the first edition of *Menopause* in the early 1980s, the major reason that scientific studies gave for prescribing progestin in opposition to estrogen was to protect the lining of the uterus (the endometrium) from developing hyperplasias. At that time, there were no documented reasons to add progestin to an HRT regimen after there was no longer an endometrium to protect. But knowledge has grown. Now, since many further research studies have been developed, we have come to the conclusion that progestin should be added to estrogen after a hysterectomy. To stimulate beta-endorphin secretions and promote a sense of well-being as well as to inhibit the development of fibrocystic breast disease and other pathology, a balanced HRT regimen appears optimal.

Although the 1990s will undoubtedly provide more information about HRT, we now understand that the benefits of a balanced estrogen and progestin regimen extend to many body systems. Thus, ERT has given way to HRT. Recently, a federally appointed "committee

---

*If a woman retains her ovaries at hysterectomy and then experiences the common reaction of an earlier menopause, we would conclude that even a hysterectomy alone caused a surgically induced menopause.

of experts" reviewing the reported state of knowledge was not fully convinced that progestational agents were warranted if a hysterectomy had been performed. This conclusion reflects a very conservative attitude, one that may be too conservative.

Summary

Although a hysterectomy can be a relatively safe operation, it is still serious surgery. If you have a noncancerous disease that may indicate the need for a hysterectomy, it would be wise to consider the surgery as a last resort. Begin by identifying the problem and the alternative treatments currently available. Then seek treatment for the disease before considering surgery. Only if these efforts fail or if the debility and alternative treatment are extreme, should you think about removing a body organ. Except in the case of pelvic cancer, uterine diseases do not urgently require immediate solution. You have the time—and you should take it—to become informed and to investigate all options.

If your uterus is incurably diseased, having the operation can enhance your well-being. But you need to be prepared. In addition to the pain of recovery, a postoperative bout of hot flashes is likely. There is also the chance of a decrease in libido and a change in your sexual response as well as a possible period of posthysterectomy depression. If you have already had a hysterectomy, there is a great deal you can do to overcome these deficits. But you must learn all you can about the subject.

10

CARDIOVASCULAR HEALTH

If you have a healthy cardiovascular system, you are fortunate, since at least 50 percent of women are not so blessed. By focusing some attention on this vital body system, we may be able to enhance its vigor.

Cardiovascular covers a lot of territory. *Cardio-* ("heart") and *vascular* ("blood vessels") describe the heart muscle plus the blood vessels to which this organ is connected. When all the parts are functioning well, the heart muscle pumps the blood, normally beating sixty to eighty times per minute, and the blood vessels, which are elastic and strong, carry the blood throughout the body. Blood is a richly complex fluid containing many elements. Some are produced in organs, others are manufactured in glands, and all are destined for use elsewhere. Oxygen-rich red blood cells give blood its color, circulating with hormones, immune substances, and fats, triglycerides, and cholesterol.

One can think of the cardiovascular system as a vast railway. The blood vessels (arteries, capillaries, and veins) form the tracks, the blood the trains. The "trains" carry passengers—hormones, fats, and other substances, and the pumping motion of the heart drives the "trains" (the blood) forward.

Each year, in over 1 million North American women, the cardiovascular system malfunctions. Sometimes it is the heart, which stops pumping. Other times it is the blood vessels, which tear and form scar tissue. Still other times it is the fats traveling in the blood that disrupt the system (too much fat can clog the circulation). When any of these problems occur, the blood circulation is in trouble and the vital capacity of the person is at risk.

In the United States, close to ½ million women per year die of a cardiovascular accident. This is eight times higher than the combined death rate from all reproductive-system cancers. And both are problems of the menopause. Until menopause, cardiovascular disease is almost never a cause of death. After menopause, the problem looms large, and it is then that the atherosclerotic process develops into the changes that lead to the enormous increase in the death rate (see Chapter 9).

Some interactive factors that influence cardiovascular health and its diseases are suggested by Figure 25. What is most apparent in this figure is the large part that a behavior can play in one's cardiovascular health.

We now know that HRT dramatically improves this picture. We also know that other actions that a woman can take may provide some protection against cardiovascular disease.

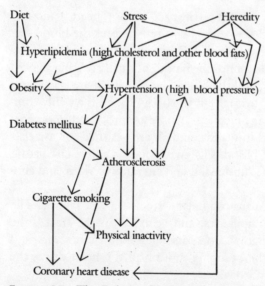

FIGURE 25 The Relationship between Controllable Risk Factors and Heredity on Coronary Heart Disease

RISK FACTORS FOR CARDIOVASCULAR DISEASE

BLOOD-BORNE SUBSTANCES

Triglycerides, cholesterol, HDL-Ch (high-density lipoprotein-cholesterol), and LDL-Ch (low-density lipoprotein-cholesterol) are measured by means of a simple, rapid blood test. The levels of each are believed to reflect risks and relationships to cardiovascular health.[13] There appear to be gender differences as well as age differences in which element causes what risk or benefit. For example, triglycerides do not seem to be relevant for either predicting or protecting the cardiovascular status in women under age fifty.[21] But men under fifty with high triglyceride levels are at an increased risk for a heart attack. The three fat substances thought to be associated with cardiovascular disease in women and that have been best studied are

- *HDL-Ch,* the beneficial lipoprotein: the higher the level, the more protected the woman (against cardiovascular accident)
- *LDL-Ch,* the dangerous lipoprotein: the higher the level, the more at risk the woman (for cardiovascular disease)
- *cholesterol,* the substance most commonly measured as a predictor of cardiovascular disease: when levels are below 180, a woman is said to be protected against most cardiovascular disease

OTHER RISK FACTORS

Other predictors of cardiovascular disease include high blood pressure, high apoprotein B levels,* lowered aproprotein A levels,* and certain diseases (diabetes mellitus, kidney disease, liver disease). Behavior habits are also strongly related to risk factors for cardiovascular disease. People who are obese, who are physically inactive, or who smoke are at much higher risk of a cardiovascular accident (heart attack or stroke, for example) than those who are physically active, trim, and do not smoke. And the relative strength of these factors shows that the behavioral ones—smoking and physical inactivity— account for most of the risk.

Because cardiovascular-disease processes can kill and because cardiovascular alterations can often be prevented, we shall focus atten-

*See the Glossary.

tion on what women can do to promote cardiovascular health. If you decide to take those actions that will promote your cardiovascular health, you may enjoy the rewards of feeling physically vigorous, which, in turn, will enhance your sense of wellness. To do this, you should focus on

- following a proper diet
- exercising regularly
- promoting emotional and spiritual wellness
- avoiding smoking (or breaking your addiction)
- regulating your blood pressure, if it is high
- considering HRT, if it is appropriate

PROPER DIET

Chapter 11 provides details on how to plan a good nutritional program for yourself. A proper diet is important for many different aspects of health, and some points are particularly relevant to cardiovascular health. In general, certain foods are known to increase the levels of cholesterol (and, with it, the dangerous LDL-cholesterol). These foods include saturated fats, diets that are high in refined carbohydrates (for instance, cake, candy, and soda), and diets that lack natural, *unprocessed* fiber, such as the fiber found in apples and in unrefined cooked oats.

To maintain a healthy cardiovascular system, you should follow a well-balanced, calorie-controlled diet that includes either an apple a day, a bowl of oatmeal, or an oat-bran muffin. These foods serve to clear cholesterol from the blood. See Chapter 11 for more details about fiber.

Vitamin C also plays a role in promoting cardiovascular health. Vitamin C deficiency leads to fat-clogged blood vessels. Because of this clogging, arterial passages narrow, thus triggering atherosclerosis.[49] Ascorbic acid (vitamin C) helps to maintain the structural integrity of the muscles that form the blood vessels. But when the ascorbic acid is depleted, the structure weakens and the vessels become more vulnerable to tears and scarring.

How much vitamin C is needed to maintain cardiovascular health? Optimal dosage depends on your levels of stress, your level of infection, your exposure to toxins, whether you smoke, whether you drink alcohol, and other variables. Smoking drastically increases the need for vitamin C; this addiction more than doubles the risk of developing cardiovascular disease.[8] Be sure to review the section on vitamin C in Chapter 11.

What about salt and other forms of potentially excess sodium in the diet? The widespread notion is that everyone should restrict her or his salt intake to prevent hypertension (high blood pressure). The facts are different. For the vast majority, salt change is irrelevant.[26] For certain groups, there is a benefit in reducing intake, especially for those individuals particularly susceptible to salt. For those people— including blacks, the elderly, and those with a family history of high blood pressure[26]—restriction will often lower blood pressure. Unless you are a member of one of these groups, it probably will not make any difference to your cardiovascular health whether or not you restrict the amount of salt in your diet.

Although we know that eating habits play a role in defining the risk of cardiovascular disease, our knowledge is incomplete. Sometimes rules that seem to work fail. For example, among 1,400 Swedish women enrolled in a twelve-year study, those who ate the least showed four times the heart-attack rate of any other group.[31] The researchers suggested that suboptimal nutrient intake might be the cause and thought that women eating so little were possibly omitting certain nutrients needed for their cardiovascular health.[31a] The other end of the spectrum (overweight women) has also been studied. And genetics play a role. In Samoa, where more than half of the female population is overweight, the obese women (66 percent of the female population) are not at any higher risk for cardiovascular disease than are the thin women.[16]

As we review the research on nutrient intake, obesity, and particular foods, we see that although a general picture forms, exceptions exist. A varied diet, rich in unprocessed, fiber-rich foods and high in vitamin C, helps. And unless you belong to a genetically overweight group, staying (or becoming) trim should help.

EXERCISE

A regular exercise program tends to lower blood pressure, prevent heart disease, lower cholesterol levels, and increase the healthy circulation of blood.[39, 14] Particularly important are aerobic exercises, the exercises that automatically cause the individual to breath deeply when she or he engages in the exercise program. For men, data suggest that to promote cardiovascular fitness, aerobic exercises be done three to four times a week for a minimum of 20 minutes for each session.[18] Unfortunately, equivalent data have not yet been collected for women. And there is no reason to believe that the number of minutes and the intensity of exercise that are appropriate for men will be comparable for women; for in most of the gender-related measures, there are large differences in levels and dosages.

In fact, in spring 1989, the first carefully controlled prospective study to evaluate physical fitness and subsequent death from either cancer or cardiovascular accident was published in the *Journal of the American Medical Association.*[8] This study followed more than 10,000 healthy men and 3,000 healthy women (that is, people without cardiovascular disease) for an average of 8 years after having first established a baseline fitness measure. Each of the 13,000 took a fitness test. He or she walked on a treadmill that would start at a level grade; with each passing minute, the grade would become steeper. The person would keep walking at the speed that the conveyor belt set and would continue to perform the increasingly more difficult task of climbing uphill until he or she could no longer do it. The fitness measure was the number of seconds an individual was able to continue performing. Using these measures, the authors were able to express the fitness level of participants still alive at the conclusion of the study and to show how this level compared to those levels of participants who had died of a heart attack or cancer.

Six facts emerged from this study:

1. Women who survived had been able to last on the treadmill a little over 10 minutes, and women who had died by the end of the study were only initially able to last for 8 minutes. The surviving men had a much higher endurance time, 17 minutes, compared to the deceased men, whose initial endurance time was 13 minutes. We

see from this that the fittest women had an endurance level (10 minutes) that was lower than that of the soon-to-be-deceased men (13 minutes). Male cardiovascular fitness levels were unnecessary for good cardiovascular health in women.

2. When individual fitness levels were divided into quintiles (five ascending levels), the group at the lowest level of fitness was more likely to die from either cancer or cardiovascular disease than everybody else. The benefit of being even mildly fit—that is in quintile 2 or 3—was profound.

3. Crossing beyond this first threshold from inactivity to some activity (that is, from no fitness to mild fitness) produced the largest increase in survival. The second increase in survival rate came from crossing from the third to the fourth quintile group. Little additional value was achieved at the highest of the fitness categories. Result: maximal fitness is not required for cardiovascular vigor.

4. The individuals who were the oldest at the start of the study benefited the most from physical fitness.

5. Both cancer and cardiovascular-disease death rates are inversely related across all fitness categories. The higher the fitness, the lower the incidence of disease. This suggests that as an individual becomes fitter her risk of death from cancer and cardiovascular accident decreases.

6. Even when cholesterol levels were high (or any other lipid level was unfavorable), highly fit individuals fared well. This means that if you monitor and improve your fitness, you will improve your health even if you cannot control your lipids by dietary planning. (See pages 288 ff.)

Chapter 13 reviews what we know about fitness and how to plan your own exercise program for fun and safety.

SPIRITUAL ATTITUDE AND RELAXATION

Attitude counts! In the early 1970s, two cardiologists, Drs. Meyer Friedman and Ray Rosenman, noticed something odd. In the waiting room of their offices, their patients with high blood pressure and other cardiovascular diseases had worn out the front edges of the upholstery on the seats. In other words, the patients tended to sit on the edge of their seat. The doctors hypothesized that a general attitude defined by impatience, explosive anger, demanding behaviors, easy irritability—that is, all the traits of what they called a "type-A personality"—formed a pattern characteristic of cardiovascular-disease patients. In their book *Type A Behavior and Your Health,* they presented the results of their discoveries. They tried to reeducate people who have a type-A personality to be calmer and gentler in their approach to life.

If you are at risk for cardiovascular disease, try to change your attitude. If you have high blood pressure, or your cholesterol levels are high, or your HDL-Ch levels are low, or if there is any other reason that your physician may have given you suggesting that you are a candidate for a cardiovascular accident, consider finding a way to bring more peace into your life. Any form of relaxation—whether it be contemplative, regularly attending a place that provides spiritual comfort, transcendental meditation, or just sitting still for 15 to 20 minutes while you count your blessings—will promote the biochemical changes in adrenaline, noradrenaline (norepinephrine), and other blood-borne substances that will help bring about a healthy cardiovascular system.

Regular physical exercise also will serve to produce relaxation and, with it, the changes in body chemistry that promote lower blood pressure.

GIVING UP SMOKING

Whenever a person breathes in smoke, either because she inhales a cigarette or because she's in a smoke-filled room, she is drawing carbon monoxide through her lungs and into her blood stream. This gas clogs the red blood cells, rendering them useless in the transporting of oxygen needed for healthy cell metabolism. The smoke also prevents the red blood cells from retrieving the carbon-dioxide waste produced by cells. Exposure to smoking upsets the cardiovascular system—it depresses it; it clogs it. And with this clogging comes the beginning of asphyxiation of all cells, which depend on blood circulation for the delivery of necessary gasses. If you smoke, you cannot have a healthy cardiovascular system. If you smoke and are receiving HRT, you should take your estrogen transdermally rather than orally to get as much beneficial lipid changes as your body will tolerate.[27] But if you want a healthy cardiovascular system—a necessity for life itself—it is critical to give up the weed. Chapter 12 provides help in overcoming the addition.

MONITORING AND REGULATING BLOOD PRESSURE

People with low blood pressure have a lower risk of heart attack than people with high blood pressure.[29] If you have high blood pressure, you should take steps to bring it down.[40] It is important to know that the first blood pressure reading in a doctor's office is not always accurate. In one recent study, investigators evaluated all of the women who were referred for hypertension by having each wear an ambulatory blood-pressure monitor that recorded blood pressure throughout a 24-hour span.[57] What the researchers found was that ambulatory (walking around) blood pressure readings of supposedly hypertense individuals were tremendously lower than the readings taken in the doctor's office. Many of these women who, at first re-cording, seemed to be hypertensive turned out not to be. If you discover that you are hypertensive and can follow this 24-hour regi-men of blood-pressure readings with ambulatory monitor, you may learn that your ambulatory blood pressure is normal. In either case, we suggest you first try the steps already outlined: to relax, adjust your diet, and exercise regularly.

If you do suffer from hypertension and your blood pressure does not respond to behavioral modifications, then you should consult with your physician about taking medication to reduce your high blood pressure. Although high blood pressure is dangerous and cer-tain drugs do correct the symptoms, drugs do not address the cause. And if the cause is related to your behavior, it is best to try to change that behavior.

CARDIOVASCULAR HEALTH AND SEX HORMONES

We know from the natural history of cardiovascular disease that men in their forties and early fifties are usually the first victims of heart attacks or strokes. Atherosclerosis and altered lipid changes that can predispose a person to hypertension, embolism,* and other cardiovascular diseases are common. Men have circulating in their blood high levels of testosterone, a concentration that is about forty times greater than that found in women. Women rarely die from cardiovascular disease before menopause. It is after menopause, when the sex hormones characteristic of young women—estrogen and progesterone—decline, that women catch up to men. This suggests that the male sex hormones—the androgens—in some way promote the risk of cardiovascular disease. And this also suggests that estrogens provide protection against cardiovascular disease. In fact, some studies of the microstructure of blood vessels tend to support this idea, but the research is a long way from yielding clear conclusions.

However, two things are clear. First, menopause greatly increases the incidence of cardiovascular disease. Second, premature menopause, induced by hysterectomy, ovariectomy, or any other medical intervention, profoundly increases the risk of cardiovascular disease—even in young women. When the ovaries are removed, the risk is immediate unless HRT begins promptly. But when the uterus is removed and the ovaries retained, the data are conflicting: some women suffer cardiovascular accident even though they still retain their ovaries. For a detailed discussion, consult *Hysterectomy: Before and After*. A cursory explanation may include the fact that about half of hysterectomized women experience an early menopause, an early shutting down of their ovaries, once the ovaries no longer have a uterus to support ovarian cycling of hormones. For chemically induced menopause due to chemotherapy for cancer, HRT may be useful unless it is contraindicated by the reason for the specific course of the chemotherapy.

HORMONE REPLACEMENT THERAPY

The increased incidence of heart attack, atherosclerosis, and stroke after menopause has led to a compilation of research data. Now, studies of the effects of different HRT regimens evaluate aspects of cardiovascular health. And with some perceptive understanding, these publications allow us to suggest that certain hormonal regi-

*See the glossary.

mens are safe while others are unnecessarily dangerous.

Studies of HRT and cardiovascular health begin with studies of estrogen, which investigate estrogen users according to incidence of heart attack, quantity of cholesterol, blood-pressure changes, and other disease or wellness aspects. The research begins with estrogen because hormone replacement therapy began as estrogen replacement therapy. In the early years of ERT, synthetic estrogens were as commonly prescribed as natural estrogens. And the doses were very high. More recently, the discovery that synthetic estrogens have a tendency to produce adverse effects on blood lipids in menopausal women has led to a swing toward the use of natural estrogens. But since this swing has occurred, one more factor has altered the picture again. As hormonal contraception for women in their late thirties and forties becomes a reality, some women will be taking synthetic estrogens because these are the modalities available for contraceptive use.

In 1989, when the Food and Drug Administration finally reversed its prior disapproval and approved the precept that women in their forties (provided that they were nonsmokers) had a right to be offered oral contraceptives, it was following what had been common practice in most of Europe for the previous two years. Women in their late thirties and forties who find themselves pregnant often suffer considerable stress. Both the prospect of late-life babies and the exhaustive energy requirements that childbearing and child raising demand create a need for effective premenopausal contraception. Since, on a global scale, oral contraceptives are the most effective and probably safest form of contraception available, we expect to see a great upsurge of oral-contraceptive use in this age group now that FDA approval has emerged, the consensus being that the many benefits of oral contraceptives greatly outweigh the risks. These benefits include:

- prevention of pregnancy
- regularity of cycles
- control of bleeding with an increase in hemoglobin (thereby preventing anemia)
- decrease in the frequency of ovarian cancer
- decrease in the occurrence of endometrial cancer
- decrease in benign breast changes

- prevention of ectopic pregnancy (that is, a pregnancy occurring in any location other than the uterus that must be terminated to save the life of the mother; the pregnancy cannot be a viable one)
- protection against osteoporosis
- reduction in myocardial infarction

Oral contraceptives contain three to five times more estrogen than HRT because that is what is required to inhibit the ovulatory processes, thus preventing conception. For women who take HRT, since the doses of estrogen (and progestin) are considerably lower, it is natural to wonder whether the positive effects listed above for contraceptive therapy will also be available to the HRT user. As data accumulate, we will pay special attention to those studies dealing with cardiovascular health in users of synthetic low-dose estrogens combined with synthetic low-dose progestins.

In general, natural estrogens are preferable to synthetic estrogen unless oral contraceptives are being considered. And it is the oral estrogens rather than the estrogens administered via patch or cream that produce the cardiovascular benefits that will be described next. When the first edition of *Menopause* was being written, the tremendous cardiovascular health benefits of oral estrogens had not yet permeated the scientific literature. At that time, therefore, we were recommending the lowest dose of estrogen that would facilitate relief of symptoms. We suggested that women consider vaginal creams (which, in today's counterpart, might be a patch) to avoid stimulating the liver. Now we know that for most women HRT stimulation of the liver produces many cardiovascular-system benefits.

HORMONAL INFLUENCES ON LDL-CHOLESTEROL

Natural oral estrogens promote cardiovascular health.[19, 42] Under normal circumstances, cholesterol levels in women rise with age;[2] the levels increase even faster in those who have had an ovariectomy.[24] However, cholesterol levels do not rise with age in women who take ERT orally.*[, 22, 42, 61]

*Women who have been on estrogens for up to three years maintain their lower (younger) cholesterol levels.[30, 58] This beneficial lowering of plasma cholesterol has been found for every estrogen so far tested, including the synthetic estrogens ethinyl estradiol at .01 mg. per day,[45] mestranol,[2] estriol succinate,[42] as well as the natural conjugated equine estrogens.[45]

For postmenopausal women who had high levels of cholesterol before taking hormones, estrogen therapy served to lower those levels.[54] And cholesterol levels have been shown to decline while menopausal women with normal levels are taking HRT.[7] At low doses, progestin added to the estrogen opposition seems to facilitate this beneficial decline in cholesterol.[15, 25, 33] Also, the dangerous LDL-cholesterol has been shown to decrease in women taking estrogen therapy.[22, 54]

Taking synthetic oral estrogens may lead to adverse effects, although these effects tend to be minor.* Nonetheless, if you have the option of taking a natural estrogen, do it. There is a growing awareness of the possible health risks involved in taking synthetic estrogen.[9, 32, 37, 38, 39, 43, 46, 47, 55] A dilemma arises if you want to take an oral contraceptive, which is only available in synthetic form. We feel that while natural estrogens are optimal when you have a choice, contraception is also critically important to the health and well-being of a woman in her forties. The risks of unwanted pregnancy are probably much greater than the risks of low-dose contraceptive adversity in the premenopausal years.

All changes in response to natural estrogen are considered beneficial, while the triglyceride changes in response to synthetic estrogens are not protective. Although triglyceride levels are not considered to be an effective risk factor for cardiovascular disease when the HDL and LDL levels of cholesterol are appropriately controlled, a study has been recently published showing that high levels of triglyceride in the blood of mature women (older than fifty) are associated with an increased risk of mortality from cardiovascular disease.[31] Dr. Leif Lapidus and colleagues, studying several thousand women in an industrial city in Sweden, followed them for 12 years. At the beginning of the study in 1968, the researchers were able to test the blood of over 1,000 of these women. Twelve years later, when the researchers

---

*In several reports,[8, 9, 31, 38, 39, 42, 43, 55, 60] synthetic estrogens increased triglyceride levels, while natural estrogens did not. A report evaluating responses to conjugated equine estrogen (natural) and ethinyl estradiol (synthetic) showed significant rises in the triglyceride levels for both high and low doses of ethinyl estradiol but no significant changes in triglyceride levels for either of two natural estrogen doses.[8] Triglyceride levels, however, do not appear to be a relevant risk factor for cardiovascular disease in women. (The only studies that have suggested that increases in triglycerides are dangerous are those that were conducted before the more-telling scores on HDL-Ch were testable.)

looked to see whether any of the baseline blood measures predicted who would be dead 12 years later, the investigators could say that women with extremely high triglyceride levels had a higher death risk. However, as the research paper pointed out, when triglyceride levels were measured, the researchers did not have the technology to measure the HDL-Ch or the LDL-Ch; and by 1980, when the death rate was known, it was too late to test for these blood lipoproteins. For that reason, the investigators were uncertain about whether high levels of triglycerides really mattered. Also, Lapidus reviewed other studies (discussed on page 233 in this book) that had shown that triglycerides are irrelevant when the other blood lipids are known. In addition, triglyceride effects produced by HRT may or may not produce similar effects in the body as natural triglyceride changes have the potential to do. Recent studies show that in monkeys the lipid alteration from hormone therapy did not lead to atherosclerosis and, therefore, may not have the same hormonal significance that the natural alteration in a genetically predisposed female may produce.[1] Nonetheless, we urge caution when thinking about using a hormonal regimen that unnecessarily increases a potentially dangerous substance.

Since the above ERT studies were undertaken, other research, showing the effects of various combinations of progestin opposed to estrogen, has appeared. This research indicates that when low-dose progestin opposition is added (in cyclic fashion, 10 to 15 days per month) to estrogen therapy, estrogen benefits remain unchanged. Only the lower doses are shown to be inobtrusive to the blood responses. The lower doses, listed in Tables 3, 4 and 5 on pages 132, 134, and 141, produce no adverse effects on any of the lipid levels that have been tested so far. The combination of natural estrogens and low-dose progestins should be beneficial in terms of your cholesterol level and blood pressure.[35, 44, 63] However, when progestin doses are high, some adverse lipid changes occur. For this reason, in Chapter 5 we recommended—and again recommend here—that you be aware of these high progestin levels so that the HRT regimen under consideration for you include low—not high—doses of progestin.

HORMONAL INFLUENCES ON HDL-CHOLESTEROL

HDL-Ch, the beneficial lipoprotein substance, has also been shown to respond well to appropriate dosages of hormone therapy. In one study of almost 5,000 women, ranging in age from twenty-one to sixty-two years, the level of HDL-Ch was (beneficially) higher in hormone users than in nonusers.[12] In this study, young women who were taking hormones were usually taking them in the form of birth-control pills (synthetic estrogen and progestins). Older women who were taking hormones were generally taking them in the form of estrogen replacement. Progestins, when added to the estrogen, reversed the beneficial effects of the estrogen: they decreased the beneficial HDL-cholesterol. But this adverse progestin influence on HDL-Ch seemed limited only to those users of very high doses of progestin (the doses that we recommended HRT users avoid).[25, 41, 50]

Menopausal women who take natural estrogens may enjoy the advantage of a higher level of these "good" high-density lipoproteins than nonusers of hormones. Several studies of different natural estrogen show this increase in HDLs.[54, 59, 60]

STUDIES AT VARIANCE WITH THE LITERATURE

There have been occasional, though infrequent, studies suggesting the opposite of the beneficial effects of hormone therapy on cardiovascular health. However, a close look at these studies generally reveals relevant variables to explain the adverse effects. One such variable is former pelvic surgery: hysterectomy increases the risk of heart attack threefold to sevenfold over age-matched nonhysterectomized women, a phenomenon described in Chapter 9. When researchers fail to distinguish between hysterectomized women and those who have not had pelvic surgery, the investigators sometimes conclude (incorrectly) that hormone-therapy users show higher risks of cardiovascular accident. In the United States, a woman has close to a 50-percent chance of having a hysterectomy, and for this reason, unless a study collects surgical data on its population, hysterectomized women are likely to comprise a large percentage of any menopausal group. Hysterectomized women also tend to use HRT. Different publications concerning the Framingham Study, which has been following an aging population over a great many years, provide an example of this kind of "confounding" of variables. In 1985, in a report of a study of 1,200 postmenopausal women, estrogen therapy was shown, as is consistent with the literature, to produce positive blood-lipid changes: estrogen lowered both the total plasma cholesterol and the LDL-Ch levels, while simultaneously increasing the HDL-Ch.[63] In this study, however, the authors concluded that ERT increased the risk of cardiovascular disease. But the same authors, in 1976, looking at the same population, had come to opposite conclusions,[46] and in 1978 they concluded that ERT increased the risk of nonfatal heart attacks.[28] We believe that the contradictory conclusions revolve around the problem of differentiating between hysterectomized women and those who have not had pelvic surgery. For details on the rationale that led to this conclusion, the reader is referred to our medical textbook.[17]

CYCLIC VERSUS CONTINUOUS HORMONE THERAPY

Every study described above on the role that progestin-opposed HRT plays in cardiovascular health used a cyclic regimen of 10 to 15 days per month, as opposed to either a constant regimen of estrogen or a cyclic regimen of estrogen. The results just described about the safety of administering natural estrogen with a low-dose of synthetic progestin apply to low-dose progestins that are given for less than 16 out of every 28 days. As the evolution of hormone therapy progresses, a number of physicians have recently been prescribing continuous HRT regimens in which a low-dose progestin opposition to estrogen is given every day for 21 to 29 days of the month. Physicians prescribe this regimen because women like the effect that it has on their menstrual pattern: within 4 to 7 months of having taken constant estrogen and progestin, all bleeding stops. These regimens do not mimic the natural hormonal cycle of younger ovaries and, as of 1989, had not been thoroughly tested to determine whether there are any adverse lipid responses to them.

The first report (a negative one) appeared in 1989 in the *British Journal of Obstetrics and Gynaecology*. Dr. Elizabeth Farish and co-investigators evaluated both the lipoprotein and the apolipoprotein levels in women who were on continuous estrogen/progestin therapy.[20] Because this is the first report of its kind, its conclusions are, at best, tentative.

Farish's group studied 38 postmenopausal women, 28 of whom had previously had a hysterectomy with removal of both ovaries and 10 of whom had not had pelvic surgery. In the 48-week double-blind study, the women were given continuous estrogen (a daily dose of 2 mg. of 17β estradiol, a natural estrogen) opposed to a synthetic progestin (the low dose of 1 mg. of norethisterone acetate). The researchers found no changes in triglyceride levels and only minor and transient changes in the lipids that have just been discussed. Their results are consistent with previous studies. However, the investigators did find adverse changes in the protein molecules of the lipoproteins. The level of apoprotein B, the one associated with LDL-cholesterol, rose. This kind of effect is adverse because, as other studies have shown, apoprotein B levels are the best discriminator for coronary artery disease in both men and women.[51] In men, it is well documented that survivors of heart attacks, particularly those with atherosclerosis, have a tendency to show increased levels of apoprotein B, even when their blood cholesterol is normal.[5] And again, in studies of men, it has been shown that apoprotein B is the best discriminator for coronary artery disease in those who are under fifty years of age, although after fifty, another blood element, VLDL-cholesterol (very low-density lipoprotein-cholesterol), is a better discriminator for coronary artery disease in men.[62] The same studies for women have not yet been done. When compared to the other lipid molecules that could be tested, Farish's study shows that the levels of the other apoproteins, AI and AII, fell; this is also considered an adverse change.[11]

In conclusion, in Farish's study, the protein changes that occurred after constant estrogen was taken with constant progestin are all considered dangerous because one of them, the apoprotein B reduction, has been associated with the increased risk of atherosclerosis and the other, increased apoprotein AI, has been associated with increased risk of coronary artery disease and increased risk of peripheral vascular disease.

We cannot tell from Farish's study whether (1) previous pelvic surgery accounted for most of these changes, (2) the form of progestin used—a 19-nortestosterone, which we described earlier—is not the optimal progestin to take, or (3) the continuous regimen in which progestin was given was the reason for the changes. This situation—three potential causes of a possible adverse effect all confounded into one research study—illustrates the kinds of problem that investigators face when they are committed to improving the quality of health care for women. It takes an enormous amount of time, energy, and money to do this type of research, as well as dedicated scientists and willing participants, before sufficient data can be assembled to optimize the regimens.

By November 1990, a second study had been published of three groups of women on 24 weeks of HRT.[64] In all three groups of postmenopausal women, the estrogen administered was in conjugated equine form and at a moderately low dose of .625 mg. In group 1 cyclic, a high dose of Provera (10 mg.) for 13 days of each cycle was coupled with 25 days of the estrogen each month. Groups 2 and 3 took the same moderately low dose of estrogen with a medium (5 mg.) or a high (10 mg.) dose of Provera every day (that is, continuously) for both hormones. All groups showed an absence of adverse lipid response in cholesterol, HDL-Ch, and LDL-Ch measurements. But unlike the women on the other two regimes, the women on the constant high dose of Provera did not show any beneficial changes in their LDL-Ch or HDL-Ch levels. All groups showed the potentially adverse declines in apolipoprotein A1 but no reduction in apolipoprotein A2; these, however, were dose-dependent. Cyclic users who took high doses of Provera showed the least decline in apolipoprotein A1; continuous users who took the highest dose of Provera had the sharpest decline.

Again, the results are difficult to interpret. The authors did not state how many of the women were surgically menopausal, but the age range of this postmenopausal group was forty-one to sixty-seven. The women in their forties probably were postsurgically menopausal and may have reacted differently than the others.

For now, we suggest that you select those regimens that have been best studied in terms of protecting cardiovascular health. Why? Because cardiovascular disease is the most pervasive health problem in mature women. If you reduce your risk of heart disease, you will promote your health. HRT (administered cyclically) drastically reduces cardiovascular death.

It is comforting to know that two recent studies have confirmed that women who take estrogen, thereby balancing their lipids, suffer less cardiovascular disease and have a lower mortality rate due to cardiovascular causes than women who do not take the hormone: the higher the estrogen dose—when opposed by 10 days of low-dose progestin (1 mg. norethisterone acetate)—the greater the lipid benefits. In the first study, the lipids that were scrutinized included cholesterol, HDL-Ch, and LDL-Ch. In this investigation, the beneficial lipid (HDL-Ch) rose, and the potentially dangerous lipids (cholesterol and LDL-Ch) declined in proportion to the amount of estrogen taken.[27] An eight-year follow-up study showed that women who took estrogen had a 41-percent reduction in mortality rate compared to age-matched contemporaries who did not take estrogen. In addition to this reduction in the death rate, there was also a 29-percent reduction in the rate of cardiovascular illness and disease.[23]

COAGULATION FACTORS IN BLOOD

The ability of your blood to coagulate properly is an essential health requirement. However, excess clotting can be dangerous. Studies have been conducted to test whether the relevant blood factors are impaired by estrogen or progestagen use. This coagulation effect appears to be dose-related. ERT uses a very small fraction of the dosage level where coagulation effects have been reported. Most laboratory studies reflect a less dynamic situation than exists in the body. Even so, results show no impairment on natural estrogens,[33, 37] and at least one investigator has suggested that natural estrogens are the most sensible estrogens to use.[37] Not everyone agrees with these conclusions.[52]

In 1988, a European group compared the patch and the oral conjugated equine estrogen.[3, 16] The researchers noted an elevated (but trivial) change in blood-coagulation factors in the oral conjugated estrogen but showed that the difference was not substantial. When, in 1974, the Boston Collaborative Drug Surveillance Program concluded that ERT does not affect thromboembolic events (those caused by clotting),[10] it was the first of several research teams to do so.[6, 38, 48, 53, 56] By 1986, investigators reporting in the *New England Journal of Medicine* also concluded that there were "no clotting factor changes" with any dose of any preparation when they compared oral estrogen in the conjugated equine form to transdermal estrogen.[14]

And the good news continues. In one study, in 10 women who had been ovariectomized and later treated with estradiol valerate (a synthetic), no significant changes emerged in any of 17 coagulation factors during a 1-month period of estrogen use.[48] In another report, estriol succinate, in doses titrated (adjusted in small increments) to that minimum level necessary for relief of menopausal-distress symptoms, was shown to have no significant effects on plasma coagulation factors in 10 women who were followed for 12 months.[56] Apparently, natural estrogens do not alter blood coagulation factors. Progestin in combination with estrogen has also been tested and shows no dangerous effects on these blood coagulation factors.[6]

Synthetic estrogens appear to be different from natural ones.[6, 56, 34] At this writing, a difference of opinion leads to confusion concerning synthetic versus natural estrogens. We tend to lean toward the use of natural estrogens because they seem less risky. However, the final word has not been written.

SUMMARY OF HRT STUDIES AND CARDIOVASCULAR HEALTH

In conclusion, we see that

- orally delivered natural estrogen protects against those risk factors known to promote cardiovascular disease
- progestin opposition to estrogen, in low doses for less than 16 days per month, produces no adverse effects
- progestin opposition to estrogen, in high doses, has been shown to have adverse effects on cholesterol, HDL-Ch, and LDL-Ch
- synthetic estrogens lower plasma cholesterol
- synthetic estrogens, in some studies but not in others, have been shown to increase plasma triglyceride levels
- triglyceride levels have not been implicated as cardiovascular risk factors for women when lipid levels are healthy, although they have been shown to be risk factors for young men
- HRT tends to lower the blood pressure although, in less than 4 percent of women, it may elevate it

SUMMARY

If you take appropriate actions to promote your cardiovascular health, you may reap tremendous benefits in terms of your overall health and well-being. The combination of factors with which you should be concerned include adequate nutrition, regular exercise, proper aerobic lung function (in other words, no smoking), and possible HRT (if you have reached that stage in life where you are at risk for cardiovascular disease). You should be aware that the heavier you get, the lower your protective HDL-Ch will be.[12] The principles of eating well-balanced meals, overcoming dangerous habits, and regularly exercising comprise the next three chapters.

11

NUTRITION

In a real sense, we are what we eat. Fortunately, an increasing amount of data on nutrition and food chemistry are being gathered. A great deal of information is now available to guide the woman who wants to learn about and alter her eating habits to promote her own long-term wellness. Yet we do not know everything. For example, although genetics seem to play a role in determining the appropriateness of particular diets, little research has been published on the ways in which different genetic groups respond to similar dietary nutrients. For this reason, when you do plan your nutritional program, you should consider not only those foods that agree with you, but those to which you react badly, your ethnic group, and your eating habits.

As we age, our nutrient needs seem to change. During our growing years, we build body mass from the foods that we eat. Later, if we continue to eat the same amount of food, we get progressively fatter. However, there is one exception to this rule: if a person exercises regularly and sensibly, she probably will not need to reduce her calories drastically as she gets older.

Protein, fat, and carbohydrate make up the three principal classes of food that we eat. These foods contain varying amounts of minerals (such as calcium) and vitamins (such as vitamin C or A). Each of these food classes serves an important role in a balanced diet, and none should be entirely avoided. For optimum health, your total calories should not be more than 25 percent to 30 percent fat-derived. As for protein, for most Americans this dietary building block is already in abundant supply. What tends to be underrepresented in the daily diet is the carbohydrate.

The pages that follow offer a short synopsis on nutrition, including a discussion of protein, fats, fiber, minerals, and vitamins. Because no two people are alike, we will not propose a nutritional program for all women but, rather, will explain the background research to show some of the variables that trigger different needs.

Two considerations are relevant as you make up a healthy nutritional plan. First is the *power of habit.* People tend to enjoy the foods they continue to eat. If you change the foods that you eat, you may not like them at first. For example, if you shift from foods that have a lot of refined sugar, such as candy bars and ice cream, to foods that contain natural and wholesome forms of sugar, such as apples and bananas, at first you will probably crave the candy bars. Within a few days, however, your tastes will change.

There was an old (and apparently true) story of English sailors washed ashore in Japan. These men had been accustomed to the high-fat, very rich English diets and found themselves forced to eat the relatively spartan fare of the Japanese, rich in raw fish and raw vegetables. What was particularly interesting was that the sailors grew to love these foods, to like the way their bodies felt when they ate them, and later found it very difficult to adjust to their old diet when they were finally rescued, returned home, and permitted to eat whatever they wanted. Habits are powerful, and changing your habits *will* change your desires.

Second is the *power of relaxation.* The stress that you bring to your meal will affect the way you digest your food. In 1989, investigators published a remarkable study in which they manipulated (through the directions they gave their research subjects) the state of relaxation and stress in their subjects; they also defined the amount of time that the subjects spent chewing each mouthful.[60] What they found has applications for all of us. They showed that, in determining the secretion of digestive enzymes in her mouth, it didn't so much matter how the person chewed but how much she relaxed. They concluded that if the relaxation component of the autonomic nervous system becomes activated, this will trigger a saliva high in volume and bicarbonate content, freely flowing, and rich in the enzyme amylase. In sum, this set of actions decreases the bacteria in the mouth and promotes proper digestion of the food. When you eat, you would be wise to tend to your needs for relaxation. Do not permit stressful emotions to override your need for good digestive practices. Perhaps this recently discovered reflex accounts for the continuing practice of saying Grace (with such pleasure) among the people who say it at the beginning of a meal: while giving thanks for the food and causing one to reflect, one does relax; and when one relaxes, one's digestive juices flow.

PROTEIN, THE BODY'S BUILDING BLOCK

Protein forms the building block for most of the parts of our body but is especially important to the muscular structure. Although fat will be found throughout the body (especially within the nervous system as well as surrounding the skeleton and sometimes marbled within the muscle), it is protein that forms the basic nonbony structure of the body. Muscles are largely built of protein.

We need protein on a regular basis, although how much we need is unclear: depending upon which nutritionist you follow, the amount will vary from 30 grams to 70 grams a day. But unless you are vegetarian, you probably do not need to worry about your protein intake. If you eat 4 ounces of meat or fish or chicken a day with 1 glass of milk or 2 eggs, you are probably getting more than enough. However, if you eat too much protein, you are likely to be either at risk for overweight or missing other important dietary elements, outlined below.

You should be aware of research that shows that calcium metabolism is affected differently by different kinds of protein. Women need a combination of protein, calcium, and phosphorus to promote bone mineralization and maintenance.[77, 87, 88] Meat is helpful to the overall calcium-balance metabolism.[24] However, other forms of protein, particularly soy and those high in dietary nitrogen, tend to weaken bone strength by increasing the amount of calcium spilled into the urine.[1, 2, 13, 37, 38, 55a] Either phosphorus or sulphur, in combination with protein, are helpful for bone metabolism.[97, 102] Perhaps because meat protein is relatively high in phosphorus, the bone metabolism is better served by meat rather than by soy sources of protein.[77, 87, 88] Fish, chicken, and eggs are high in sulphur, beef is high in phosphorus, and all provide good sources of protein. We do not know of any published research that deals with whether the soy-eating peoples of the world are small-boned because of high urinary calcium loss. But we can see that those Oriental peoples who follow a diet high in soy tend to have small bones. If you are at risk for osteoporosis, perhaps you should avoid soy protein such as tofu until more is known.

CONTROL OF DIETARY FATS

The fats that we eat affect our cholesterol level and other cardiovascular-health-associated lipids that travel in our blood. Confusion arises as to the use of terms, which tends to overlap. *Dietary* fats are different from *plasma* fats. For example, a diet high in cholesterol does not necessarily affect the plasma cholesterol; but a diet high in saturated fatty acids will more often increase the cholesterol levels in the blood, and high plasma cholesterol is believed to be related to increased risk for cardiovascular disease.

Since the Framingham Study showed that people with high HDL levels and low cholesterol levels have the lowest risk for coronary heart disease, it becomes especially appropriate to review how your choice of diet can affect your plasma levels of cholesterol and HDL-Ch.[10] Although the data are not yet complete and most of the studies have been conducted solely on men or primarily on men, several issues should be addressed. First, the studies that have so far been published deal with people who had cardiovascular disease and their prior or current plasma levels of the lipids. Until studies follow women across many years, monitoring the changes in their lipids and how these changes relate to cardiovascular disease, we cannot reach any definite conclusions. Nonetheless, since we have to take action now, it would be prudent to do those things that the data are beginning to suggest will be healthful.

If you want to establish eating habits that keep your plasma cholesterol down and your HDL-Ch up, you should know several things—most importantly, which foods contain which fats. Tables 12 and 13, which show the major sources of dietary fats and cholesterol, respectively, are useful when you want to check your own eating patterns.

TABLE 12   Major Sources of Dietary Fats*

SATURATED	MONOUNSATURATED	POLYUNSATURATED
Butter, butter fat	Avocado, avocado oil	Cottonseed oil
Cheese	Olives, olive oil	Corn oil
Chocolate, cocoa butter	Margarines with	Fatty fish
Coconut, coconut oil	hydrogenated oil as first	Margarines with oil from
Hydrogenated solid fats	ingredient	this group listed as first
Lard	Lightly hydrogenated	ingredient
Meat fat (from beef,	shortening	Mayonnaise
lamb, pork, veal,	Nuts such as almonds,	Safflower oil
poultry)	Brazil nuts, pecans,	Salad dressing made from
Palm oil	filberts, macadamia nuts	oil in this group
	Peanuts, peanut butter,	Soybeans, soybean oil
	peanut oil	Sunflower seeds,
	Rice-bran oil	sunflower-seed oil
		Walnuts, walnut oil
		Wheat germ, wheat-germ
		oil

Source: C. J. W. Suitor and M. F. Crowley, *Nutrition Principles and Application in Health Promotion,* 2d ed. (Philadelphia: Lippincott, 1986).

*Fried foods, pastries, and other foods that are cooked in or made with fat are important sources of fatty acids. Which category they should be placed in depends on which fat is used in their preparation.

Research has shown that when plasma cholesterol rises, there is a simultaneous rise in the LDL-Ch; and when plasma cholesterol levels drop, the LDL-Ch levels drop, too. HDL-Ch (the beneficial one) is unpredictable with respect to changing cholesterol levels: sometimes it moves in the same direction; at other times, it moves in the opposite direction.

To optimize your plasma lipids by means of dietary control, consider these principles:

- Limit your fats to no more than 25 percent to 30 percent of the total calories of your diet.
- Adjust your diet so that the fats you do consume are relatively high in polyunsaturated and low (less than half) in saturated forms.[21a, 96a] See Table 12.
- Some studies have indicated that monounsaturated fats such as olive and peanut oils do not seem to affect the plasma lipids. So if you eat them, reduce some of the saturated fats such as butter and

TABLE 13 Cholesterol Content of Some Foods

FOOD	CHOLESTEROL (MG. PER 100 G.)*
Egg yolk, dried	2,950
Brains, raw	2,000
Egg yolk, fresh	1,500
Egg, whole	500
Kidney, raw	375
Caviar or fish roe	300
Liver, raw	300
Butter	250
Sweetbreads	250
Oysters	200
Lobster	200
Heart, raw	150
Crabmeat	125
Shrimp	125
Cheese, cream	120
Cheese, Cheddar	100
Lard and other animal fat	95
Veal	90
Cheese (25% to 30% fat)	85
Milk, dried, whole	85
Beef, raw	70
Fish, steak	70
Fish, filet	70
Lamb, raw	70
Pork	70
Cheese spread	65
Margarine (2/3 animal fat, 1/3 vegetable fat)	65
Mutton	65
Chicken, flesh only, raw	60
Ice cream	45
Cottage cheese, creamed	15
Milk, fluid, whole	11
Milk, fluid, skim	3
Egg white	0

Source: see reference 20.

*Most standard kitchen scales measure in grams as well as in ounces. If you weigh the food and note its gram content, you can then compute its cholesterol content from this chart.

palm oil. Be alert to rigorous research in this area of nutrition because monounsaturated fats, aside from tasting good, may, in moderation, be beneficial to cardiovascular health when substituted for polyunsaturated fats.[21a, 96a]

- Be aware that cholesterol in food will not necessarily hurt you, particularly if you belong to a genetic group that is not at risk for cardiovascular disease and/or if your diet is low in saturated fat.[26, 84, 98]

- Although eggs may lead to an increased level of cholesterol, they usually do not.[22, 44] Eggs provide a rich, low-calorie source of protein, iron, and other nutrients. An egg, hard- or soft-boiled, provides 6 grams of protein and only 70 calories. If your diet is low in saturated fat, eggs can be important in maintaining and elevating your HDL-Ch level.[36, 45, 63, 64]

- Fish is rich in PUFA (polyunsaturated fatty acid) oils and is believed to be protective against heart and cardiovascular diseases.[61] It appears that the PUFAs decrease the formation of blood clots. But while fish oils in capsule form are high in polyunsaturated fat, they are not yet safe unless they are taken under the supervision of a medical professional. There is the risk of contamination from excess vitamins A and D since the oils are concentrated during the manufacturing process.[8, 40] We believe it is best for you to eat fish but avoid fish-oil capsules.

- A diet rich in soluble fiber will lower plasma lipids (see pages 259–261).

- Relatively high levels of dietary vitamin C also lower plasma cholesterol (see pages 272–275).

- As Table 12 shows, beef fat is a saturated fat. If you limit your total quantity of fat as described, beef fat itself is unlikely to alter the cholesterol level in your blood. As was discussed earlier, the meat form of protein helps to maintain a positive calcium balance, while the soy form of protein increases the urinary loss of calcium. Therefore, meat is an important part of the diet of most women and should not be automatically deleted from a healthy nutritional plan. In fact, meat, in moderation, will help build your strength, energy, and muscle mass.*

*Additional studies of dietary fats and dietary cholesterol include the following: 4, 56, 63, 64, 90.

One way to learn whether your nutritional regimen is adequately controlling your plasma fats is to have annual or twice-annual assays of your fasting blood for its cholesterol and HDL-Ch levels. In some areas of the eastern part of the United States, mobile units provide tests with results within 3 minutes. The fees are modest—from $7 to $12. Alternatively—and for more money—your physician can take blood at your annual exam, send it out for testing, and provide you with results 1 to 2 weeks later. Regardless of how you take the tests, the results will be useful in guiding your nutritional planning.

There is another benefit to lowering the amount of fat that you eat. Investigators in Israel, evaluating 850 women who had benign breast disease, compared this group to a group of disease-free women who lived in the same neighborhood and were the same age.[54]

A careful study of the eating habits of the two groups revealed that the women with benign breast disease tended to eat more, particularly those foods containing saturated fats (which are inadvisable for your health). Therefore, it is reasonable to assume that if you not only lower the fat content in your diet, but lower as well that portion which is saturated, you may lower your risk of benign breast disease and perhaps breast cancer.

DIETARY FIBER AND GOOD HEALTH

Fiber is a term used to describe substances in the diet, principally derived from plant cell walls, that do not get absorbed into the blood stream.[86, 92] When you swallow food, it goes from the mouth into the esophagus, down into the stomach, from there into the intestines; finally, whatever is not digested and absorbed (across the walls of the intestines) passes out as stool. Fiber in your diet serves many vital functions. When passing through the intestines, it provides the bulk that stimulates the motion of the bowels; and the more frequent the motion, the lower the risk of intestinal diseases, including cancer of the colon and diverticulitis. Fiber attracts water, softening the stools and preventing constipation and hemorrhoids. Fiber provides the bulk (without the calories) that leads to a pleasant sense of fullness.

Dietary-fiber sources from plants derive from three broad groups:

• cereals (such as oats, corn, wheat), which are low in fat and rich in starch

- legumes (such as lima beans, peas), which are highest in fat and rich in starch
- fruits and other vegetables (such as apples, oranges, cabbage), which are low in fat and high in water

Soluble fiber dissolves in water to form a gel; insoluble fiber does not dissolve. Most foods contain a combination of each. If you are looking for soluble fiber, you can be guided by foods containing oats and barley, and by fruits like apples, which are high in pectin. Insoluble fibers can be thought of as those that are woody or composed of older vegetables that are getting tough. Also, the fiber in wheat bran is insoluble.

Table 14 shows the fiber content of a number of commonly available foods, and can provide a basis for planning your own nutrition regimen.

Modern civilization has witnessed a new phenomenon in food processing that has promoted a number of contemporary "western" diseases. This phenomenon, known as *fiber depletion,* is used in the production of candy bars, ice cream, cakes, and other sweet and rich nonbulky foods that taste delicious but are not satisfying: the high calories that these foods contain do not provide a correspondingly big nutritional wallop. Instead, the nutritionally poor fiber-depleted foods increase the appetite for more of the same; as we satisfy our hunger for these products, we get fatter.

Lack of fiber has caused other health problems in the West, especially since about 1900,[66] as the following list of diseases that are significantly related to a fiber-depleted diet indicates:

- diverticular disease of the colon[7, 66]
- hiatal hernia[79]
- diabetes mellitus[55, 83]
- lipid-metabolism and cardiovascular health problems that emerge in some studies[10] but not in others[29]
- gallstones[35]
- bowel cancer[15]
- varicose veins and hemorrhoids (a specialized form of varicose veins)[7]
- deep vein thrombosis (clots in a vein) and pelvic phleboliths (stone-like substances)[7]
- kidney stones[5]

Each of these diseases has been studied by nutritionists specializing in fiber and its role in the physiology and prevention of these diseases. For a more complete description of each disease as it relates to fiber depletion and to a high-fiber diet, see the references cited above. For our purposes, being aware of the disease-prevention benefits of fiber should stimulate you to include it in your nutritional planning.

Although fiber is important to our diet and we should probably consume as much as we can handle, a daily minimum of about 30 grams is sensible. Fiber-based laxatives should not be relied on since fiber itself is abundantly available in delicious natural foods and since laxatives are less desirable than wholly natural approaches. If you ingest enough natural fiber, there should be no reason to take laxatives, which themselves tend to be habit-forming. It is much better to form the habits of a nutritionally sound high-fiber diet. However, if, after establishing a high-fiber diet and regular exercise regimen, you still need help, discuss laxatives with your physician—but only as a last resort.

One warning: women (and men) must eat their fiber-rich foods appropriately. High-fiber foods tend to prevent the absorption of certain minerals such as calcium and iron across the wall of the intestines.[23, 30, 19, 18, 32, 95]

If, for example, you eat a high-fiber cookie while you drink a glass of milk, you may not benefit from the calcium in the milk because the cookie will bind the calcium molecules in the milk and pass calcium out with the feces. And, although spinach has been shown to be rich in calcium, recently it also has been shown to act as a high fiber, binding the calcium and preventing its absorption into the blood stream.[34] So the use of fiber should be prudently added to one's planning: eat it abundantly, but not with your calcium. And if you want fiber with your iron (wheat toast with eggs), be sure to consume a vitamin C–rich component (see pages 272 ff.) at the same time in order to facilitate the iron absorption.

CALCIUM AND VITAMIN D

Although our bones store 99 percent of the calcium in our bodies, the 1 percent that circulates in the blood stream and adjacent to nerves and muscles powerfully influences our body functions. Muscle contraction demands calcium; nervous-system function demands cal-

TABLE 14   Fiber (NDF)* Content of Some Foods

FOOD	SERVING SIZE (G.)	FIBER PER SERVING	GRAMS PER SERVING	WATER (%)†
FRUITS				
Apple, fresh	180 (1 medium)	1.1	0.6	91
Apple, cooked, peeled	122 (½ cup)	0.7	0.6	91
Banana	175 (1 medium)	1.1	0.7	74
Blueberries, frozen	83 (½ cup)	1.5	1.8	83
Cantaloupe	136 (¼ melon)	0.7	0.5	88
Grapes, green seedless, fresh	80 (½ cup)	0.4	0.5	78
Orange, fresh	160 (1 medium)	1.2	0.8	87
Peach, fresh	115 (1 medium)	0.6	0.6	91
Peach, canned	122 (½ cup)	0.7	0.6	88
Peach, cooked	122 (½ cup)	1.1	0.9	90
Pear, fresh	180 (1 medium)	3.6	2.0	84
Pineapple, canned	123 (½ cup)	1.2	1.0	83
VEGETABLES				
Beans, green, canned	120 (½ cup)	1.6	1.3	92
Broccoli, cooked	73 (½ cup)	1.5	2.1	87
Cabbage, fresh	45 (½ cup)	0.5	1.1	89
Carrot, fresh	81 (1 medium)	0.8	1.0	88
Carrots, canned	73 (½ cup)	0.5	0.7	92
Celery, fresh, diced	67 (½ cup)	0.5	0.7	94
Corn, whole-kernel, canned	83 (½ cup)	1.2	1.4	78
Corn, whole-kernel, frozen	88 (½ cup)	1.3	1.5	68
Lettuce, fresh	70 (⅛ head)	0.4	0.6	95
Mushrooms, fresh	35 (½ cup)	0.6	1.7	90
Onion, fresh, chopped	43 (¼ cup)	0.5	1.1	87
Potatoes, boiled, peeled	76 (½ cup)	1.2	1.2	71
Spinach, frozen, cooked	100 (½ cup)	1.2	1.2	90
Squash, zucchini, fresh	65 (½ cup)	0.5	0.8	93
Tomato, fresh	135 (1 medium)	0.8	0.6	95
Tomato, cooked	120 (½ cup)	1.0	0.8	94
LEGUMES				
Beans, kidney, canned	93 (½ cup)	3.9	4.2	39
Beans, lima, mature, cooked cooked	95 (½ cup)	3.3	3.5	74
Peas, canned	79 (½ cup)	2.2	2.8	83

FOOD	SERVING SIZE (G.)	FIBER PER SERVING	GRAMS PER SERVING	WATER (%)†
REFINED GRAIN PRODUCTS				
Bread, white	25 (1 slice)	0.5	2.0	31
Corn Flakes	21 (²⁄₃ cup)	0.3	1.4	5
Cornmeal, cooked	120 (½ cup)	0.6	0.5	87
Cream of Wheat	163 (²⁄₃ cup)	0.7	0.4	87
Macaroni, cooked	65 (½ cup)	0.5	0.8	57
Rice cereal, puffed	11 (⅓ cup)	0.1	0.9	4
Rice, white, cooked	100 (½ cup)	0.5	0.5	70
Rice Krispies	18 (²⁄₃ cup)	0.1	0.6	5
Special K	18 (²⁄₃ cup)	0.2	1.1	4
White flour	30 (¼ cup)	0.3	1.0	1
Popcorn	6 (1 cup)	0.5	8.0	4
UNREFINED GRAIN PRODUCTS				
Barley, pearled, cooked	100 (½ cup)	1.0	1.0	84
Bran Buds	28 (⅓ cup)	6.4	22.8	5
Bran Chex	23 (²⁄₃ cup)	3.9	17.0	4
Bread, rye	25 (1 slice)	1.2	4.8	36
Bread, wheat	28 (1 slice)	1.3	4.5	8
Bread, whole-wheat	25 (1 slice)	1.8	7.2	7
40% Bran Flakes	23 (²⁄₃ cup)	3.2	13.9	3
Granola	28 (¼ cup)	0.8	3.0	6
Oatmeal, cooked	160 (²⁄₃ cup)	1.1	0.7	86
Shredded Wheat	25 (1 biscuit)	2.6	10.0	6
Wheat bran	30 (½ cup)	11.2	37.3	8

Source: see reference 20.

*NDF represents the neutral-detergent-fiber method of testing fiber. Several different methods are currently available, and each yields different values. This method appears to be useful.

†Foods with higher percentages of water provide bulk without calories. As the concentration of water diminishes, the concentration of calories, fiber, and nutrients tends to increase.

cium; and bone metabolism demands calcium. Meanwhile, we lose calcium every day in urine, feces, and sweat; this calcium must be replaced, even after we have stopped growing. Calcium deficiency can lead to both osteoporosis and periodontal disease.[23] The amount of calcium that we need varies, depending on a number of factors unique to each individual. Probably, somewhere between 750 and 1,500 mg. per day is the right amount of calcium for you: the more estrogen circulating in your blood, the more you can move toward the lower end of the requirement;[32, 51] the less estrogen circulating in your blood, the more calcium you need. Table 15 gives the calcium values of some commonly available foods.

Ideally, your calcium should come from a natural diet combining dairy foods and other calcium-rich sources. But if your diet does not provide enough calcium, consider taking calcium tablets. Be aware, however, that calcium tablets do not necessarily dissolve in the stomach, nor do they necessarily get absorbed in the intestines (see pages 98–99).*

Another problem with calcium is that a calcium-rich meal should not be the same one in which you are deriving your dietary iron: calcium reduces the retention of iron from food.[21] Therefore, if you are going to take a nonacid form of calcium, you need to get it from a meal that is not providing your iron source.† And only supplement that by the use of tablets as needed.

Vitamin D and the kind of protein in your diet also influence the way your body uses calcium. Both were reviewed earlier (see pages 96 f. and 254 f.). Likewise, caffeine will have a slight effect on increasing urinary loss of calcium,[33] but the effect is so trivial that you can probably disregard caffeine as a critical element in planning your calcium intake.

Research studies consistently show that it is the combination of foods that we eat, in addition to what those foods are, that determines the value of the nutrients. For example, vegetarians have significantly lower levels of estrogen as compared to nonvegetarians,[27, 82] and lower estrogen means higher calcium requirements. Middle-aged women would also be expected to have greater needs for calcium in their diet since the lower the estrogen level, the more calcium they need to promote bone health. If you are aware of these combinations of factors, you can plan to include all the elements you need to promote your good health.

A majority of the world's peoples suffer from *lactose intolerance*—that is, if they drink milk, they shortly afterward suffer from intestinal gas pains and, usually, diarrhea. The reason for the discomfort has re-

---

*Dr. Ralph Shangraw, chairman of the Department of Pharmaceutics, University of Maryland School of Pharmacy.

†Our review of the research on calcium pills uncovered so many problems of this kind that we concluded that it would be best to obtain calcium from food, if possible.

cently been uncovered and explained. In 1988, the American Society for Clinical Nutrition devoted an entire journal supplement to the subject of the acceptability of milk and milk products in populations with a high prevalence of lactose intolerance.[78] These researchers explained that the digestion of dairy products begins with the enzyme lactase, which converts lactose, the principal sugar in milk, into two simpler sugars that the intestines are able to absorb. These absorbed sugars provide the body with energy and calories. The lactase enzyme is gradually lost after infancy by most humans and other mammals. Although a few genetic groups have experienced a mutation that allows them to retain the lactase enzyme, this preservation of lactase after childhood is the *abnormal* condition rather than the normal one.

People naturally wonder whether, in the face of this gastric distress, it does them any good to drink milk. Would an inability to digest the milk sugar interfere with the ability to digest and absorb the milk calcium? The results are *not* obvious. It turns out that people with lactose intolerance actually digest *more* calcium from milk than people who don't have the problem.[28] When you drink a glass of milk, your stomach and intestines must break the milk down into its principal parts and absorb the parts that your body requires. The most important requirement is the calcium, and the irritability of the intestines that lactase-deficient people experience in some unknown way promotes the absorption of calcium. For this reason, even if you do suffer from lactose intolerance, try to drink milk. Many sufferers discover that by drinking the milk in small doses at a time—say, 4 ounces separated by at least 1 hour—they are able to enjoy the milk without much gastric distress. But if you cannot tolerate regular milk, you might consider either LactAid, which contains lactase, or LactAid drops, which you add to your milk. Yogurt is another good alternative because it is rich in calcium and is usually easier to digest than other dairy products.

One further note: since high fiber should not be consumed with milk taken for purposes of calcium absorption, the ideal time to eat a fiber-depleted piece of junk food (such as a superrich cookie) would be with your milk. We don't expect that anybody follows the perfect diet, one totally lacking in all fiber-depleted food. But a prudent course of action would be to consume these fiber-depleted very rich foods with the milk as a snack.

TABLE 15 Calcium Values of Some Foods

FOOD	PORTION	CALORIES	CALCIUM (MG.)
Breads and cereals			
Cream of Wheat, Instant	1 cup, cooked	130	185
Pabulum cereal			
Barley or rice	¾ cup, cooked	108	188
Oatmeal or mixed	¾ cup, cooked	110	188
Thomas Protein Bread	1 slice	45	78
Dairy products			
Cheese			
American	1 ounce	107	195
Cheddar	1 ounce	112	211
Cottage, creamed	1 cup	239	211
Edam	1 ounce	87	225
Swiss	1 ounce	104	259
Ice Cream (Chocolate)	⅙ quart	174	131
Ice Milk (Vanilla)	⅙ quart	136	189
Milk			
Buttermilk, from skim	1 cup	88	296
Skim	1 cup	89	303
Whole, fat 3.5%	1 cup	159	288
Vanilla pudding	½ cup	139	146
Yogurt from skim with nonfat milk solids	1 cup	127	452
Goat milk	1 cup	163	315
Eggs			
Scrambled, milk and fat	1 medium	112	52
Fish and shellfish			
Flounder	3 ounces	61	55
Mackerel, canned	3½ ounces	192	194
Oysters, raw	5–8 medium	66	94
Sardines, canned	8 medium	311	354
Scallops, cooked	3½ ounces	112	115
Shrimp, raw	3½ ounces	91	63
Fruits and seeds			
Figs, dried	5 medium	274	126
Orange	1 medium	73	62
Sunflower seeds	3½ ounces	560	120

FOOD	PORTION	CALORIES	CALCIUM (MG.)
Syrups and sweets			
Blackstrap molasses	1 tablespoon	43	116
Maple sugar	4 pieces ($2 \times 1 \times 1/2$ inches)	348	180
Chocolate candy	1 bar (2 ounces)	296	52
Vegetables			
Artichoke	edible portion (base and soft end of leaves)	44	51
Beans			
Lima, green, cooked	6 tablespoons	111	47
Snap, green, cooked	1 cup	31	62
Wax, yellow, cooked	1 cup	22	50
Beet greens, cooked	1/2 cup	18	99
Broccoli			
Raw	1 stalk (5 inches long)	32	103
Cooked	2/3 cup	26	88
Cabbage, savoy, raw	2 cups shredded	24	67
Chard, cooked	3/5 cup	18	73
Chicory	30–40 inner leaves	20	86
Collards, cooked	1/2 cup	29	152
Endive	20 long leaves	20	81
Escarole	4 large leaves	20	81
Fennel, raw	31/2 ounces	28	100
Leeks	3–4 (5 inches long)	52	52
Lettuce, romaine	31/2 ounces	18	68
Mustard greens, cooked	1/2 cup	23	138
Parsley, raw	31/2 ounces	44	203
Parsnips, raw	1/2 large	76	50
Rutabagas, cooked	1/2 cup	35	59
Spinach			
Raw	31/2 ounces	26	93
Cooked	1/2 cup	21	83
Sweetpotatoes, baked	1 large	254	72
Watercress, raw	31/2 ounces	19	151

Source: A. Bowes and C. Church, *Food Values of Portions Commonly Used* (Philadelphia: Lippincott, 1970, 1980).

IRON FOR ENERGY

Iron serves our body in critical ways. One of its functions is to form the core of the hemoglobin molecule in our red blood cells. Hemoglobin (from *hemo,* for "blood," and *globin,* for "globule") is the critical oxygen-bearing pigment of our red blood cells. In the normal process of blood circulation, hemoglobin delivers oxygen to the body cells and carries away their carbon dioxide. The oxygen that the hemoglobin delivers provides the basic capacity for all the body cells. Oxygen itself is *not* a fuel. It supports combustion of other substances. When we are iron-deficient, there isn't enough oxygen circulating throughout our body to support the metabolism of our cells; thus, we feel fatigued, a condition called anemia. Without sufficient oxygen, our cells cannot receive the energy that they need. So be sure to provide iron in your nutritional planning.

Major sources of iron include

- liver
- prune juice
- red meat (rare is best)
- dried beans (providing that vitamin C is ingested with them to enable the iron to be extracted)[23]

Most multivitamins contain adequate daily iron. But remember that whenever you bleed (menstruate), you need substantially more iron to maintain the same energy level because you are losing iron.

ABOUT VITAMINS

By the early 1990s, much significant information had become available showing the importance of vitamins in maintaining a healthy, vibrant existence.

WHAT ARE VITAMINS?

The word *vitamin* has an interesting history. It was first used in 1912 by C. Funk, a Polish biochemist, who conflated the words *vita* ("life") and *amine* (he mistakenly believed that these vital substances contained amino acids, the building blocks of protein). Today, according to *Webster's New World Dictionary, vitamin* means "any of a number of unrelated, complex organic substances found variously in most foods or sometimes synthesized in the body, and essential in small amounts, for the regulation of the metabolism and normal growth and function of the body." In other words, our body needs these essential substances to do its work. And while some of these substances are manufactured by the body, others can only be obtained through diet or in pill form.

Since nutritionists and chemists who do vitamin research are constantly discovering new things about vitamins, we are still learning about vitamins and the role that they play in maintaining a healthy body. But one thing we do know: vitamins are vital to life—we need them.

WHY TAKE VITAMIN SUPPLEMENTS?

The question of whether taking vitamins is advisable has plagued us for many years. In the United States, one-third of the adult population takes vitamin and mineral supplements regularly, and on average the amount they take is three times higher than the RDA (recommended daily allowances).[8, 70a] Should you do this? Is it beneficial? Is it risky? And why even bother? There are some good answers, but the research is incomplete.

As we age, our needs for vitamins and nutrients change. And even when we carefully design our diet, the amount of energy and effort it would take to make sure that we are ingesting a balanced regimen of vitamins and minerals may be beyond what people want to do with their time. Certain responsible vitamin manufacturers have already done the research and have put together sensible multivitamin tablets—One-A-Day, Centrum, and Within. These vitamin pills attempt to provide a balanced regimen without megadosing. We think that a daily vitamin supplement makes sense, provided it is from a trusted and honest pharmaceutical house or vitamin company. Since, as we age, our caloric needs may decline while our vitamin and mineral needs increase, a daily multivitamin will go a long way in providing the insurance that we are properly nourished.

If you decide to take vitamins, consider these three critical questions:

1. How much of a particular vitamin is beneficial to health?
2. Is there any danger in taking too much of a particular vitamin?
3. Is there any danger in taking too little of a particular vitamin?

Although the RDAs that were originally set were based on the discovery that lower levels of these amounts produced serious deficiency diseases, more recent research has shown that optimal levels of vitamins are linked to healthy functioning and to energetic living. In other words, more than avoiding disease, optimal concentrations of vitamins can promote good health. However, overdoses of the fat-soluble vitamins (for example, A, D, and E) can be dangerous. Water-soluble vitamins (the B vitamins and C, for instance) have consistently shown a lack of such danger. Why? Apparently, this has to do with the body's ability to store fat-soluble vitamins in the fat cells of the body and the body's inability to store water-soluble vitamins, which pass out in the urine when we take in more than our body can use. Since vitamins A and E are fat-soluble, it makes sense to be particularly careful. Are they needed? And, if they are, what amount is appropriate? Because of the complexity and the limitations of current knowledge, what follows is a brief review of the relevant recent research on vitamins.

FRUIT IN BALANCING VITAMINS AND MINERALS

In 1989, investigators published a study in which they concluded that the ability of the body to retain a positive balance of particular minerals and vitamins (versus spilling them out into the urine and feces) could be analyzed in accordance with the balance of other elements in the diet. The investigators, evaluating men only (although the results could hold true for women), studied calcium, magnesium, iron, manganese, zinc, and copper, and found that people who ate a balanced diet in which at least 20 percent of their calories came from either fructose carbohydrates (fruit sugars) or cornstarch carbohydrates (the grains) showed a great difference in their mineral and vitamin balance. The fructose-rich diet led to a positive balance in all of the elements they studied; the grain-rich diet led to a negative balance in all of these same elements except one.[41]

One other benefit of fruit has been demonstrated. Boron, a mineral that may be found in abundance in apples and other noncitrus fruits, appears to help menopausal women. Although we only have data from one study, the results are worth noting. Twelve post-menopausal women not taking HRT were fed diets either rich in boron or poor in boron. Their estrogen levels were twice as high on the boron-rich diet (that is, at levels equivalent to low levels of HRT), and their urinary loss of calcium was lower.[62] Both of these effects would well serve metabolic bone health as well as general well-being.

What does this mean to us? Probably that an apple a day is sensible, although we will need more studies to be sure that this result is universal. For now, there is some evidence in favor of having fruit every day—and for more than simply achieving the positive mineral balance of the above study. People can eat, without gaining weight, about 10 percent more calories when, as its carbohydrate source, their diet contains the fructose element rather than the cornstarch element. What this means is that you can probably eat more and stay thinner if you include fruit as a regular part of your diet.

VITAMIN A

Vitamin A is fat-soluble; the liver stores the excess.[3] Although vitamin A is essential for the proper development of our bones, for the maturation of a baby in the womb, for the maintenance of healthy skin and vision in both children and adults, we generally do not need to take it as we age. The reason for this has to do with the storage component. Our liver can store it for up to 2 years before depleting what is already there.[3] If you are deficient in vitamin A, you will suffer from night blindness. The RDA, set at 5,000 IU per day, is now considered to be too high by some investigators working in the field of vitamin A research.[47] These investigators found, in their study of close to 600 healthy people between the ages of sixty and ninety-eight, that biochemical evidence of liver damage kept showing up in the people who had been taking supplemental megadoses of this vitamin, and the longer they took these supplements, the greater the incidence and degree of liver damage. For this reason, it is believed that vitamin A should not be taken unless you have reason to believe that you are deficient—and, then, only under medical supervision.

THE B VITAMINS

The B vitamins are water-soluble, and, unless extremely large megadoses (6,000 or more mg. per day) are taken, they are not likely to be dangerous. Be warned, however, that excessively high levels (6,000 mg. per day) have been shown to produce nerve damage. Dr. Linus Pauling has thoroughly reviewed the scientific literature on the B vitamins and presents a good case against maintaining the present RDA levels of these vitamins, which he feels, have been set unreasonably low.

There are five B vitamins currently understood, and all of them are essential to various body functions, including emotional wellness. Table 16 lists each one by number and name, the RDA, and Pauling's recommendations. For the logic of Pauling's reasoning, complete with scientific references, you might find his book useful.[67]

VITAMIN C

Vitamin C is probably the most widely publicized and researched of the vitamins. Studies have suggested that megadoses of vitamin C are highly beneficial to human health.[50] There is ample proof that vitamin C has positive effects on the following:

- healing of wounds[70]
- cardiovascular health and reduction of the risk of atherosclerosis[24a, 42, 67, 80]
- strengthening of the bones[24]
- overcoming the toxic effects of benzene, phenol, alcohol, ozone, and textile dust[12, 49, 59, 85, 101]
- prevention of certain cancers[9, 72, 73, 93, 96, 52, 89, 99]

TABLE 16   Vitamin B Dosages

	VITAMIN	RDA (MG.)	DR. PAULING'S RECOMMENDATIONS (MG.)
B_1	(thiamine)	1.5	50–100
B_2	(riboflavin)	1.7	50–100
B_3	(niacinamide)	18.0	300–600
B_6	(pyridoxine)	2.2	50–100
B_{12}	(cobalamin)	0.003	0.1–0.2

Source: see reference 67.

- prevention of cataracts (for review, see reference 67, page 208)
- central-nervous-system disease functioning[25, 46, 50]
- absorption of iron[31]

Cancers that have been studied and that have been inhibited by, been prevented by, or have beneficially reacted to vitamin C include the following:

- leukemia[9, 58]
- advanced breast cancer[9]
- cervical dysplasia[72, 73, 96, 99]
- intestinal cancer[89]
- lung (precursors to) cancer[12, 49, 59]
- immune system (opponents to) cancer[93]

In 1987, the New York Academy of Sciences held its second convention (twenty years after its first) on the subject of vitamin C. Researchers from all over the world contributed the results of their studies of the effects of different doses of vitamin C on wound healing, cardiovascular health, overcoming toxins, and so forth. The conclusion of the researchers was overwhelmingly in favor of the value of megadoses of vitamin C. The scientists also showed that in the dose range of 500 mg. per day to 10,000 mg. per day, *no untoward side effects* had been discovered.

Pauling, a long-time advocate of megadoses of vitamin C and a two-time Nobel Prize winner, has provided critical clues in helping individuals to decide how much vitamin C to take. In general, his principles work as follows. When you take too much vitamin C, the signal that your body sends is a mild diarrhea. Vitamin C in doses of 500 mg. or 1,000 mg. can be taken every 4 hours for most people (that is, between 3,000 mg. per day and 6,000 mg. per day)—and up to 10,000 mg. per day, if an individual is under stress—without any diarrhea ensuing. If you take the megadoses of vitamin C and have no accompanying diarrhea, you will know that the body needs the vitamin and is consuming it. If, however, you take the megadoses and have mild diarrhea, you will know that your body cannot absorb that much that fast, and that lowering the dose will rapidly relieve the problem.

When does your body "burn up" vitamin C? When you are under

stress, when you have a wound, when your cholesterol level is high, when you are exposed to toxins such as ozone or smoke or those in red wine. At these times, your body needs more vitamin C to handle the stress. For example, if you drink red wine at a meal in which red meat is served, the tannin in the wine will inhibit the iron absorption from the meat—unless you have taken a reasonable amount of vitamin C during the course of that meal. The less wine you drink, the less vitamin C you need for the iron to be absorbed from the meat. This seems to work like the combination of high-fiber cookie and milk that was described earlier: the fiber attaches the calcium molecules and prevents them from being absorbed. Here, the tannin attaches the iron and prevents it from being absorbed. In any event, research has shown that 250 mg. of vitamin C is the most you would need to ingest in a meal with red wine, 25 mg. if only a small amount of wine is consumed. (A tomato salad would provide enough vitamin C, if your wine consumption were moderate—as it should be for your general good health.) Another benefit of taking vitamin C if you drink alcohol is that this vitamin helps to eliminate the toxic effects of the alcohol and to promote mental clarity the next day.

Dietary vitamin C is destroyed when foods are stored after they have been cooked. The foods must be eaten immediately after cooking.

Vitamin C is so important to us, its benefits so profound, that people naturally wonder why our diets are incapable of providing it in sufficient quantity.* For instance, you would have to drink 4 quarts of freshly squeezed orange juice immediately after it comes out of the juicer to get the same amount of vitamin C that a 500 mg. tablet provides. When vitamin C–rich foods sit for a few minutes, the vitamin C evaporates.

Since the vitamin is so fragile and so beneficial, we recommend that you take significantly more than the current RDA of 60 mg. that is usually found in multivitamin pills and that you change the dose according to your changing needs: when you are under stress, take more but divide the doses; when you are calm, take less. Finally, it is important to increase or decrease the doses of vitamin C gradually— not more than 500 mg. a day, gently building and lowering.[65]

---

*Some have suggested that a genetic mutation early in evolution altered our ability or need for the vitamin.

VITAMIN E

Fat-soluble vitamin E, according to research, has no effect on sexual desire, aging processes, and the risk of cancer and mortality. It is ineffective in treating hot flashes and other menopausal signs, according to carefully controlled double-blind studies.[39, 48] But it may increase your level of energy when combined with exercise, thus protecting your cardiovascular system.[39] It may also help to protect against arterial disease.[67, 80] This vitamin is abundantly available in both saturated fats and eggs. So if you are eating either, you probably do not need to take vitamin E supplements. To avoid toxicity, do *not* ingest more than 400 units per day as a supplement.

ALCOHOL AND BREAST CANCER

A number of frightening stories appearing in the media in late 1989 and in 1990 suggest that there is proof that alcohol increases the risk of breast cancer. The facts are actually quite different. And eleven studies, published between 1989 and 1990, have helped to clarify the picture.

The prospective studies* report "no association between alcohol and breast cancer." For example, the Framingham Study enrolled 2,600 women, thirty-one to sixty-four years old, and followed them for up to 32 years. In this group, 143 (.5 percent) developed breast cancer, and no association between alcohol and breast cancer could be shown.[76]

Other (case/control) studies in which breast-cancer patients were compared to controls use smaller groups and are, therefore, much more limited in what they are capable of proving. Some recently published case/controls studies tend not to support an association between moderate wine consumption and breast cancer;[74, 14, 57] but two other case/control studies have shown that when the alcohol intake was higher than 40 grams per day—the equivalent of about half a bottle of wine—a slightly increased risk of breast cancer did emerge in northern Italy[91] and the Netherlands.[94]

The possibility that moderate alcohol use may be protective has

*Those carefully designed studies that begin with healthy individuals, then follow their health and behavior patterns for long periods of time.

also been raised. One study in Japan compared women with breast cancer to those with uterine, ovarian, and no cancer, and showed a slightly increased incidence of daily alcohol use in the breast-cancer patients. But in this study, a lower incidence of alcohol use among patients with both uterine and ovarian cancer suggested that alcohol might lower the risk of these pelvic cancers if subsequent prospective studies could confirm the relationship.[43] Since these associations are so weak, we cannot recommend that a woman alter her behavior.

The possibility that there is an increased risk of postmenopausal breast cancer in women who start drinking at a young age—less than twenty-five years old—found some support in two studies.[94, 100]

Perhaps the most powerful analysis of published studies was undertaken by an investigator at the National Cancer Institute who showed that, while there was some correlation between increased alcohol use and increased incidence of breast cancer (mortality and morbidity), when the data were controlled for a woman's level of dietary-fat consumption, what had been a positive alcohol–breast-cancer relationship then dissolved.[76]

We conclude from our analysis of the abstracts of these studies that there are no data sufficiently profound to suggest that moderate use of alcohol will increase the risk of breast cancer.

CONCLUSION

Putting together a healthful nutritional plan takes hard work and intelligent study. To do this, you must measure what you eat (with spoons, with cups, and on a food scale) not only to define your quantity, but to know that you are getting the right amount. You may need to buy a calorie chart that includes the vitamins and minerals of standard portions of food. One such manual that we use can be found as reference.[6]

Move slowly in planning a new nutritional program. Avoid megadoses of vitamins unless you have scientific support (as with vitamin C) of their safety. We suggest you begin by learning what your current habits are. If you record everything that you eat, including the quantity, for a week or two, you may be surprised. Once you have that information, you can analyze how many calories you are consuming and the kind of nutrients you are taking in. Then you can calculate where you are deficient and where you are getting too much. Armed with the information on your own habits and the information in this chapter, you will be equipped to make plans for your own health. The rewards of such an effort will be translated into longevity, the quality of life, and your feeling of well-being.

12

OVERCOMING SMOKING AND OBESITY

If you smoke or if you think you are too heavy, you are suffering from a problem that deserves attention. Many women suffer from one or both. Fortunately, there is good news for those who want to change their habits. Both overweight and smoking are hazardous to your health. Both have in common a behavior that leads a person to ingest substances that are detrimental to her well-being and then to feel uncomfortable about herself.

Probably the majority of women consider themselves overweight. Some of them may truly be obese, having disregarded the signals of progressive weight gain. Obesity is dangerous. And the fatter a woman is, the more dangerous it is. When should you seek medical attention? If you are unable to control your weight; if you are nauseous; if you vomit; if you have a compulsive, ravenous appetite. Behavior-modification treatment is often helpful. As bad as obesity is, smoking is even more dangerous to the health, promoting and triggering diseases in just about every body system that has ever been investigated. If you want to overcome these health hazards, you can. But it will not be easy.

The power of habits is immense. Changing behavior is painful—usually, one cannot avoid experiencing distress. Both physiological and emotional discomfort occur when one tries to break a bad habit. But once the habit is broken, rewards follow: a healthier, more vigorous life.

How to Stop Smoking

Consider the following statistics brought to light by recent research studies on the effects of smoking:

- In one study of women with osteoporosis, 94 percent of those who had had a spinal fracture before the age of sixty-five "happened to be" cigarette smokers.[3]
- In another study, smokers were shown to have less bone mass than nonsmokers of the same age.[12]
- The results of yet another study indicated that the risk of hip fracture is greater in smokers who are thin than in nonsmokers who are thin.[23]
- For nonsmokers who do not take hormones, there is a 12 percent loss in bone mass to osteoporosis 15 years after menopause; but for smokers who do not take hormones, almost twice as much—23 percent—of their bone mass is lost 15 years after menopause.[10]
- Cancer victims who do not smoke have a much better prognosis for nonrecurrence of the disease after surgery.[4]
- Heart, lung, and peripheral vascular diseases are all accelerated drastically by smoking.
- Smokers age faster, entering menopause earlier.[18a]

If you smoke, you do not need these grim statistics as a reminder of why you should quit. Probably what you do need is the impetus to do it, coupled with the information that might help make it less painful to accomplish.

Once you have become addicted to cigarettes and you attempt to stop smoking, you will suffer. And there is no way around this suffering during the early stages of your withdrawal from the addiction. One way to help yourself get through the discomfort is to prepare yourself in advance. You should know that the pain of nicotine withdrawal is relatively tiny compared to the pain of cancer, the pain of broken bones, the pain of seeing yourself rapidly and prematurely age every time you look in the mirror, and the pain of the shortness of energy and breath as you move through the day.

Although there are many approaches, ours, which works, indicates that smoking should not be stopped gently. An addiction that strong is best overcome by a total and sudden withdrawal from it. The nature of the withdrawal is to produce intense cravings for the cigarettes that have been given up. Before you stop smoking, you should prepare yourself spiritually, psychologically, and intellectually for the enormous effort you are about to undertake. You should know that the cravings for the cigarette can be fought. You can win the fight by doing several things when the cravings occur.

- Drink plenty of liquids, particularly high-acid liquids such as orange juice or diluted soda water with orange or other citrus flavors in it. Taking vitamin C will probably help.[15]
- Do breathing exercises that mimic smoking, but in which you inhale air rather than the carbon-monoxide weed: every time you crave a cigarette, pretend that you are smoking—by deeply inhaling the air, holding the air for several seconds in your lungs, and then deeply exhaling it. If, whenever you crave a cigarette, you "pretend to smoke an entire cigarette of air," you will be fighting back. You will be telling your body and brain that you are now giving them oxygen, not carbon monoxide. Your body will get the message. The brain will respond. One of the immediate responses will be an increased burst of physical and mental energy.
- Expect to be irritable and energetic. What is important here is that you take that burst of energy and spend it. What an ideal time to do all the really hard cleaning that you have been putting off, or outdoor work, or any other job requiring intense physical effort.

The first week will be your worst; and the power of prayer, if it is part of your life, should be used freely and fully as you fight the nemesis of tobacco addiction. If prayer is not a part of your life, try affirmations. Write out, before you even start this enormous task of giving up smoking, a series of positive statements about what giving up smoking means to you, comments like "I am choosing to provide my body with healthful oxygen. No more poison. No more carbon monoxide!" or "I am choosing life and health and vigor. I can do it!"

Whatever giving up smoking means to you, write it out before you start the withdrawal. Place these aphorisms throughout your home: on the refrigerator, in the bathroom in front of the mirror, in your car, and anywhere else you are accustomed to smoking. They will help.

Some people join smoking-cessation groups, but research has

shown that the failure rate in these is much higher than among people who stop smoking on their own.[20] We don't know why but surmise that it has something to do with dependency on the group rather than the independent decision to overcome the habit.

In 1988, when the then surgeon general of the United States, Dr. C. Everett Koop, made his announcement about cigarette smoking, his comments were shocking as well as true. He said that cigarette smoking (and other tobacco use) produced an addiction that was as powerful as that of heroin. He said that for an individual to give up smoking, he or she could expect to go through as severe and unpleasant a withdrawal as heroin-addicted people do when they give up heroin. We believe that he is right. The data that he cited to marshal arguments in his favor were voluminous. But that doesn't matter for you if you are a smoker. What you need is to understand the power of the addiction and that once you have gotten used to smoking, smoking controls you. What you need to know is that every time you inhale cigarette smoke, you are drawing carbon monoxide into your lungs. That gas is permeating the walls of your lungs and entering into your blood stream. Once carbon monoxide gets into the blood stream, it makes its way to the red blood cells—those carriers of oxygen and carbon dioxide discussed earlier (see pages 238–239). The carbon monoxide binds tightly, attaching itself to the red blood cells and preventing them from transporting the life-giving oxygen to the body and from taking away the carbon-dioxide wastes. Thus, a smoker is interfering with the ability of her red blood cells to nourish and cleanse all the cells of her body. And this seems to be one of the major dangers of smoking. Although smoking as a cause of lung cancer is well known, what is much less appreciated is the pervasive poisoning of the entire body that smoking produces. This is why smoking has been so heavily linked to almost every disease of every body system that has been studied. People who do not smoke tend *not* to get osteoporosis bad enough to break their spine and hip. They tend *not* to get breast cancer. They tend *not* to have atherosclerosis. Since, unlike our behavior, our genetic endowment is something that we cannot control, this information may help empower you to take action now.

Women who give up smoking show an average weight gain of 5 to 7 pounds. Why? We do not know for certain, but we can suggest the following. Androgen levels are higher in smokers, a hormonal change that appears to increase the metabolic rate.[18a] If you convert the early bursts of extra energy that breaking the smoking habit produces, you can increase your activity and rapidly overcome this gain in weight.

What about nicotine gum (available by prescription) or biofeedback? We find, both from experience and the literature, that these methods have a lower success rate than the self-contained plan that we have already described.

The sooner you take action, the sooner you allow the organs and cell structures of your body to begin to heal. Hopefully, if you give up smoking now, the oxygen that the red blood cells bring to the stricken tissue will allow that tissue to begin to regenerate itself. Hopefully, you will increase your health, your vigor, and your life span. Giving up smoking is tough. Continuing to smoke is tougher because of what it will do to you.

How to Lose Weight

There is diversity of opinion about the benefits of being very slim, moderately rounded, or somewhere in between. Fat cells serve as miniature factories, converting the androgen hormones produced in both the adrenal glands and the maturing ovaries into estrogens. Thus, as women age, those who maintain some padding will have more natural estrogen circulating throughout their body compared to those who are more slender. However, too much fat, is extremely dangerous to your health. The question, then, is: Exactly how much is too much? The National Cholesterol Education Program quotes a relative weight of 130 percent of ideal weight as being obese.

We know that obesity—particularly gross obesity—is associated with all kinds of dangers, including

- increased risk of cholesterol gallstones[21, 18]
- increased risk of endometrial cancer[7, 14, 24]
- increased risk of breast cancer
- increased risk of diabetes
- increased risk of heart attack

DRASTICALLY

If you undergo a modified high-protein fast, reducing your daily calories to 300 and supplementing the protein with multivitamins, you could lose an enormous amount of weight rapidly.[6] However, the problem with this kind of approach is that not only is it physiologically dangerous to the cardiovascular system, but often the body responds to this abrupt and shocking denial of food by lowering its metabolic rate. If the rate is lowered, then the body conserves its weight even while calories are restricted. Be forewarned: dieting lowers the resting metabolic rate most drastically when the calories are reduced most drastically.[6, 22] In the research that had the most drastic caloric restrictions, the metabolic rate of the women studied remained depressed 8 weeks after the dieting had stopped and massive weight loss (25 percent of the body's weight) had been achieved. The problem with this kind of dieting is that these formerly obese women who had lost a great deal of weight were at risk for gaining it back if their metabolic rate stayed low.

Metabolic rate measures how much energy your body is burning per minute or per hour. The higher the metabolic rate, the more food you can eat without gaining weight; the lower your metabolic rate, the more weight you will gain on even a low-calorie diet. If your goal is to lose weight, you should embark on a sensible weight-loss program that does not lower your metabolic rate. Apparently, the reduction of metabolic rate is the body's attempt to maintain itself in the face of a loss of nourishment. We know that thin people who are force-fed very high quantities of food tend to gain only a little bit of weight; shortly thereafter, they can handle all of those extra calories without any further weight gain.

Another problem with rapid weight loss is the frequent occurrence of a "rebound" effect—that is, a regaining of the lost weight plus extra, leaving the person fatter than when she started to diet.[2] In 1989, several research studies were published explaining some of the elements that caused these effects. And with those studies come discoveries that you can use effectively to lose weight and keep it off.

Research now reveals that the kind of diet that you follow will have profound effects on your hormonal environment as well as your metabolic processes. For instance, in young women, vegetarian diets tend to abolish several different elements of their fertility.[16, 17, 19] The most vulnerable part of their fertility cycle appears to be the luteal phase—those two weeks in between ovulation and the next menstruation[19]—and this closely matches the experience of perimenopausal women, whose luteal phase is the one most vulnerable to destruction.

SENSIBLY

Although diet studies have mostly been conducted using younger women, there is much to suggest that most of the principles of effective weight loss hold true for all ages. For example, in 1989, investigators published studies that evaluated two different diets: those diets in which individuals consumed about 840 calories a day and those in which individuals consumed 1,450 calories a day. These studies showed that any form of diet that produces less energy going out than coming in produces weight loss.[22, 8]

If you go on a diet, make it a point to become physically active. Most people who are reasonably active will burn anywhere from 1,800 to 2,500 calories a day. Calories are one measure of energy. Calorie restriction is one of the elements that causes the body to give up its fat. When the total caloric intake is less than the total calories burned, weight loss follows. But some diets are healthier than others. And some diets are more dangerous than others.

Low-fat diets coupled to high complex-carbohydrate intake appear to be the best way to promote weight loss because the body may burn more calories than it consumes as it digests the carbohydrates (particularly if the carbohydrates are high-fiber food).

Dieting hurts. There is pain, both physical and psychological, in giving up some of our body, and dieting is a process in which we are attempting to "melt down" a part of ourselves—particularly the fat part. Pain is a signal of danger, and the mind experiences losing weight as dangerous because losing a part of the self may endanger the entirety. The "pain signals" that our nervous system is structured to produce appear to have evolved to serve the organism. Your determination to lose weight involves a decision to overcome automatic maintenance structures built into the machinery of your physiology. Changing a habit is stressful. Consequently, you will feel pain when you first start dieting. Fortunately, once a diet is under way, another adjustment occurs: that painful sense of hunger is lost within a short period of time—often in just a few days. The objective of a good diet plan should be to develop a new way of eating that allows you to lose weight gradually in order to minimize the pain of changing the pattern from that of a fat person to that of a thin one. Your objective should be to replace a set of bad eating habits with a set of good eating habits so that, ultimately, you don't consider dieting as a denial of self, but, rather, as a contribution to your own well-being. Once good dietary habits are in place, food becomes a pleasure rather than a distressful part of one's existence.

You might want to join one of the excellent and helpful diet groups. Weight Watchers International is renowned for its ability to help dieters establish new eating habits that are sensible, promote good health, and build self-esteem as weight is lost. Other successful organizations include Jenny Craig and TOPS, an acronym for Take Off Pounds Sensibly. You might want to read your local newspaper ads because these groups advertise in them. The organizations cover every aspect of formulating a new, healthful diet: what kinds of foods to buy; how to prepare them; how to measure them; how to consume them sensibly; how to minimize the pain and maximize the pleasure of adjusting your own eating habits. But be warned: some groups advocate diets that are extreme and unbalanced, and these could be dangerous.

"RULES" FOR EFFECTIVE WEIGHT LOSS

The principles of good and healthful eating habits emerge from a knowledge of nutrition coupled with an understanding of what it takes to lose weight. Sensible weight loss involves the following:

- Plan and follow a regular exercise program (see Chapter 13).
- Eat foods that are high in fiber and low in fat—for example, popcorn, bran, bread and potatoes without butter, and lots of steamed (not sautèed) vegetables. These foods will produce a feeling of satiety—that is, they will fill you up without stuffing your fat cells. And instead of drinking fruit juice, eat the whole fruit because the fiber that comes with the fruit contains no extra calories but adds the bulk that you need in order to feel satisfied.[5]
- Remember that the habits you form train your brain. As you diet, you change your habits; it will take awhile for your brain to go

along with this new pattern. Until you have triggered the change, you may want to use affirmations, much like the ones for cessation of smoking, described earlier. You can jot down notes to yourself and post them on the refrigerator, the mirror, or wherever else you may find yourself thinking about eating nondiet-related foods. Before starting your diet, write out what your purposes and goals are. Affirmations such as "I am going to be trim and slim" or "I am going to be healthy and vigorous as I lose weight and create a better shape for myself" will help.

- Drink lots of water to help flush out toxins and promote a sense of fullness.
- Aim to lose weight slowly and steadily. About a pound a week is plenty, if you are embarking on a lifetime change in eating habits. Fifty-two weeks of such a loss equal 52 pounds, and very few of us need to lose that much. But in the process of losing weight at such a slow, steady pace, you will form habits that will make it easier and easier to lose and keep off that weight.
- Avoid high-fat as well as high-protein reducing diets because they are very dangerous. Although they trigger weight loss, they do it at the expense of your cardiovascular health.[9] Avoid them like the poison they create in your blood stream.
- Buy or borrow from the library the several books you will need to plan your diet, including a calorie-counting book and a nutrient-evaluation book.[1] You will also need measuring implements such as a small kitchen scale, measuring cups, and measuring spoons. Initially, you should measure and record the calories and food values of what you eat *before* you sit down to eat it.
- Join a support group, if you can afford it. You will probably benefit enormously from it. Typically, there is an initial fee of about $25 and a weekly meeting fee of about $8. But find out who is running the program. A psychologist specifically trained in weight-control behavior, a registered dietitian, or a trained leader in Weight Watchers or TOPS should be good for you. If funds are limited, you could do without a support group or you could create your own support group with some friends.

Many good cookbooks are available to help you learn how to prepare food with little added fat. The Weight Watchers International group produces a new cookbook about every year; each book is filled with delicious recipes that are low in calories, high in fiber, and provide for well-balanced meals. Jane Brody's *Good Food Book, Jane Brody's Good Food Gourmet,* Ron and Nancy Goor's *Eater's Choice, Cooking Light* magazine, Sonia and William Connor's *The New American Diet,* and a host of others add to the excitement of planning a healthy diet—they allow for tremendous creativity in working out meals. A good daily menu plan would probably help you to stay with your diet. But the menu should be varied and should include all the food groups (proteins, carbohydrates, and fats); and the dishes should be as low in fat as you can handle, but should not eliminate fat entirely. The reason for severely restricting dietary fat is that you have excess body fat that you are trying to lose. As that fat melts down, it will supply your body with the elements that the dietary fat would have contributed. Fat is the one thing that you can most afford to restrict as you develop your dietary regimen because you already have plenty stored.

13

EXERCISE

The benefits of regular and systematic exercise are nothing less than magical. When a woman exercises on a regular basis, the entire physical and mental aspect of her being changes. People who are physically active are healthier than those who aren't physically active; and in aging populations, people who are healthier tend to exercise about twice as much as those who are chronically ill.[14]

Many physiological systems reap the benefits of exercise. When we regularly exercise, we breathe better, we feel better, and our blood circulates more efficiently—that is, the waste gas, carbon dioxide, traveling in the blood is more rapidly eliminated, and the fuel gas, oxygen, is carried in greater quantity to the cells. When we regularly exercise, we burn more calories, we have greater reserves of energy, we age more slowly, and we have a lower "functional aerobic age," which indicates how biologically young we are. And when we regularly exercise, our breathing improves, as does our lung function.

BREATHING FOR WELL-BEING

Although most of us take for granted the automatic (reflex) processes of breathing, the cultures of the East have long recognized that proper breathing is fundamental to a healthy life. As the first lesson in being well, Eastern teachers instructed (and continue to instruct) their students how to breathe. And their approach is correct.

If you were enrolled in a fitness and health course at the local Y or an adult education center, the first lessons would probably begin with principles of proper breathing. You don't need to go to a class to learn these, although it is helpful to have a teacher's feedback to make certain you are learning the techniques correctly.

Let us begin with posture. To inhale adequately, you must be able to take a deep breath; and to do that, you must sit up straight rather than slouch. Once you are sitting up straight, mouth closed, deliberately and slowly (for 7 seconds) inhale as you silently count to 7. As you inhale, first fill with air the lower portion of your lungs—the area close to the diaphragm, producing the correct "breathing noises" as the air hits the back of your throat (a deep, strong sound similar to wind rustling through a leafy tree). After air has filled the diaphragm, it should begin to fill the upper air passages of the lungs until, at the end of the 7 seconds, the air has reached the top of the throat. Having filled the airway passages with fresh air, hold your breath for a slow count of 3 or 4. Then, begin exhaling by slowly forcing out the top air. Moving downward, let yourself feel the motion of the air as it passes out of the airway until finally the diaphragm region flattens.

If you do this simple breathing exercise 4 or 5 times in a row, you will discover how energized you feel afterward. Correctly done, this exercise will provide a profound exchange of oxygen and carbon dioxide, refreshing the cells of your body by removing the carbon dioxide that may have been building up and replenishing the cells with fresh oxygen. Exhilaration is the usual response to having completed the exercise correctly. This breathing exercise can replace a cup of coffee for a sudden burst of energy and can be repeated as often as you wish throughout the day, especially for relaxation, energy, and the clearing of your mind. Try it. You will probably like it.

The benefits of breathing properly are usually obvious to anyone who completes a breathing exercise such as the one that was just described. However, if you are a nonsmoker, as soon as you engage in any form of "aerobic" (air-burning) exercise, your reflex processes will stimulate changes in the way you breathe that will automatically increase the quantity of oxygen brought into your body as well as increase the quantity of carbon dioxide removed from your body. Thus, you will prevent the pooling of fetid air in the base of your lungs, thereby preventing the growth of bacterial infection.

INTELLIGENT EXERCISE PROGRAMS

People who regularly exercise without overtraining (pushing the body beyond its healthy limits) generally experience good health. By contrast, overtraining has been associated with an increased incidence of minor infection.[11] The reason for this is not well understood but appears to be related to the stress and subsequent suppression of certain immune-fighting globulins in the blood.

One of the repeating themes of any intelligent plan for good health revolves around moderation: extremes of exercise can be dangerous; moderate and intelligent exercise is tremendously beneficial.

Systematic research on human exercise programs and fitness patterns is relatively limited. What we do know has begun to form a cohesive picture, but many blanks in our knowledge remain to be filled in as scientists conduct experiments, measure results, and publish their discoveries. Each sport that has been studied seems to have a different incidence of injury, benefit, likelihood of preventing particular diseases, and general effectiveness. Several examples may show the variations in exercise choice.

Experiments have been conducted to evaluate aerobic dancing. Are all the aerobic dance classes one sees advertised in the yellow pages, in the newspaper, and at the local Y good for you? Is there an inordinately high incidence of injury among users of this form of exercise? The answers to both questions combine a bit of uncertainty with a bit of meaningful data. We do know that when aerobic dance is both high-impact (with both feet leaving the floor and bouncing back) and high-intensity, it provides maximum cardiovascular benefits for young women.[25] But it also seems to be associated with a high rate of injury among both students who take the courses and instructors who give them.[5] In fact, injury rates of 43 percent to 44 percent of all students are common. And injury rates are significantly higher for instructors: 75 percent to 77 percent. This sport is so strenuous that very few peri- or postmenopausal women engage in it. But the studies are valuable to peri- and postmenopausal women because they illustrate how an exercise that may be good for the breathing and cardiovascular functions (which aerobic dance definitely is) can be injurious to the overall well-being of the body. If you are engaging in an exercise program to increase your well-being, fitness, and cardiovascular health, it will be less valuable if you are injured. (The newer low-impact aerobic exercises will probably avoid these risks.)

Exercise requires disciplined, consistent activity. Injury requires you to stop exercising for at least as long as it takes to heal. Therefore, injury interferes with your ability to reap the benefits of regular exercise. It is important to select exercise programs that you will be able to follow routinely, without "downtime" for injury repairs.

Swimming has been studied and appears to be an ideal exercise in terms of cardiovascular and pulmonary (lung) benefits. It is known that the lung function in swimmers, particularly competitive swimmers, is very different from the lung function in all other athletes:[3] more oxygen gets into the blood; more carbon dioxide is removed. However, investigators could not conclude whether the improved lung functions of swimmers was a result of swimming or whether it was simply a matter of people with very good lung functions choosing swimming as their sport.

Walking, dancing, and other exercises that allow you to alter the pace at your own initiative are probably ideal. But the fact is that any regular physical activity in which you engage, providing that it aerobically alters your breathing by causing you to breathe more deeply for a sustained duration, will probably serve you equally well in optimizing and then maintaining a general pattern of excellent health. What should that duration be? We cannot say with certainty. For men, a 20-minute period of sustained exercise 3 to 5 times per week appears optimal; equivalent studies of women are not yet available. Gender differences in muscle mass, blood volume, and bone strength are all documented; and these gender differences may apply to optimal exercise patterns as well.

TRAINING TO BUILD STRENGTH

Another term for *training effects* is *conditioning*. Both refer to the fact that practice increases the ability of the body to work. If you are unable to walk 5 blocks right now, start with 1 block. The more you walk, the more conditioned your body will become and the easier it will be for you to increase the distance as well as the intensity of the effort. One of the remarkable aspects of human biology is that by working the machine, the machine gets stronger; and with increased strength comes better breathing, improved cardiovascular health, and a host of other health benefits.

EXERCISE AND EATING

If you exercise before a meal rather than immediately after a meal, evidence suggests that you will burn more fat.[18] But regardless of when you exercise—providing you do it correctly—you will increase your metabolic rate and alter a variety of metabolic processes.[1, 22]

As women age, their ability to metabolize glucose declines. As a result, women start to be at risk for increased insulin and sometimes even diabetes. One recent study investigated whether a systematic fitness program would improve the metabolism of the sugar consumed by older women. The answer was yes. It appeared as if the early response to a sugar overload—comparable to what happens when one eats a candy bar—in women who were in the fitness program was optimal. Trained women showed lower levels of insulin than those who were untrained.[22] Although this is the first study of its kind and would need to be replicated and expanded before broader conclusions could be drawn, for now we can say that in aging women exercise helps keep insulin levels down after a sugar overload.

EXERCISE AND THE SENSE OF WELL-BEING

People who exercise feel better than people who don't, and people who exercise regularly discover that they are dependent upon the exercise in order to maintain this sense of well-being. If you have friends who exercise regularly or are one of those who has already developed that habit for herself, you are probably familiar with the body's response when regular exercise is missed: a sluggish feeling, a mild depression. Why? Or, better yet, why does regular exercise promote a feeling of well-being?

Although simply having better circulation of the blood, better muscle tone, greater strength, and more vigor is enough to promote well-being, recent investigations have begun to look for blood-borne elements associated with this good feeling. A prime candidate for this feeling of well-being is the beta-endorphin, discussed earlier (see pages 131, 135). In fact, we do not know much about beta-endorphin response to exercise, but some information shows that when a person exercises to a certain point, beta-endorphins in the blood increase. What remains unresolved is the duration and intensity of the exercise required to produce this increased secretion of beta-endorphins. Athletes appear to have a different beta-endorphin response to exercise than nonathletes, and young women who have fertile-type cycles appear to show differences in their beta-endorphin reaction to exercise when compared to young women who are not menstruating.

Some of the results that are beginning to emerge include the following:

- Athletes (highly conditioned and trained individuals) must exercise at close to maximum volume of oxygen consumption in order to produce a beta-endorphin response.[9, 16, 17, 21]
- Some studies of men and women indicate what the different oxygen-consumption levels of each gender must be before beta-endorphins are secreted.
- Several studies maintain that there is no gender difference in oxygen-consumption levels needed to secrete beta-endorphins—men and women react the same way.[13, 17]
- Other studies have shown that while men must work at 80 percent to 100 percent of their maximum oxygen-consumption capacity to produce an increase in the beta-endorphin level in their blood, women will show a comparable increase when they work at significantly less than maximum.[23]
- Young women who have become amenorrheic (nonmenstruating) show less of a beta-endorphin response than those who menstruate.[9]
- No research has yet been done on whether nonmenstruating postmenopausal women show a blunted beta-endorphin response to exercise similar to that of young amenorrheic women, or what role hormone therapies play.
- Research indicates that for people who are not athletes, when they begin an exercise program, they start to show surges in beta-endorphins.[10]
- And some studies show that the more exercise training an individual gets, the larger the beta-endorphin reward when exercising.[2]

Exercise, therefore, affects the blood level of the beta-endorphins; we look forward to research that will tell us how.

Exercise also affects the sex hormones of athletes who have been studied. Extreme exercise—the kind that produces Olympic-caliber young women—has been shown to lower the circulating levels of estrogen and progesterone in these young women,[19] and the women have been clearly shown to be at increased risk of becoming amenor-rheic.[6] Again, we find that moderation seems to promote optimal health.

THE MEANING OF MUSCLE SORENESS

ACUTE MUSCLE SORENESS

If, while you are taking your long walk or riding your bicycle, your muscles begin to ache, this probably indicates that they have begun to build up lactic acid—a metabolic waste—and that they are almost exhausted. The buildup is not dangerous, nor is the soreness damaging.[15] The soreness indicates that you have reached the limit of the amount of exercise you should be doing and that you should stop. But you should stop slowly. If you are running, for example, stop running and begin walking. This will help circulate the blood throughout the sore area, hastening the removal of the lactic acid that has built up. You will feel better faster if you do this.

DELAYED MUSCLE SORENESS

The other kind of muscle soreness, that which occurs 8 to 24 hours after you have finished exercising, is different. This soreness usually reflects injury, generally some local damage to the tendons near the muscle that was overworked.[4] If you are suffering from this delayed muscle soreness, the best thing to do is to rest that area until it heals. If you exercise the area that is experiencing delayed muscle soreness, you can increase the injury, further damaging the tendons or muscles and further delaying your return to vigorous exercise.

WARMING UP TO PREVENT INJURY

One way to lessen the likelihood of delayed muscle soreness and to increase the amount of exercise that you can do without injury is to warm up before beginning your exercises. You can do this in several ways, but all of them have in common increasing the temperature of the region of the body that is going to be engaged in exercise. Warming up will probably prevent tearing of the muscle fibers.[15]

You can warm up by being in a warm environment, such as a sauna or a steam room, before going off to run or swim. You can wear extra clothing such as leg warmers before you begin to exercise. Or you can warm up by bringing blood circulation to the region via gentle stretching of the relevant muscles that will be worked. When you stretch these muscles, don't bob or bounce because this action can tear the tendon. Just stretch slowly and easily, and hold the position for 5 to 10 seconds.

If you live in a warm region or if it is summertime, you will need less of this warming process before beginning your exercise. But if you are exercising in a cold climate, swimming in an ice-cold lake, or otherwise exposed to cold temperatures, then take the precaution of warming up. Although recently some investigators have suggested that warming up is not necessary, others have provided equally strong arguments for engaging in it. Why take the risk?

A PROGRAM FOR GENERAL FITNESS

Although there are plenty of attractive actresses and others who will sell you their method for building a level of fitness to match theirs, you should not be fooled by the appearance of the salesperson. What works for one may not work for another, and there is little research available to define the elements of a safe, effective exercise program. One thing is certain, however. Pain is your signal that you are damaging yourself. Do not exercise if you begin to feel pain. Stop immediately. If you are in a class and your teacher tells you to "go for the burn" or "exercise through the pain," get out of that class because the teacher is incompetent. Our bodies are designed in such a way that if we are hurting ourselves or are being hurt, pain will be the signal. Respect the signal that your body sends you.

TIMING

As you begin an exercise program, build up strength at a pace that suits your nature. Probably the most important thing you can do is to establish a regular time. Make a plan by deciding *in advance* how much time you will reserve for your exercise program.

Setting aside the time to exercise is an extraordinary gift that you are giving to yourself. And, incidentally, this is a gift that you pass on to others: when you give it to yourself, you simultaneously give it to all of the people who care about and depend on you because you will get sick less often, you will feel better, you will be more pleasant and cheerful, and you will work more efficiently.

HOW OFTEN?

If your life is a sedentary one, it would not be unreasonable to set aside at least 11 hours a week for regular physical activity. In fact, individuals who do this are shown to be much healthier than those whose total physical activity is less than this.[15, 14] We suggest that you select two or three kinds of exercise that you like—perhaps walking, tennis, and dance—and plan a weekly schedule that includes some of each at regular intervals. The setting aside of time for exercise should be a priority in your life. Exercise is at least as important as keeping a doctor's appointment, eating your meals, resting, or any thing else you are currently spending your time on. When you realize this, you will find time for it. Exercise should be on the top of the list of anyone who wants to be healthy and to age well.

Your body will tell you how much exercise you can handle at each session if you have taken the opportunity, the space, and the time to engage in it.

EXERCISE AND CLOTHING

What to wear for your exercise and fitness sessions is important. Your clothing should be loosely fitted, comfortable, warm enough so that you do not feel chilled, and layered so that as you get warm you can peel the layers off. The choice of fabrics also matters. If you think of the plastic wraps that we use to seal freshness in foods, you will see why some fibers such as certain polyesters should not be worn when you are exercising. These nonbreathing fibers will prevent your sweat from evaporating. Likewise, the socks and shoes that you wear should protect you, should have thick soles to cushion your feet, and should be large enough so that your bones are not cramped.

SUMMARY

If you remember these principles, you should be able to put together a fitness program uniquely designed for your needs, one that will promote your health and well-being. Here is a checklist:

- Regular exercise is fun. Once you start, you will be doing something that should make you feel good and happy even as you are doing it.
- Regular, *routine* exercise can be boring. To overcome that possibility, take action: add music, or vary your program so that it is not boring.
- Exercise must not be painful if the goal is good health and well-being. Remember that pain is a signal that you are at risk for injury. So stop doing what hurts.
- Exercise needs to be engaged in on a regular basis. Set your schedule, and keep to it—make it a routine part of your life.
- A varied set of exercises will probably be easier to maintain than a monotonous program. Plan several different exercises into your routine.
- Although exercise should not be too intense, you will want some intensity. Even low-intensity exercises have been shown to improve oxygen consumption.[7] Do as much as you can, and don't quit even if what you can do appears to be a small amount. Your ability to exercise more per session will, inevitably, increase because of your disciplined efforts.
- Don't take foolish risks that may lead to injury. Remember that injury will force you to stop exercising.
- Choose carefully whose advice to follow. If your trainer tells you to do something that hurts, seek another trainer. Experts are out there.
- Eat properly before you exercise.[24] If you are on a diet while you

are engaging in an exercise program, you must have a high-carbo-hydrate component in order to provide the fuel that you will need to burn during the exercise. Fats will be burned off from your own body fat, but carbohydrates must be supplied from your diet.

- Dress properly during exercise. Wear comfortable shoes and un-constricting, layered clothing that will allow you both not to catch a chill and to remove layers when you begin to feel warm from the exertion.

Exercise is a great joy to those who engage in it on a regular basis. Once you start, the experience is delightful. The hardest part is in getting started while honoring a sensible pace. Exercise can be, for some, a mountain that needs to be climbed in order to attain the joyous experience that people who regularly exercise have. Try it for 2 weeks. You will find out for yourself why so many people make regular exercise a fundamental part of their lives.

14

ALTERNATIVES TO HORMONE REPLACEMENT THERAPY

Personal and professional experience combined with our review of some 3,000 research studies have convinced us that hormonal changes inevitably produce other changes in a woman's life. Beginning in her forties, these hormonal changes are made visible as signs of aging. Hormone replacement therapy (HRT) is just what it says it is—a replacement of the natural hormones that the body normally manufactures in abundance when it is younger. HRT, when appropriately applied, greatly enhances the quality of life for most women. But it is not for everyone. There is a small percentage of women who do not need HRT. They have plenty of estrogen; they do not have hot flashes; their bone and cardiovascular health stays vigorous. For the rest of us, our hormone levels decline so much that an HRT supplement is very beneficial to health.

HRT, as we know, can maintain bone mass, promote cardiovascular health, keep the sexual systems going, and give us a sense of well-being. However, there are alternatives to HRT that we should know about so that they may be used appropriately, if we wish.

If you are suffering from any of the signs of aging characteristic of a reduction in hormones, you should know that HRT has been brought into the same realm as heating for a house or processing for food. Although these products of civilization are imperfect, they have promoted good health and welfare. HRT especially has extended the healthy life span of the women who use it. Even though, in the Third World, the life span is significantly shorter than that in more technologically advanced countries and the high-quality products of civilization are lacking, studies show that certain aspects of Third World countries—high-fiber diets, for example—prevent many diseases. Perhaps the course of greatest wisdom is to try to learn from both worlds.

FOR HOT FLASHES

If you suffer from hot flashes and either cannot or do not want to take estrogens, there are still things that you can do. Progestagen therapy has been shown to help reduce the severity and incidence of hot flashes by about 50 percent.[3, 17, 18, 21] Although progestagen will help reduce the hot flashes, it has some negative side effects when it is given without accompanying estrogen. Why? Because progestagen taken alone reduces the body's natural level of estrogen and tends to produce vaginal thinning and dryness.

If you do take progestagen, you should know that different progestagens have different properties with respect to blood-lipid responses. Cholesterol, HDL-Ch, and LDL-Ch seem relatively unaltered by the ingestion of medroxyprogesterone acetate, when likened to other progestagens taken at comparable doses.[27] Thus, if you take unopposed progestagens, try to limit yourself to medroxyprogesterone acetate.

Other studies have evaluated nonhormonal drug treatments for hot flashes. Clonidine, an antihypertensive drug, has had mixed results. Although one study showed it to be no better than a placebo,[16] two studies showed that it could reduce hot flashes.[5, 28] Another drug used to combat hypertension, propranolol, also was beneficial in reducing hot flashes.[6] Attempts to use LH RH analogs (newly developed drugs—see the glossary) were not successful in reducing hot flashes.[7] Another drug, Bellergal Retard, was also studied and shown to be beneficial:[2] short-term severe hot flashes were reduced substantially—from 90 percent of the women to 5 percent of the women after 12 weeks on the drug. This was in contrast to only 20 percent of women who benefited from a placebo.[2] Unfortunately, the drug produced adverse reactions in about one-third of the women who took it, reactions severe enough to cause them to drop out of the study before the drug had had a chance to be effective.

The autonomic nervous system plays a significant role in the hot flashes that women experience, and the beneficial response of all of these drugs appears to work by means of changes in the autonomic nervous system.[28] Autonomic-nervous-system drugs are being studied in Belgium, where one—a benzamide derivative—has been proven to be effective.[29] This drug alters hormone levels—raising prolactin, lowering LH and FSH—acting somewhat like estrogen.

Remedies are available for you if you suffer from hot flashes but do not want to take any drugs. First, do not get overheated. Hot flashes occur more frequently during the summer than the winter. Second, carry a fan to cool you rapidly, thereby reducing the severity of the hot flashes. Third, meditation, whether through religion or, less formally, taught in classes (widely available at local Y's and schools), calms the autonomic nervous system. Although currently unstudied with respect to hot flashes, meditation may prove helpful in reducing both the severity and the incidence of the flashes.

Also, you should know that a fright produces a "cold" sweat. It is a reflection of changes (both increasing and decreasing) in the flow of blood through the skin. This is similar to a hot flash. The decrease in estrogen produces less efficient control of skin blood flow, leading to hot and cold episodes similar to the "fright" effect. Although the initial cause of the hot flash is felt to be in the central nervous system, the ultimate reaction of the hot flash is this change in skin blood flow.

For Sexual Problems

Certain sexual problems occur early in the perimenopausal period. Others occur as late onset signs of the menopause. Whenever they occur, they are distressing.

In 1990, oral estriol, initially administered at 3 mg. per day, then, in the fourth week, tapering to 2 mg. per day, was proved effective in lessening the effects of poor sexual lubrication. It reduced vaginal pain, fecal-type bacteria, and potential for urinary-tract infections. Blood estrogen levels were not reported in this Swedish study.[17a]

For poor sexual lubrication, unopposed progesterone therapy will increase the problem. If you are unable to take estradiol and are suffering from vaginal dryness, vaginal atrophy, or pain or bleeding at intercourse, ask your physician about vaginal estriol cream. As early as 1978, Dr. Isaac Schiff and colleagues reported on the benefits of estriol (.5 mg.) applied to the vagina.[22] More recently, investigators in Europe have reported on routine use of vaginal estrogen cream for the treatment of postmenopausal vaginal atrophy.[13] Vaginal tissue responds well to estriol cream when the cream is either spread on the skin's surface or is inserted as a vaginal suppository.[1a]

Since none of these creams is available in the United States, if you get a prescription for one of them, it will have to be custom-made by your pharmacist. Once this is done, the cream will probably solve your vaginal problem without altering the estradiol levels in the blood. Dosages will vary, depending on the woman. The several studies in the literature do not yet provide enough data to allow us to recommend a specific dosage. Your physician may want to read the references cited in this paragraph, if consideration of this form of treatment seems appropriate.

Local manual massage (masturbation) of the vaginal area will also help to maintain vaginal tissue and prevent or reverse deterioration of the skin lining. Massage stimulates the epithelial cells, encouraging them to multiply. When they multiply, they form a cushion that protects against injury and bleeding, thus reducing the incidence of painful intercourse. Lubricants will also help. The use of lubricants will overcome vaginal dryness and will allow for coitus without the discomfort of a "dry vagina." Subsequent coital activity with the lubricant will allow for a healthier vagina, which, when maintained, will in turn allow for coitus without the need for prior lubrication. In other words, once you get the system going, it usually continues on its own without the need for any external lubricant. A vaginal moisturizer that is effective is Replens® (Columbia Laboratories, Miami), which helps to maintain a healthy vagina by retaining normal acidity.

FOR DEPRESSION AND PMS

During the menopausal transition years, usually from about ages forty-three to forty-nine, the premenstrual week is commonly difficult. Hormonal changes during this time probably account for a substantial part of the problem. In the Stanford Menopause Study, women would frequently complain that their premenstrual discomfort was getting worse as they were getting older. The forms of discomfort most often mentioned were irritability, depression, and other emotional plummets. Since, for women entering their forties, the monthly estrogen peaks at ovulation are rising and the troughs premenstrually are moving lower, this increasing premenstrual emotional distress closely parallels the changing hormonal experience. If you suffer from this, you should know that there are remedies other than hormone therapy.

Exercise is an important part of any health program. Chapter 13 describes how to set up a sensible exercise program. Likewise, good nutritional habits can help reduce the severity of such problems. Chapter 11 discusses nutritional planning, and Chapter 12 contains information on how to lose weight. Combining exercise and good nutrition with adequate rest and interesting work will serve to reduce the depression at this stressful time of life.

Meaningful and productive work forms an important part of a well-rounded existence. It is never too late to get a job, although many women in their menopausal years have expressed fear of the search process. Fortunately, a number of universities, colleges, junior colleges, and public-service programs now offer courses that help women hone their skills so that they can seek productive work. Being connected to the outside world through the contributions you make it (whether for pay or as a volunteer) will go a long way toward preserving your well-being.

FOR PROTECTING BONES

For the 65 percent of women at risk for osteoporosis, hormone therapy offers a major and significant boon when combined with adequate dietary calcium and vitamin D as well as a good exercise program. If your sex-hormone levels are declining—a characteristic of the menopausal years—and you are unable to take HRT, there is help available.

First, be sure to read about your calcium needs (page 261). Without estrogen, you should probably aim for a daily intake of 1,500 mg.

Second, exercise will keep your muscles strong and help prevent the common problem of falling and then breaking fragile bones.

Third, if you do become osteoporotic, calcitonin treatments can be used as a substitute for estrogen/progesterone therapy. Research in this area has begun to explore the beneficial effects of calcitonin on bone health. Osteoporotic women, in one recent study, were shown to have a calcitonin deficiency when they were contrasted to women of the same age who did not have osteoporosis.[26] Long-term use of calcitonin therapy in postmenopausal osteoporosis has been reported to be beneficial.[4, 11]

Calcitonin seems to work in several ways. It helps the kidneys convert vitamin D into its active form, thereby increasing calcium absorption from the diet.[23] It decreases the breakdown of bone without changing the formation rate of bone.[11, 19] This combination of effects should increase bone mass. Calcitonin stops the reduction of bone loss at the spine, decreases the loss of calcium in the urine, and serves as a pain killer for bone pain.[9, 14, 19, 25]

If you take calcitonin, you must still do the same things that an HRT user does: you must exercise, eat right, and have vitamin D in your diet or from sunshine. Although calcitonin is currently available only by injection and only at highly sophisticated medical centers in the United States,[24] its use by other methods of administration is being developed.

Calcitonin is a second-choice hormone regimen. Although it helps maintain healthy bones, it has significant side effects (when administered by injection of the synthetic salmon form), and it does not help reduce the other effects of hormone deficiency that are characteristic of menopausal women.

Last but not least, avoid smoking because it increases the problems associated with osteoporosis for those at risk.

FOR IMPROVING THE QUALITY OF SLEEP

If you cannot take hormone therapy and are not sleeping well, thereby suffering from the exhaustion so common to women who are in the acute stages of hormone deficiency, exercise will help. Take a long walk or engage in some other aerobic form of exercise an hour before bedtime, and the quality of sleep should noticeably improve.

Warm milk at bedtime works for many insomniacs. Perhaps it is the action of the calcium on the nerves that elicits the desired result. We have not seen any double-blind studies, but anecdotal feedback is positive. You might as well try it and perhaps be pleasantly surprised.

FOR PROMOTING CARDIOVASCULAR HEALTH

The single largest cause of disease and death in women after menopause is from cardiovascular accidents. Heart attacks, strokes, and atherosclerosis increase dramatically at the menopause and reach levels in excess of those of age-matched men. Although cardiovascular health will greatly benefit from HRT (see Chapter 10), if you cannot take hormones there are still steps that you can take to help protect your cardiovascular system.

First, you must eat correctly. Follow a diet low in saturated fats and high in fiber. Chapter 11 provides the details.

Then, you must exercise to promote stamina and strength. People who are fit have healthier cardiovascular systems. Chapter 13 will help you plan your fitness program.

HRT AND GALLSTONE SUFFERERS

For individuals at high risk of gallstone attacks, oral HRT should be avoided. Prior to 1989, no studies had been conducted that evaluated whether an alternative approach such as the patch (in the United States) or cream (in Europe) might be effective in reducing hormone-deficiency signs without stimulating cholesterol crystals in the bile duct. In 1989, the first such study appeared as a result of an opportunity to study one seventy-four-year-old woman 22 years after her menopause. Because she had been previously operated on for gallstones and because of other reasons, investigators were able to study whether different forms of estrogen therapy had different prognostic values in promoting or preventing gall-bladder attacks. The results indicated that the nonoral route of hormone administration is successful in preventing the formation of cholesterol crystals in the bile duct.[8] Therefore, if you suffer from gallstones and decide to take HRT, consider taking your hormone via patch or vaginal cream.

FOR MUSCULAR-SYSTEM CHANGES

With advancing years and a decline in sex-hormone production, the muscular system loses strength and size. The average person of advanced age has little muscle mass and is, therefore, at risk for a variety of problems. If you have strong muscles that are regularly exercised, your gracefulness and gait will be improved. This, in turn, will keep you from falling; and, if you do trip, it will help you to fall with more grace. If you do fall, however, then the way you fall can affect your bones. Ideally, you should aim to "break your fall" with the parts of your body least vulnerable to crippling, should those parts break. Rolling, crouching, or sitting down, rather than breaking your fall with your hand or hip, can prevent fractures. Since the hip and the wrist are the bones most vulnerable to fracture in osteoporotic women, these are the body regions you should protect if you feel yourself falling. Regular strength building and fitness conditioning can maintain a strong muscular system. Anyone who wants a healthy old age should begin a fitness program now (see Chapter 13).

FOR GENITOURINARY ATROPHY

Just as the general musculature of the body tends to lose mass with the decline of sex-hormone production, the genitourinary system suffers similar effects of aging. Estrogen replacement therapy (even weak estrogen—estriol—applied locally as a cream) rebuilds this wasting tissue. Locally applied weak estrogens can be given in doses low enough to help the genital tissue without altering the blood levels of the hormone. But not everyone can take even these mild locally applied hormones. If you are one of these women, then regular exercise and proper eating will be even more important to the maintenance of your genitourinary system than to the hormone user. Also, the Kegel exercises described in Chapter 3 will help to maintain the genitourinary system.

GINSENG

Ginseng, an herbal substance (root) that has been cultivated for centuries in the Orient, is said to have medicinal or aphrodisiacal properties.[12] We caution against its use either as a face cream or by other routes because of its tendency to promote abnormal bleeding in women.[10, 20] The literature is meager, but the consistency of three different reports suggests that if you are ingesting ginseng or using it in a face cream, you should be aware that it seems to have some form of hormonelike property. The real danger is that we do not know what its effects are, and to take it without knowing is as dangerous as taking any drug that alters one's function that has not yet been adequately tested for side effects.

CONCLUSIONS

Good health and well-being derive from a combination of attitude, actions, and genetic endowment. Every woman can learn about proper nutrition and integrate it into her life. Every woman can learn about exercise and build up her aerobic fitness. It is never too early to begin; it is also never too late to start. Within a week, you will notice significant improvement once you establish your own plan of action. Smoking, whether cigarettes or other forms of tobacco, is probably the most significant disease-producing agent available in the marketplace. Smoking negatively affects bones,[15] the cancer-prevention systems, cardiovascular health, and general well-being. If you smoke, give yourself the gift of life by withdrawing from this addiction (see Chapter 12).

One final point. Your personal connectedness to other people should be a major consideration in your plan for a healthy life. In order to serve your own health, you must serve others. There are countless ways in which you can be of service to other people. And when you are, you reap rich rewards in increased self-esteem, vigor, and attitude. Somehow, when you help others, you end up truly appreciating the gift of your own life.

APPENDIX 1
The Studies on Hormone Replacement Therapy and Hot Flashes

The studies are consistent with each other in showing the relief that estrogen and opposed estrogen provide to women suffering from hot flashes.[5, 7, 10, 13] A few examples are detailed in this appendix.

One report[2] evaluated 369 patients with menopausal distress who were given "titrated" doses of estrogens (17β estradiol). In other words, if a particular dose did not work, the dose was increased until it did. By using this method, excellent relief of symptoms was reported by 96 percent of the women studied, with 76 percent of the women reporting that their hot flashes had totally disappeared. Total disappearance of sweating was reported by 80 percent of the women, of tingling by 91 percent, and of genital atrophy by 88 percent. Estriol, even in its lowest doses (2 mg. per day), was also usually effective at relieving menopausal flashes.[13] When the lowest doses of estriol failed to provide total relief, higher doses increased the beneficial response.

Double-blind studies that compare placebo to estrogen therapy have also been reported. One study compared the effects of Premarin (1.25 mg. per day taken 3 out of 4 weeks) to placebo (using the same schedule) on women who were experiencing severe menopausal distress.[3] Premarin was significantly more effective than placebo in relieving hot flashes, insomnia, irritability, anxiety, urinary frequency, general well-being deficits, and memory loss. There was no evidence that Premarin helped backache, joint aches, or libido. Interestingly, there was a highly significant placebo effect on problems of vaginal dryness, memory loss, urinary frequency, and skin appearance; but the placebo effect (on vaginal dryness, memory, etc.) was not as pronounced as the effect recorded when hormones were taken. We can conclude that although some distress can be reduced by faith in the treatment, hormones work more reliably.

Double-blind studies that compared placebos, sedatives, and antihypertensive drugs to different brands of estrogen among women with menopausal hot flashes have also been published.[4, 5, 9, 11] They show that hormones are most effective, placebos are least effective, and the other drugs fall somewhere in between. For example, in one study of 30 women given placebos, 29 percent said that things had improved although none reported disappearance of her flashes. Sedatives eliminated the flashes in 28 percent of a different group of 56 women. In contrast, between 68 percent and 92 percent of the women taking different regimens of hormone therapies found total relief from hot flashes. This seemed to be a function of the particular hormone given. Even when total disappearance of symptoms failed to occur on estrogen therapy, every woman given these hormones noticed some improvement. Although conjugated equine estrogen was the most effective agent tested in this study, others were also helpful—estradiol valerate and estriol in several different doses.[9]

Vaginal cream—both Estrace (.2 mg.) and Premarin (1.25 mg.)—as well as sublingual tablets (.5 mg. every other day) have all been tested and shown to relieve hot flashes.[12] Synthetic and natural estrogens eliminate hot flashes.[1, 8, 10] For 22 weeks in one study,[6] estrogen (100 mg.) implants, a form of hormone that is surgically inserted via a tiny incision, also were effective. Implants are less desirable than other forms of administration because surgery is required. But they work as well as other forms of estrogen therapy.

The results are unambiguous. Estrogen therapy relieves hot flashes.

APPENDIX 2

The Studies on Cardiovascular Health and Hormones

A number of investigators have evaluated different aspects of heart disease with respect to hormone use. It is important to understand that while estrogen replacement therapy has been common for many years, progestin opposition to estrogen therapy has not been common. Because progestin has only relatively recently become widely used and studies to evaluate it require several years to complete, there is less information available on the effects of progestin on the cardiovascular health of menopausal women than there is on the effects of estrogen. Moreover, biomedical investigators are only now working to determine the appropriate dose of progestin to prescribe. Therefore, it is critically important in evaluating the association between hormones and heart health to note the doses of particular hormone therapy regimens. For example, even if a high dose of progestin were harmful, a low dose could be helpful.

Viewed from this perspective—that estrogen treatment came first, then a lowering of estrogen doses, then the addition of progestin opposition, followed by a new trend toward lowering the doses and increasing the number of days that progestins are taken each month—the studies discussed below will clarify an issue that has long appeared confusing because specific attention has not always been paid to the details of dosage.

HORMONES AND BLOOD PRESSURE

Blood-pressure changes have been evaluated before, during, and after HRT regimens, and results suggest no bad effects for the vast majority of women.[14] There are exceptions, however, and if you do take hormones, it is important to have your blood-pressure levels checked regularly.

In one double-blind study comparing Premarin (1.25 mg.) to a placebo, no elevation in either systolic or diastolic blood pressure was noted in association with hormone use. In fact, there was a fall in the systolic blood pressure in both conditions.[6]

In another study, 50 women, forty-five to fifty-five years old, were placed on estrogen therapy (estradiol valerate) or placebo 6 months after having had their ovaries removed. Blood pressure was measured before the treatment began, then 3, 6, and 9 months later. For 48 of the 50 patients, there were no significant changes in diastolic blood pressure on any treatment. Two of the 50 patients were exceptions: they showed a marked elevation in diastolic blood pressure.[34] In another study, women taking estrogen or estrogen opposed by progestin were followed before, during, and after HRT, and these women were compared to a third group who took a placebo. Both systolic and diastolic blood-pressure levels were significantly lower during either hormone regimen, with a return to the higher pretreatment level after stopping the hormones. Placebo users did not show significant changes in diastolic pressure, although their systolic pressure did drop a little while taking the placebo.[15] Diastolic pressure appears to be the most critical pressure measure in terms of the risks that hypertension poses for heart disease, and diastolic pressure seems to be unimpaired by hormones.

Another group of researchers studied 570 women, all of whom had high blood pressure. Five of the 570 hypertensive patients had passed their menopause, and each of the 5 were also taking estrogens. Each of these 5 menopausal women was taken off the estrogens, and the blood-pressure level of each returned to normal, taking from 1 to 7 months to normalize.[8]

How do we interpret these apparently conflicting studies? You should realize that only 1 percent of these hypertensive patients were menopausal. Since there were so few women to study (5), it would be foolish to draw any sweeping conclusions about all menopausal women from this investigation—particularly in light of the studies that evaluate large groups of hormone users. The only thing we can say is that if you develop high blood pressure on hormone therapy, stop taking the hormones and have your hypertension evaluated. If it persists or returns on HRT, then HRT is not for you. These exceptions suggest that women who take hormones should routinely have their blood pressures checked just to be on the safe side.

ATHEROSCLEROSIS AND HEART ATTACK

Atherosclerosis (hardening of the arteries, which predisposes a person to heart disease) does not appear to be increased by hormone therapy. One prospective study of 1,900 women could find no association between the use of estrogen and the subsequent development of atherosclerotic heart disease.[16]

Possible relationships between hormone use and myocardial infarction (heart attack) have also been considered. For 11 years, 15,500 women residents in a retirement community were evaluated. Of these women, 220 suffered a heart attack for the first time. Analysis of the records showed that the heart-attack victims were no more likely to have used HRT than the other age-matched women in the retirement community.[23] Another retirement-community study reached similar conclusions.[28]

Myocardial infarction was also studied in detail in the Framingham Study (an ongoing prospective evaluation of a population in Massachusetts). With respect to menopause and coronary heart disease, 2,873 Framingham women were followed for 24 years. No premenopausal woman developed a myocardial infarction or died of coronary heart disease. Such events were more common among postmenopausal women over age forty-five, regardless of whether the menopause began naturally or was the result of a hysterectomy.[10]

The Framingham investigators then looked at those women who took estrogens (but they did not describe the brand or dose) and compared these women to those who did not take estrogens to see if hormone use influenced the rates of death or the rates of heart attacks. Death rates were not affected by estrogen use. Just as the retirement community described earlier showed, about 7 percent of the postmenopausal women died from coronary heart disease, and this occurred whether or not hormones were used. Heart-attack rates also were not affected by the use of estrogens.

A third evaluation of natural-estrogen use in postmenopausal women also showed that estrogens do not increase—and may actually reduce—the likelihood of heart attack. Among 7,000 healthy menopausal women studied, 5 percent were found to be users of HRT; among 336 menopausal patients who had suffered a heart attack, only half as many, 2.5 percent, used these menopausal hormones. Duration of treatment and age of the women were equivalent in both groups.[27] This study suggests that estrogen may provide some protection against heart attack.

There are probably exceptions to the general rule that hormones are not involved in increased risks of heart attacks at the menopause, and regular blood-pressure checkups might help distinguish those women at risk from those who can safely take hormones. The increased risk, for those at risk, is very small. If your blood pressure is higher than normal, you might consider not taking hormone therapy. If your blood pressure is normal when on hormone therapy, you probably will not be at risk of heart disease.[23]

STUDIES OF COAGULATION FACTORS IN BLOOD

The ability of your blood to coagulate properly is essential to your health. Studies have been conducted to test whether the relevant blood factors are impaired by estrogen or progestin use. Most laboratory studies reflect a less dynamic situation than that which exists in the body. Nonetheless, results show no impairment on natural estrogens,[15, 20] and at least one investigator has suggested that natural estrogens are the most sensible estrogens to use.[20]

In one study, 10 women who had been ovariectomized and later treated with estradiol valerate showed no significant changes in any of 17 coagulation factors during a 1-month period of estrogen use.[29] In another report, estriol succinate, in doses titrated to that minimum level necessary for relief of signs of menopausal distress, was shown to have no significant effect on plasma coagulation factors in 10 women who were followed for 12 months.[33] Apparently, natural estrogens do not alter blood coagulation factors. Progestin in combination with estrogen has also been tested and shows no dangerous effects on these blood coagulation factors either.[1]

Synthetic estrogens appear to be different from the natural ones. One investigator claimed that there were "profound risks" for those women who took ethinyl estradiol, a synthetic estrogen, and these risks persisted for 9 months after hormone therapy stopped.[1] Other investigators also commented on these risks.[33] For a fuller discussion of synthetic-hormone risks, see pages 145–146, "Avoiding Synthetic ERT."

STUDIES OF SERUM CHOLESTEROL, LIPID BALANCE, AND SERUM TRIGLYCERIDES

Women who have unusually high levels of low-density lipoproteins in their blood are those who are most likely to have heart disease.[13] High-density lipoproteins, in direct contrast, have been shown to be beneficial to coronary health.[18] High-density lipoprotein is so named because the molecule (protein coupled to a kind of fat droplet called a lipid) has a higher proportion of protein than lipid. Apparently, when the lipid is balanced by relatively high protein concentration (i.e., high density), there is greater protection against clogged arteries. Estrogens have been shown to increase the levels of these beneficial high-density lipoproteins.

Among 4,978 women ranging from twenty-one to sixty-two years, at each age the average level of the high-density lipoprotein was higher in hormone users than in nonusers.[4] Young hormone users are usually taking birth-control pills. Older hormone users are generally taking estrogen replacement. Progestagens, when added to the estrogen, had the reverse effect; but it appears that this adverse progestagen influence on high-density lipoprotein is limited to much higher doses of progestin than were recommended in Chapter 6.[11, 19, 24, 30]

Studies have shown that the fatter you get, the lower your high-density-lipoprotein level will be.[4] So here lies another danger in being fat.

Menopausal women who take natural estrogens may enjoy the advantage of a higher level of these beneficial high-density lipoproteins than nonusers. Several studies of different natural estrogens showed this increase.[31, 35, 36] Synthetic estrogens also produced increases in the level of these beneficial lipoproteins.[36]

Cholesterol levels (another predisposing factor for heart disease) have been shown to decline while menopausal women are on hormone therapy, thereby producing another beneficial effect.[2] And one group of researchers reported positive results after giving estrogen (estradiol valerate) to women to reduce their excessively high cholesterol levels.[31] Progestin opposition seems to facilitate this beneficial decline in cholesterol.[8, 11, 15]

Serum triglycerides (fats traveling in blood that also can cause heart disease) are increased in menopausal women who take synthetic estrogens, but they are not increased when menopausal women take natural estrogens.[15, 19, 36] Progestin effects depend on the dose. In one study using high doses of norgestrel (1.8 mg. per day), progestins were shown to increase certain triglycerides.[31] Lower doses (levels corresponding to recommendations listed in Chapter 6) and other types have not been implicated as causing triglyceride increases.[15, 19, 31]

One estrogen that has been evaluated, (seminatural) estradiol valerate (2 mg. per day), produced no increases in blood cholesterol or triglycerides in one group of 10 ovariectomized women being given hormone replacement.[29] Another study showed that neither estradiol (2 mg. per day) nor estriol (1 mg. per day) produced any significant changes in cholesterol or triglycerides when compared to placebo in one group of 49 postmenopausal women who were taking hormones for relief of menopausal distress.[37] Confirmation has been reported.[9] A third approach compared three natural estrogen brands—Premarin (high and low doses), Harmogen (a brand name for piperazine oestrone sulfate, packaged in Great Britain), and estradiol valerate—and evaluated three different serum (blood) lipids.[17] None of the hormones produced any significant changes in any of the serum lipids measured, and none of the lipids increased when progesterone was added. Another recent report has provided data that support these comforting findings.[7] However, because the higher doses of progestins sometimes caused triglyceride and cholesterol changes,[11, 30] the newer lower doses may be more desirable.

NATURAL VERSUS SYNTHETIC ESTROGENS

In general, heart and blood health seems to be increased or unaffected by natural estrogens, as the studies just described have detailed. However, synthetic estrogens sometimes appear to have some dangerous side effects. In several reports,[3, 19, 25, 26, 36] synthetic estrogens increased triglyceride levels while natural estrogens did not. A report evaluating responses to conjugated equine estrogen (natural) and ethinyl estradiol (synthetic) described significant rises in serum triglyceride levels on both low and high doses of ethinyl estradiol (20 or 50 micrograms per day) but no significant change on either of two natural estrogen doses (.625 or 1.25 mg. per day).[3] Here, 17 ovariectomized women had been treated with each of 4 hormonal doses at different times. There is a growing appreciation of the possible risks of synthetic estrogen on menopausal heart health.[3, 14, 19, 20, 21, 24, 26, 27, 28, 32] Until these questions are fully resolved, we prefer natural estrogens.

ESTROGENS IN YOUNG WOMEN

Young women appear to be physiologically different from mature postmenopausal women. And although in some cases estrogens (as oral contraceptives) have been associated with increased risks of various heart-disease factors, natural estrogens among older women have not been related to these risks. One unresolved area concerns the young woman who is hysterectomized and then wants to know whether estrogen therapy will do for her what it does for other menopausal women or whether it will work on her body as the oral contraceptives do on other young women.

HYSTERECTOMY AND HORMONES

Young women who become menopausal have an increased risk of heart disease. This appears to be true for those who take HRT as well as for those who do not take HRT, although the evidence is inconclusive since there are so few detailed studies. If you are younger than forty-eight and have become menopausal because of a hysterectomy (regardless of whether your ovaries were removed), you should monitor your cardiovascular health. You should also exercise regularly, stay slim, and follow a sensible diet. The large-scale studies of thousands of hysterectomized women on HRT showed no increased risk of heart disease.[5, 22] One small study that looked at women with heart disease who were taking HRT found that in almost all the cases the women were under forty-eight years old and had been hysterectomized.[12] This probably means that hysterectomy at a premenopausal age, not the hormones that were given in compensation, increased the risk of heart disease. But because of this study, we recommend that young hysterectomized women who take HRT schedule regular checkups of their cardiovascular system.

If you are older than forty-eight, the best evidence to date suggests that even if you have been hysterectomized, you are not at any more risk of death from heart disease if you take hormones than if you don't take hormones. Still, you should have your blood pressure and low-density-lipoprotein levels monitored as a precaution. Blood pressure is easy to monitor. The low-density-lipoprotein analysis requires your health-care specialist to draw a bit of blood for analysis in the laboratory. If either of these two measures shows you are above normal, then you will have to balance your decision about future hormone use by comparing the risks and benefits that your situation demands.

APPENDIX 3
The Breast Self-Exam

1. The self-exam should always be performed in good light. Stand or sit in front of a mirror, arms at your sides. Look for dimpling or puckering of the breast skin, retraction (or pushing in) of the nipples, and changes in breast size or shape. Look for the same signs with your hands pressed on your hips and then with your arms raised high.

2. Lie on your back with your left hand under your head. With your right hand, gently feel your left breast, using small, circular motions. Begin at the top of your breast and move around the outside in a large circle (see below). When you return to the top, move your hand closer to the nipple and make a smaller circle. Repeat until you have examined all of the breast tissue, then repeat the procedure for your right breast.

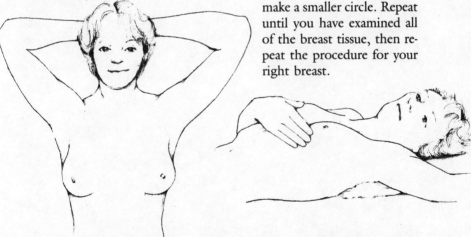

"The Breast Self-Exam" is reprinted courtesy of The American College of Obstetricians and Gynecologists, "Mammography," ACOG Patient Education Pamphlet AP076 (Washington, D.C.: © 1987).

3. Examine the nipple areas in the same way and check for any discharge. Also be sure to examine the areas below the armpits, which also contain breast tissue.

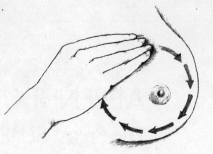

BIBLIOGRAPHY

Reference citations in the biomedical sciences follow a commonly accepted, abbreviated format. Should you wish to locate any citation and are unfamiliar with the notation form used, the reference librarian will be able to direct you. The abbreviations used are listed below.

Acta Diabetol Lat   (Acta Diabetologica Latina)
Acta Endocrinol   (Acta Endocrinologica)
Acta Med Scand [Suppl]   (Acta Medica Scandinavica [Supplement])
Acta Obstet et Gynecol Scand or **Acta Obstet Scand**   (Acta Obstetricia et Gynecologica Scandinavica)
Acta Physiol Scand   (Acta Physiologica Scandinavica)
AIM   (Annals of Internal Medicine)
Am J Clin Nutr   (American Journal of Clinical Nutrition)
Am J Clin Pathol   (American Journal of Clinical Pathology)
Am J Epidemiol   (American Journal of Epidemiology)
Am J Med   (American Journal of Medicine)
Am J Obstet Gynecol   (American Journal of Obstetrics and Gynecology)
Am J Prev Med   (American Journal of Preventive Medicine)
Am J Psychiat   (American Journal of Psychiatry)
Am J Roentgenology   (American Journal of Roentgenology)
Am J Surg   (American Journal of Surgery)
Am Physiol Soc   (American Physiological Society)
Am Soc Clin Nutr   (American Society of Clinical Nutrition)

Ann Chir Gynaecol   (Annales Chirurgiae et Gynaecologiae [Helsinki])
Ann Clin Res   (Annals of Clinical Research)
Ann Int Med   (Annals of Internal Medicine)
Ann NY Academy of Sciences   (Annals of the New York Academy of Sciences)
Ann Surg   (Annals of Surgery)
Ann Intern Med   (Archives of Internal Medicine)
Arch Phys Med Rehabil   (Archives of Physical Medicine and Rehabilitation)
Arch Sex Beh   (Archives of Sexual Behavior)
Aust N Z J Med   (Australian and New Zealand Journal of Medicine)
Aust N Z J Obstet Gynaecol   (Australian and New Zealand Journal of Obstet-
   rics and Gynaecology)
Bone Miner   (Bone and Mineral)
Brit Med J   (British Medical Journal)
Br J Cancer   (British Journal of Cancer)
Br J Derm   (British Journal of Dermatology)
Br J Exp Pathol   (British Journal of Experimental Pathology)
Br J Obstet Gynaecol   (British Journal of Obstetrics and Gynaecology)
Br J Prev Soc Med   (British Journal of Preventative and Social Medicine)
Br J Radiol   (British Journal of Radiology)
Br J Urol   (British Journal of Urology)
Calcif Tiss Int   (Calcified Tissue International)
Calcif Tiss Res   (Calcified Tissue Research [Berlin])
Cancer Res   (Cancer Research)
Clin Biomech   (Clinical Biomechanics)
Clin Chem   (Clinical Chemistry)
Clin Chim Acta   (Acta Chimica Clinica)
Clin Endocrinol or **Clin Endocrinol (Oxf)**   (Clinical Endocrinology [Ox-
   ford])
Clin Endocrinol Metab   (Clinics in Endocrinology and Metabolism)
Clinics in Obstet & Gynaecol   (Clinics in Obstetrics and Gynaecology)
Clin Orthop or **Clin Orthop and Rel Res**   (Clinical Orthopaedics and Related
   Research)
Clin Res   (Clinical Research)
Clin Sci   (Clinical Sciences)
Contem OB/GYN   (Contemporary Obstetrics and Gynecology)
Curr Med Res Opin   (Current Medical Research and Opinion)
Endocrinol   (Endocrinology)
Eur J Clin Invest   (European Journal of Clinical Investigation)
FASEB J   (Journal of the Federation of American Societies of Experimental
   Biology)
Fertil Steril   (Fertility and Sterility)
Front Horm Res   (Frontiers in Hormone Research)

Geront Clin   (Gerontologica Clinica)

Gynec Invest   (Gynecological Investigation)

Gynecol Oncol   (Gynecologic Oncology)

I J Fertil   (International Journal of Fertility)

Int Arch Allergy Appl Immunol   (International Archives of Allergy and Applied Immunology)

Int J Cancer   (International Journal of Cancer)

Int J Epidemiol   (International Journal of Epidemiology)

Int J Health Services   (International Journal of Health Services)

Int J Obstet Gyn   (International Journal of Obstetrics and Gynecology)

Invest and Cell Path   (Investigative and Cell Pathology)

Israel J Med Sci   (Israeli Journal of Medical Sciences)

JAMA   (Journal of the American Medical Association)

J Am Geriatr Soc   (Journal of the American Geriatrics Society)

J Am Pharm Assoc   (Journal of the American Pharmaceutical Association)

J Appl Physiol   (Journal of Applied Physiology)

J Biosoc Sci   (Journal of Biosocial Science)

J Bone Joint Surg (AM)   (Journal of Bone and Joint Surgery [American])

J Chron Dis   (Journal of Chronic Diseases)

J Clin Endocrinol Metab   (Journal of Clinical Endocrinology and Metabolism)

J Clin Invest   (Journal of Clinical Investigation)

J Endoc   (Journal of Endocrinology)

J Endocrinol Invest   (Journal of Endocrinological Investigation)

J Geriatr Psychiatry   (Journal of Geriatric Psychiatry)

J Geron   (Journal of Gerontology)

J Kentucky Med Assn   (Journal of the Kentucky Medical Association)

J Lab Clin Med   (Journal of Laboratory and Clinical Medicine)

J Natl Cancer Inst   (Journal of the National Cancer Institute)

J Nutr   (Journal of Nutrition)

J Ob Gyn of the Br Commonwealth   (Journal of Obstetrics and Gynaecology of the British Commonwealth)

J Physiol (Lond)   (Journal of Physiology [London])

Jpn J Clin Oncol   (Japanese Journal of Clinical Oncology)

J Reprod Med   (Journal of Reproductive Medicine)

J Sex Res   (Journal of Sex Research)

J Soc Cosmetic Chemists   (Journal of the Society of Cosmetic Chemists)

J Steroid Biochem   (Journal of Steroid Biochemistry)

J Toxicol Environ Health   (Journal of Toxicology and Environmental Health)

Life Sci   (Life Sciences)

Mayo Clin Proc   (Proceedings of the Mayo Clinic)

Med J Aust   (Medical Journal of Australia)
Med Sci Sports and Exercise   (Medicine and Science in Sports and Exercise)
Med Times   (Medical Times)
Metab Bone Dis & Rel Res   (Metabolic Bone Disease and Related Research)
Metab Clin Exper   (Clinical Experimental Metabolism)
NEJM   (New England Journal of Medicine)
Neuroendocrinol   (Neuroendocrinology)
Nutr Cancer   (Nutrition and Cancer)
NY State J Med   (New York State Journal of Medicine)
Ob/Gyn News   (Ob. Gyn. News)
Obstet Gynecol   (Obstetrics and Gynecology)
Obstet Gynecol Clin NA   (Clinics in Obstetrics and Gynecology of North America)
Obstet Gynecol Surv   (Obstetrical and Gynecological Survey)
Physiol & Behav   (Physiology and Behavior)
Postgrad Med   (Postgraduate Medicine)
Postgrad Med J   (Postgraduate Medical Journal)
Proc Natl Acad Sci USA   (Proceedings of the National Academy of Science [USA])
Proc Royal Soc of Med   (Proceedings of the Royal Society of Medicine)
Royal Soc of Health J   (Royal Society of Health Journal)
S Afr Med J or S A Med J   (South African Medical Journal)
Scott Med J   (Scottish Medical Journal)
Soc Biol   (Social Biology)
Soc Sci Med   (Social Science and Medicine)
South Med J   (Southern Medical Journal)
Surg Gynecol Obstet   (Surgery, Gynecology and Obstetrics)
Tex Med   (Texas Medicine)
Thromb Haemostasis   (Thrombosis and Haemostasis)

CHAPTER 1.   THE SEX HORMONES

1. Abraham, G. E.; Lobotsky, J.; and Lloyd, W. 1969. Metabolism of testosterone and androstenedione in normal and ovariectomized women. *J Clin Invest* 48:696–703.
2. Ballinger, C. B.; Browning, M. C. K.; and Smith, A. H. W. 1987. Hormones profiles and psychological symptoms in peri-menopausal women. *Maturitas* 9:235–51.
3. Barret, I.; Cullis, W.; Fairfield, L.; Nicholson, R.; MacNaughton, M.; Williamson, C. F.; and Sanderson, A. E. 1933. Investigation of meno-

pause in 1000 women. Subcommittee of the Council of Medical Women's Federation of England. *Lancet* 106–8.

4. Bengtsson, C., and Lindquist, O. 1977. Coronary heart disease during the menopause. *Clinics in Obstet & Gynaecol* 4:234–42.

5. Carlstrom, K.; Brody, S.; Lunell, N. O.; Lagrelius, A.; Mollerstrom, G.; Pousette, A.; Rannevik, G.; Stege, R.; and von Schoultz, B. 1988. Dehydroepiandrosterone in serum: differences related to age and sex. *Maturitas* 10:297–306.

6. Crilly, R. G.; Marshall, D. H.; and Nordin, E. E. 1979. Effect of age on plasma androstenedione concentration in oophorectomized women. *Clin Endocrinol* 10:199–201.

7. Edman, C. D., and MacDonald, P. C. 1978. Effect of obesity on conversion of plasma androstenedione to estrone in ovulatory and anovulatory young women. *Am J Obstet Gynecol* 130:456–61.

8. Frumar, A.; Meldrum, D.; Geola, F.; Shamonki, I.; Tataryn, I.; Deftos, L.; and Judd, H. 1980. Relationship of fasting urinary calcium to circulating estrogen and body weight in postmenopausal women. *J Clin Endocrinol Metab* 50:70–75.

9. Grodin, J. M.; Siiteri, P. K.; and MacDonhald, P. D. 1973. Source of estrogen production in postmenopausal women. *J Clin Endocrinol Metab* 36:207.

10. Jick, H.; Porter, J.; and Morrison, A. D. 1977. Relation between smoking and age of natural menopause: report from the Boston Collaborative Drug Surveillance Program, Boston University Medical Center. *Lancet* 1:1354–55.

11. Judd, H. G.; Judd, G. E.; Lucas, W. E.; and Yen, S. S. C. 1974. Endocrine function of the postmenopausal ovary: concentration of androgens and estrogens in ovarian and peripheral vein blood. *J Clin Endocrinol Metab* 39:1020.

12. Judd, H. L.; Davidson, B. J.; Frumar, A. M.; Shamonki, I. M.; Lagasse, L. D.; and Ballon, S. C. 1980. Serum androgens and estrogens in postmenopausal women with and without endometrial cancer. *Am J Obstet Gynecol* 136:859–71.

13. Korenman, S. G.; Sherman, B. M.; and Korenman, J. C. 1978. Reproductive hormone function: the perimenopausal period and beyond. *Clin Endocrinol Metab* 7:625–43.

14. Lenton, E. A.; Sexton, L.; Lee, S.; and Cooke, I. D. 1988. Progressive changes in LH and FSH and LH:FSH ratio in women throughout reproductive life. *Maturitas* 10:35–43.

15. Longcope, C.; Franz, C.; Morello, C.; Baker, R.; and Johnston, C. C., Jr. 1986. Steroid and gonadotropin levels in women during the peri-menopausal years. *Maturitas* 8:189–96.

16. Longcope, C.; Hunter, R.; and Franz, C. 1980. Steroid secretion in the postmenopausal ovary. *Am J Obstet Gynecol* 138:564–68.

17. McNatty, K. P.; Makris, A.; DeGrazia, C.; Osathanondh, R.; and Ryan, K. J. 1979. The production of progesterone, androgens and estrogens by granulosa cells, thecal tissue and stromal tissue by human ovaries in vitro. *J Clin Endocrinol Metab* 49:687–99.

18. Monroe, S. E., and Menon, K. M. J. 1977. Changes in reproductive hormone secretion during the climacteric and postmenopausal periods. *Clin in Obstet & Gynaecol* 20:113–22.

19. Rannevik, G. N.; Carlstrom, K.; Jeppsson, S.; Bjerre, B.; and Svanberg, L. 1986. A prospective long-term study in women from pre-menopause to post-menopause: changing profiles of gonadotropins, oestrogens and androgens. *Maturitas* 8:297–307.

20. Reyes, F. I.; Winter, J. S.; and Faiman, C. 1977. Pituitary-ovarian relationships preceding the menopause. I: A cross-sectional study of serum follicle-stimulating hormone, prolactin, estradiol and progesterone levels. *Am J Obstet Gynecol* 129:557–64.

21. Rosenberg, S.; Bosson, D.; Peretz, A.; Caufriez, A.; and Robyn, C. 1988. Serum levels of gonadotropins and steroid hormones in the post-menopause and later life. *Maturitas* 10:215–24.

22. Sherman B. M., and Korenman, S. G. 1975. Hormonal characteristics of the human menstrual cycle throughout reproductive life. *J Clin Invest* 55:699–704.

23. Treloar, A. E.; Boynton, R. E.; and Cowan, D. W. 1974. Menarche, menopause and intervening fecundability. *Human Biology* 16:89–107.

24. Trevoux, R.; DeBrux, J.; Castanier, M.; Nahoul, K.; Soule, J. P.; and Scholler, R. 1986. Endometrium and plasma hormone profile in the perimenopause and post-menopause. *Maturitas* 8:309–26.

25. Vermeulen, A. 1980. Sex hormone status of the postmenopausal woman. *Maturitas* 2:81–89.

26. Vermeulen, A., and Verdonick, L. 1978. Sex hormone concentration in post-menopausal women: relation to obesity, fat mass, age, and years post-menopause. *Clin Endocrinol* 9:59–66.

27. Wyshak, G. 1978. Menopause in mothers of multiple births and mothers of singletons only. *Soc Biol* 25:52–61.

ADDITIONAL RECOMMENDED READINGS

Abraham, G. E. 1974. Ovarian and adrenal contribution to peripheral androgens during the menstrual cycle. *J Clin Endocrinol Metab* 39:340–46.

Abraham, G. E.; Odell, W. D.; Swerdloff, R. S.; and Hopper, K. 1972. Simultaneous radioimmunoassay of plasma FSH, LH, progesterone, 17 hydroxypro-gesterone and estradiol 17β during the menstrual cycle. *J Clin Endocrinol Metab* 34:312–18.

Adashi, E. Y.; Rakoff, J.; Divers, W.; Fishman, J.; and Yen, S. S. C. 1979. The effect of acutely administered 2 hydroxyestorone on the release of gonadotro-pins and prolactin before and after estrogen priming in hypogonadal women. *Life Sci* 25:20–51.

Anderson, D. C. 1976. The role of sex hormone binding globulin in health and disease. In *The endocrine function of the human ovary,* ed. V. H. T. James, M. Serio, and G. Giusti, pp. 141–58. London: Academic Press.

Balog, J. 1980. Obesity and estrogen. *Am J Obstet Gynecol* 138:242.

Calanog, A.; Sall, S.; Gordon, G.; and Southern, A. 1977. Androstenedione metabolism in patients with endometrial cancer. *Am J Obstet Gynecol* 129:553–56.

Carlstrom, K.; Damber, M.; Furuhjelm, M.; Joelsson, I.; Lunell, N.; and Von Schoultz, B. 1979. Serum levels of total dehydroepiandorosterone and total estrone in post-menopausal women with special regard to carcinoma of the uterine corpus. *Acta Obstet et Gynecol Scand* 58:179–81.

Chakravarti, S.; Collins, W. P.; Forecast, J.; Newton, J.; Oram, D. H.; and Studd, J. W. 1976. Hormonal profiles after the menopause. *Brit Med J* 2:784–86.

Dor, P.; Muquardt, C. L.; Hermite, M.; and Borkowski, A. 1978. Influence of corticotrophin and prolactin on the steroid sex hormones and their precur-sors. *J Endoc* 77:263–64.

Flickinger, G. L.; Elsner, C.; Illingworth, D. V.; Muechler, E. K.; and Mikhail, G. 1977. Estrogen and progesterone receptors in the female genital tract of humans and monkeys. *Ann NY Academy of Sciences* 286:180–89.

Grattarola, R.; Secreto, G.; and Recchione, C. 1975. Correlation between uri-nary testosterone or estrogen excretion levels and interstitial cell stimulation hormone concentrations in normal postmenopausal women. *Am J Obstet Gynecol* 121:380–81.

Gurpide, E. 1978. Enzymatic modulation of hormonal action at the target tis-sue. *J Toxicol Environ Health* 4:249.

Hutton, J. D.; Jacobs, H. S.; James, V. H. T.; Murray, M. A. D.; and Rippon, A. E. 1977. Episodic secretion of steroid hormones in post menopausal women. *J Endoc* 73:25P.

Jacobs, H. S.; Hutton, J. D.; Murray, M. A. D.; and James, V. H. T. 1977. Plasma hormone profiles in postmenopausal women before and during oestro-gen therapy. *Br J Obstet Gynaecol* 84:314.

Judd, H. L., and Yen, S. S. C. 1973. Serum androstenedione and testosterone levels during the menstrual cycle. *J Clin Endocrinol Metab* 36:475–81.

Judd, S. J.; Rakoff, J. S.; and Yen, S. S. C. 1978. Inhibition of gonadotropin and prolactin release by dopamine: effect of endogenous estradiol levels. *J Clin Endocrinol Metab* 47:494–98.

Kwa, H. G.; Bulbrook, R. D.; Cleton, F.; Verstraeten, A. A.; Hayward, J. L.; and Wang, D. Y. 1978. An abnormal early evening peak of plasma prolactin in nulliparous and obese postmenopausal women. *Int J Cancer* 22:691–93.

Larsson-Cohn, U.; Johansson, E. D.; Kagedal, B.; and Wallentin, L. 1977. Serum FSH, LH and oestrone levels in postmenopausal patients on oestrogen therapy. *Br J Obstet Gynaecol* 85:367–72.

Longcope, C. 1971. Metabolic clearance and blood production rates of estrogens in postmenopausal women. *Am J Obstet Gynecol* 111:778–81.

Longcope, C.; Pratt, J. H.; Schneider, S. H.; and Fineberg, S. E. 1978. Aromatization of androgens by muscle and adipose tissues in vivo. *J Clin Endocrinol Metab* 46:146–52.

MacDonald, P. C.; Edman, C. D.; Hemsell, D. L.; Porter, J. C.; and Siiteri, P. K. 1978. Effect of obesity on conversion of plasma androstenedione to estrone in postmenopausal women with and without endometrial cancer. *Am J Obstet Gynecol* 130:448–55.

Medina, M.; Scaglia, H. E.; Vazquez, G.; Alatorre, S.; and Perez-Palacios, G. 1976. Rapid oscillation of circulating gonadotropins. *J Clin Endocrinol Metab* 43:1015–19.

Milewich, L.; Gomez-Sanchez, C.; Madden, J. D.; Bradfield, D. J.; Parker, P. M.; Smith, S. L.; Carr, B. R.; Edmanb, C. H.; and MacDonald, P. C. 1978. Dehydroisoandrosterone sulfate in peripheral blood of premenopausal, pregnant, and postmenopausal women and men. *J Steroid Biochem* 9:1159–64.

O'Dea, J. P.; Wieland, R. G.; Hallberg, M. C.; Lerena, L. A.; Zorn, E. M.; and Genuth, S. M. 1979. Effect of dietary weight loss on sex steroid binding, sex steroids and gonadotropins in obese postmenopausal women. *J Lab Clin Med* 93:1007–8.

Poliak, A.; Seegar-Jones, G.; and Goldberg, I. V. 1968. Effect of human chorionic gonadotropin on postmenopausal women. *Am J Obstet Gynecol* 101:731–39.

Rader, M. D.; Flickinger, G. L.; de Villa, G. O.; Mikuta, J. J.; and Mikhail, G. 1973. Plasma estrogen in postmenopausal women. *Am J Obstet Gynecol* 116:1069–73.

Sherman, B. M.; West, J. H.; and Korenman, S. G. 1976. The menopausal transition: analysis of LH, FSH, estradiol, and progesterone concentrations during menstrual cycles of older women. *J Clin Endocrinol Metab* 42:629–36.

Taylor, M. A.; Chapman, C.; and Hayter, C. J. 1977. The effect of altering thyroid hormone concentrations on plasma gonadotropins in postmenopausal women. *Br J Obstet Gynaecol* 84:254–57.

Vermeulen, A. 1976. The hormonal activity of the postmenopausal ovary. *J Clin Endocrinol Metab* 42:247–53.

Wise, A. J.; Gross, M. A.; and Schalch, D. A. 1973. Quantitative relationship of the pituitary gonadal axis in post-menopausal women. *J Lab Clin Med* 81:28–36.

CHAPTER 2.   THE CHANGE OF LIFE

1. Asch, R.; Balmaceda, J.; Ord, T.; Borrero, C.; Cefalu, E.; Gastaldi, C.; and Rojas, F. 1987. Oocyte donation and gamete intrafallopian transfer as treatment for premature ovarian failure [letter]. *Lancet* 687.

1a. Ballinger, C. B. 1975. Psychiatric morbidity and the menopause: screening of general population sample. *Brit Med J* 3:344–46.

2. Barret, I.; Cullis, W.; Fairfield, L.; Nicholson, R.; MacNaughton, M.; Williamson, C. F.; and Sanderson, A. E. 1933. Investigation of menopause in 1000 women. Subcommittee of the Council of Medical Women's Federation of England. *Lancet* 106–8.

3. Bart, P. 1971. Depression in middle aged women. In *Women in a sexist society,* ed. V. Gornick and B. K. Moran. New York: Mentor.

4. Berg, G.; Gottqall, T.; Hammar, M.; and Lindgren, R. 1988. Climacteric symptoms among women aged 60–62 in Linkoping, Sweden, in 1986. *Maturitas* 10:193–99.

5. Boyers, S. P.; Luborsky, J. L.; and DeCherney, A. H. 1988. Usefulness of serial measurements of serum follicle stimulating hormone, leutinizing hormone and estradiol in patients with premature ovarian failure. *Fertil Steril* 50, 3:408–12.

6. Bye, P. G. 1978. Review of the status of oestrogen replacement therapy. *Postgrad Med J* 54:7–10.

7. Campbell, S., and Whitehead, M. 1977. Oestrogen therapy and the menopausal syndrome. *Clinics in Obstet & Gynaecol* 4:31–47.

8. Casper, R. F., and Yen, S. S. C. 1981. Menopausal flushes: effect of pituitary gonadotropin desensitization by a potent luteinizing hormone releasing factor agonist. *J Clin Endocrinol Metab* 53:1056–58.

9. Casper, R. F.; Yen, S. S. C.; and Wilkes, N. M. 1979. Menopausal flushes: a neuroendocrine link with pulsatile luteinizing hormone secretion. *Science* 205:823–25.

10. Chakravarti, S.; Collins, W. P.; Thom, M. H.; and Studd, J. W. 1979. Relations between plasma hormone profiles, symptoms and response to oestrogen treatment in women approaching the menopause. *Brit Med J* 1:983–85.

11. Coope, J.; Williams, S.; and Patterson, J. S. 1978. A study of the effectiveness of propanolol in menopausal hot flushes. *Br J Obstet Gynaecol* 185:472–75.

12. Coulam, C. B.; Adamson, S. C.; and Annegers, J. F. 1986. Incidence of premature ovarian failure. *Obstet Gynecol* 67:604–6.

13. Crawford, M. P., and Hooper, D. 1973. Menopause, aging and family. *Soc Sci Med* 7:469–82.

14. Daw, E. 1975. Duration of effect of treatment of menopausal symptoms by oestrogen fraction. *Curr Med Res Opin* 3:22–25.

15. Flint, M. 1975. The menopause: reward or punishment. *Psychosomatics* 16:161–63.

16. Gambrell, R. D. 1977. Postmenopausal bleeding. *Clinics in Obstet & Gynaecol* 4:1.

17. Gamst, F. 1969. *The Quemant, a pagan hebraic peasantry of Ethiopia.* New York: Holt, Rinehart and Winston.

18. Guyton, A. C. 1986. *Textbook of medical physiology.* 7th ed. Philadelphia: Saunders.

19. Herold, E.; Mottin, J.; and Sabry, Z. 1979. Effect of vitamin E on human sexual functioning. *Arch Sex Beh* 8:397–403.

20. Hostetler, J., and Huntrington, G. E. 1967. *The Hutterites of North America.* New York: Holt, Rinehart and Winston.

21. Huggins, G. R., and Zucker, P. K. 1987. Oral contraceptives and neoplasia: 1987 update. *Fertil Steril* 47, 5:733–61.

22. Hung, T. T.; Ribas, D.; Tsuiki, A.; Preyer, J.; Slackman, R.; and Davidson, O.W. 1989. Artificially induced menstrual cycle with natural estradiol and progesterone. *Fertil Steril* 51, 6:968–71.

23. Jaszmann, L. J. B. 1973. Epidemiology of climacteric and post climacteric complaints. In *Aging and Estrogens,* ed. P. A. Van Keep and C. Lauiritzen. *Front Horm Res* 2:22–34.

24. Kaufert, P. N. A.; Gilbert, P.; and Tate, R. 1987. Defining menopausal status: the impact of longitudinal data. *Maturitas* 9:217–26.

25. Kinsey, A.; Pomeroy, W.; and Martin, C. 1953. *Sexual behavior in the human female.* Philadelphia: Saunders.

26. Kronenberg, F.; Carraway, R.; Cote, L. J.; Linkie, D. M.; Crawshaw, L. I.; and Downey, J. A. 1981. Changes in thermoregulation, immunoreactive neurotensin, catecholamines and LH during menopausal hot flashes. In *Proceedings of the sixty-second annual meeting of the American Endocrine Society,* 141, abst. no. 236.

27. Kupperman, H. S.; Wetchler, B. B.; and Blatt, M. H. G. 1959. Contemporary therapy of the menopausal syndrome. *JAMA* 171:1627–37.

28. Leiblum, S. R., and Swartzman, L. C. 1986. Women's attitudes toward the menopause: an update. *Maturitas* 8:47–56.

29. Lock, M.; Kaufert, P.; and Gilbert, P. 1988. Cultural construction of the menopausal syndrome: the Japanese case. *Maturitas* 10:317–32.

30. McKinlay, S. M.; Bifano, N. L.; and McKinlay, J. B. 1985. Smoking and age at menopause in women. *Ann Int Med* 103:350–56.

31. McKinley, S. M., and Jeffrey, M. 1974. The menopausal syndrome. *Br J Prev Soc Med* 28:108–15.

32. Marks, R., and Shahrad, P. 1977. Skin changes at the time of the climacteric. *Clincs in Obstet & Gynaecol* 4:207–26.

33. Meldrum, D.; Tataryn, I.; Frumar, A.; Erlet, J.; Lu, K.; and Judd, H. 1980. Gonadotropins, estrogens, and adrenal steroids during the menopausal hot flash. *J Clin Endocrinol Metab* 50:685–89.

34. Metcalf, M. G. 1979. Incidence of ovulatory cycles in women approaching the menopause. *J Biosoc Sci* 11:39–48.

35. Molnar, G. W. 1975. Body temperatures during menopausal hot flashes. *J Appl Physiol* 38:499–503.

36. Molnar, G. W. 1980. Menopausal hot flashes: their cycles and relation to air temperature. *Obstet Gynecol* 57:52S–55S.

37. Pedersen, S. H., and Jeune, B. 1988. Prevalence of hormone replacement therapy in a sample of middle-aged women. *Maturitas* 9:339–45.

38. Punonen, R. 1972. Effect of castration and peroral estrogen therapy on the skin. *Acta Obstet et Gynecol Scand* suppl 21:1–44.

39. Punonen, R., and Rauamo, L. 1977. The effect of long-term oral oestriol succinate therapy on the skin of castrated women. *Ann Chir Gynaecol* 66:214–15.

40. Rabinowe, S. L.; Ravnikar, V. A.; Dib, S. A.; George, K. L.; and Dluhy, R. G. 1989. Premature menopause: monoclonal antibody defined T lymphocyte abnormalities and antiovarian antibodies. *Fertil Steril* 51, 3:450–54.

41. Reyes, F.; Winter, J.; and Faiman, C. 1977. Pituitary ovarian relationships preceding the menopause, *Am J Obstet Gynecol* 129:557–64.

42. Riphagen, F. E. 1988. Contraceptive behavior of women aged over 35. *Maturitas* suppl. 1:51–61.

43. Ryan, T. J. 1966. The microcirculation of the skin in old age. *Geront Clin* 8:327.

44. Ryan, T. J., and Kurban, A. K. 1970. New vessel growth in the adult skin. *Br J Derm* 82, suppl. 5:92.

45. Schiff, I.; Regestein, Q., Tulchinsky, D.; and Ryan, K. J. 1979. Effects of estrogens on psychological state of hypogonadal women. *JAMA* 242:2405–7.

46. Schurz, B.; Wimmer-Grienecker, G.; Metka, M.; Heytmanek, G.; Egarter, C. H.; and Knogler, W. 1988. Endorphin levels during climacteric period. *Maturitas* 10:45–50.

47. Semmens, J. P., and Wagner, G. 1982. Estrogen deprivation and vaginal function in postmenopausal women. *JAMA* 248:445–48.

47a. Sherwin, B. 1988. Estrogen and/or androgen replacement therapy and cognitive functioning in surgically menopausal women. *Psychoneuroendocrinology* 13:345–57.

47b. ———. 1988. The role of androgens in menopausal women. In *Androgens in the menopause,* ed. Leon Speroff. Marietta, Ga.: Reid-Rowell.

48. Stadel, V., and Weiss, N. 1975. Characteristics of menopausal women: a survey of King and Pierce Counties in Washington, 1973–1974. *Am J Epidemiol* 102:209–16.

49. Studd, J.; Chakravarti, S.; and Oram, D. 1977. The climacteric. *Clinics in Obstet & Gynaecol* 4:3–29.

50. Sturdee, D. W.; Wilson, K. A.; Pipili, E.; and Crocker, A. D. 1978. Physiological aspects of menopausal hot flush. *Brit Med J* 2:79–80.

51. Tataryn, I. V.; Meldrum, D. R.; Lu, K. H.; Frumar, A. M.; and Judd, H. L. 1979. LH, FSH and skin temperature during the menopause hot flash. *J Clin Endocrinol Metab* 49:152–54.

52. Teichmann, A. T. 1988. Age, metabolism and oral contraception. *Maturitas* suppl. 1:117–30.

53. Thompson, B.; Hart, S. A.; and Durno, D. 1973. Menopausal age and symptomatology in a general practice. *J Biosoc Sci* 5:71–82.

54. Thomson, J.; Maddock, J.; Aylward, M.; and Oswald, I. 1977. Relationship between nocturnal plasma oestrogen concentration and free plasma tryptophan in perimenopausal women. *J Endoc* 72:395–96.

55. Thomson, J., and Oswald, I. 1977. Effect of oestrogen on the sleep, mood and anxiety of menopausal women. *Brit Med J* 2:317–19.

56. Treloar, A. E. 1974. Menarche, menopause and intervening fecundability. *Human Biology* 16:89–107.

57. ———. 1981. Menstrual cyclicity and the premenopause. *Maturitas* 3:249–64.

58. Treloar, A. E.; Boynton, R. E.; Behn, D. G.; and Brown, B. W. 1967. Variation of the human menstrual cycle through reproductive life. *I J Fertil* 12:77–126.

59. Treloar, A. E.; Boynton, R. E.; and Cowan, D. W. 1974. Secular trend in age at menarche, USA 1893–1974. In *Excerpta Medica international congress series no. 394, biological and clinical aspects of reproduction.* Amsterdam: Excerpta Medica.

60. Vollman, R. F. 1977. *The menstrual cycle.* Major Problems in Obstetrics and Gynecology. Philadelphia: Saunders.

CHAPTER 3.   BODY CHANGES AT THE MENOPAUSE

1. Brodie, B. L., and Wentz, A. C. 1987. Late onset congenital adrenal hyperplasia: a gynecologist's perspective. *Fertil Steril* 48, 2:175–88.

2. Brown, A. G. 1977. Postmenopausal urinary problems. *Clinics in Obstet & Gynaecol* 4:181–206.

3. Burgio, K. L.; Robinson, J. C.; and Engel, B. T. 1986. The role of bio-feedback in Kegel exercise training for stress urinary incontinence. *Am J Obstet Gynecol* 154:58–64.

4. Costoff, A., and Mahesh, V. B. 1975. Primordial follicles with normal oocytes in the ovaries of postmenopausal women. *J Am Geriatr Soc* 23: 193–96.

5. Cutler, W. B., and García, C.-R. 1983. Hysterectomy and sexual deficits: a reappraisal and review. Unpublished ms.

6. de Aloysio, D.; Villecco, A. S.; Fabiani, A. G.; Mauloni, M.; Altieri, P.; Miliffi, L.; and Bottiglioni, F. 1988. Body mass index distribution in climacteric women. *Maturitas* 9:359–66.

7. Dennefors, B.; Janson, P.; Knutson, F.; and Hamberger, L. 1980. Steroid production and responsiveness to gonadotropin in isolated stromal tissue of human postmenopausal ovaries. *Am J Obstet Gynecol* 136:997–1002.

8. Fedor-Freybergh, P. 1977. The influence of estrogens on the well being and mental performance in climacteric and postmenopausal women. *Acta Obstet et Gynecol Scand* 64:suppl 1–66.

9. Gaddum-Rosse, P.; Rumer, R. E.; Blandau, R. J.; and Theirsch, J. B. 1975. Studies on the mucosa of post menopausal oviducts: surface appearance, ciliary activity and the effect of estrogen treatment. *Fertil Steril* 26: 951–69.

10. Kegel, A. M. 1951. Physiologic therapy for urinary stress incontinence. *JAMA* 146:915–17.

11. Lind, T.; Cameron, E. C.; Hunter, W. M.; Leon, C.; Moran, P. F.; Oxley, A.; Gerrard, J.; and Lind, U. C. G. 1979. A prospective controlled trial of six forms of hormone replacement therapy given to post-menopausal women. *Br J Obstet Gynaecol* 86:suppl 3:1–29.

12. Longcope, C.; Hunter, R.; and Franz, C. 1980. Steroid secretion by the postmenopausal ovary. *Am J Obstet Gynecol* 138:564–68.

13. Longcope, C.; Jaffee, W.; and Griffing, G. 1981. Production rates of androgens and oestrogens in postmenopausal women. *Maturitas* 3:215–23.

14. Lucisano, A.; Russo, N.; Acampora, M. G.; Fabiano, A.; Fattibene, M.; Parlati, E.; Maniccia, E.; and Dell'Acqua. 1986. Ovarian and peripheral androgen and oestrogen levels in post-menopausal women: correlations with ovarian histology. *Maturitas* 8:57–65.

15. Ludwig, E. 1964. Diffuse alopecia in women: its clinical forms and probable causes. *J Soc Cosmetic Chemists* 15:437–446.

16. McNatty, K. P.; Makris, A.; DeGrazia, C.; Osathanondh, R.; and Ryan, K. J. 1979. The production of progesterone, androgens and estrogens by granulosa cells, thecal tissue and stromal tissue by human ovaries in vitro. *J Clin Endocrinol Metab* 49:687–99.

17. Marks, R., and Shahrad, P. 1977. Skin changes at the time of the climacteric. *Clinics in Obstet & Gynaecol* 4:207–26.
18. Mikhail, G. 1970. Hormone secretion by the human ovaries. *Gynec Invest* 1:5–20.
19. Monroe, S. E., and Menon, K. M. J. 1977. Changes in reproductive hormone secretion during the climacteric and postmenopausal periods. *Clinics in Obstet & Gynaecol* 20:113–22.
20. Novak, E. R. 1970. Ovulation after fifty. *Obstet Gynecol* 36:903–10.
21. Novak, E. R.; Goldberg, B.; and Jones, G. S. 1965. Enzyme histochemistry of the menopausal ovary associated with normal and abnormal endometrium. *Am J Obstet Gynecol* 93:669–73.
22. Novak, E. R., and Richardson, E. H. 1941. Proliferative changes in the senile endometrium. *Am J Obstet Gynecol* 42:564.
23. Perry, J. D., and Whipple, B. 1981. Pelvic muscle strength of female ejaculators: evidence in support of a new theory of orgasm. *J Sex Res* 17: 22–39.
24. Rittmaster, R. S., and Loriaux, D. L. 1987. Hirsutism. *Ann Int Med* 106: 95–107.
25. Robertson, D. M., and Landgren, B. M. 1975. Oestradiol receptor levels in the human fallopian tube during the menstrual cycle and after menopause. *J Steroid Biochem* 6:511–13.
26. Rodin, M., and Moghissi, K. S. 1973. Intrinsic innervation of the human cervix: a preliminary study. In *The biology of the human cervix*, ed. R. J. Blandau and K. Moghissi. Chicago: University of Chicago Press.
27. Ruutianinen, K.; Erkkola, R.; Gronroos, M. A.; and Irjala, K. 1988. Influence of body mass index and age on the grade of hair growth in hirsute women of reproductive ages. *Fertil Steril* 50, 2:260–66.
28. Ruutianinen, K.; Erkkola, R.; Gronroos, M. A.; and Kaihola, H. L. 1988. Androgen parameters in hirsute women: correlations with body mass index and age. *Fertil Steril* 50, 2:255–59.
29. Silva, P. D.; Gentzschein, E. E. K.; and Lobo, R. A. 1987. Androstenedione may be a more important precursor of tissue dihydrotestosterone than testosterone in women. *Fertil Steril* 48, 3:419–22.
30. Smith, P. 1972. Age changes in the female urethra. *Br J Urol* 44:667–76.
31. Stone, S. C.; Mickal, A.; and Rye, P. H. 1975. Post-menopausal symptomatology, maturation index, and plasma estrogen levels. *Obstet Gynecol* 45, 6:625–27.
32. Zussman, L.; Zussman, S.; Sunley, R.; and Bjornson, E. 1981. Sexual response after hysterectomy-oophorectomy: recent studies and reconsideration of psychogenesis. *Am J Obstet Gynecol* 140:725–29.

CHAPTER 4. THE BONES AND HOW THEY GROW

1. Adams, J. S. 1982. Vitamin D synthesis and metabolism after ultraviolet irradiation of normal and vitamin deficient subjects. *NEJM* 306:722–25.
2. Albanese, A. A. 1978. Calcium nutrition in the elderly. *Postgrad Med* 63: 167–72.
3. ———. 1977. Osteoporosis. *J Am Pharm Assoc* 17:252–53.
4. Albanese, A. A.; Edelson, A. A.; Lorenze, E. J.; and Wein, E. H. 1969. Quantitative radiographic survey technique for the detection of bone loss. *J Am Geriatr Soc* 17:142–54.
5. Albanese, A. A.; Edelson, A. H.; Lorenze, E. J.; and Wein, E. H. 1980. Osteoporosis: a new screen for asymptomatic bone loss. *Diagnosis* 2:71.
6. Albanese, A. A.; Edelson, A. H.; Lorenze, E. J., Jr.; and Woodhull, E. 1975. Problems of bone health in the elderly: a ten year study. *NY State J Med* 75:326–36.
7. Albanese, A. A.; Lorenze, E. J.; Edelson, A. H.; Wein, E. H.; and Carroll, L. 1981. Effects of calcium supplements and estrogen replacement therapy on bone loss of postmenopausal women. *Nutrition Reports International* 24:403–14.
8. Albright, F.; Smith, P. H.; and Richardson, A. M. 1941. Postmenopausal osteoporosis, its clinical features. *JAMA* 116:2465–74.
9. Alfram, P. A. 1964. An epidemiologic study of cervical and trochanteric fractures of the femur in an urban population. *Acta Orthopaedica Scandinavica* 65, suppl. 1:9–102.
10. Alhava, E. M., and Puittinen, J. 1973. Fractures of the upper end of the femur as an index of senile osteoporosis in Finland. *Ann Clin Res* 5:398 ff.
11. Aloia, J. F.; Vaswani, A.; Yeh, J. K.; Ellis, K.; Yasumura, S.; and Cohn, S. H. 1988. Calcitriol in the treatment of postmenopausal osteoporosis. *Am J Med* 84:401–8.
12. Ayalon, J.; Simkin, A.; Leichter, I.; and Riafmann, S. 1987. Dynamic bone loading exercise for postmenopausal women. *Arch Phys Med Rehabil* 68, 5:280–83.
13. Barentsen, R.; Raymakers, J. A.; Landman, J. O.; and Duursma, S. A. 1988. Bone mineral content of the forearm in healthy Dutch women. *Maturitas* 10:231–41.
14. Beals, R. K. 1972. Survival following hip fracture: long term followup of 607 patients. *J Chron Dis* 25:235–44.
15. Boucher, A.; D'Amour, P.; Hamel, L.; Fugere, P.; Gascon-Barre, M.; Lepage, R.; and Ste-Marie, L. G. 1989. Estrogen replacement decreases the set point of parathyroid hormone stimulation by calcium in normal menopausal women. *J Clin Endocrinol Metab* 68, 4:831–36.

16. Boyle, I. T. 1981. Treatment for postmenopausal osteoporosis. *Lancet* 1376.

17. Bullamore, J. R.; Gallagher, J. C.; and Wilkinson, R. 1970. Effect of age on calcium absorption. *Lancet* 2:535–37.

18. Chalmers, J., and Ho, K. C. 1970. Geographical variations in senile osteoporosis: the association with physical activity. *J Bone Joint Surg* 52b:667–75.

19. Chestnut, C. H. 1981. Treatment of postmenopausal osteoporosis: some current concepts. *Scott Med J* 26:72 ff.

20. Chestnut, C. H.; Baylink, D. J.; and Nelp, W. B. 1979. Calcitonin therapy in postmenopausal osteoporosis: preliminary results. *Clin Res* 27:85A abstract.

21. Christianssen, C., and Christensen, M. S. 1981. Bone mass in postmenopausal women after withdrawal of oestrogen/gestagen replacement therapy. *Lancet* 459–61.

22. Civitelli, R.; Agnusaei, D.; Nardi, P.; Zacchei, F.; Avioli, L. V.; and Gennari, C. 1988. Effects of one-year treatment with estrogens on bone mass, intestinal calcium absorption, and 25-hydroxyvitamin D-1α-hydroxylase reserve in postmenopausal osteoporosis. *Calcif Tiss Int* 42:77–86.

23. Crilly, R.; Horsman, A.; Marshall, D. H.; and Nordin, B. E. C. 1979. Prevalence, pathogenesis and treatment of post-menopausal osteoporosis. *Aust N Z J Med* 9:24–30.

24. Cutler, W. 1988. Single photon absorptiometry imaging as a screening method for diminished dual photon density measures. *Maturitas* 10:143–55.

25. ———. 1988. *Hysterectomy: before and after.* New York: Harper & Row.

26. Deeny, M.; Farish, E.; Tillman, J.; Dagen, M.; Hart, D. M.; and Fletcher, C. D. 1988. Changes in the bone and liver isoenzymes of alkaline phosphatase in postmenopausal women being treated with noresthisterone. *Clin Chim Acta* 171, 1:103–8.

27. Enzelsberger, H.; Metka, M.; Heytmanek, G.; Schurz, B.; Kurz, C. H.; and Kusztrick, M. 1988. Influence of oral contraceptive use on bone density in climacteric women. *Maturitas* 9:375–78.

28. Gallagher, J., and Nordin, B. E. C. 1975. Effects of oestrogen and progestogen therapy on calcium metabolism in post-menopausal women. *Front Horm Res* 3:150.

29. Gallagher, J. C.; Riggs, B. L.; and DeLuca, H. F. 1978. Effect of age on calcium absorption and serum 1,25 OH2D. *Clin Res* 26:680A.

30. Garn, S. M. 1970. *The earlier gain and the later loss of cortical bone in nutritional perspective.* Springfield, Ill.: Charles C. Thomas.

30a. Genant, H.; Baylink, D.; Gallagher, J. C.; Harris, S.; Steiger, P.; and

Herbert, M. 1990. Effect of estrone sulfate on postmenopausal bone loss. *Obstet Gynecol* 76:579–84.

31. Geola, F.; Frumar, A.; Tataryn, I.; Lu, K.; Hershman, J.; Eggena, P.; Sambhi, M.; and Judd, H. 1980. Biological effects of various doses of conjugated equine estrogens in postmenopausal women. *J Clin Endocrinol Metab* 51:620–25.

32. Gordan, G. S. 1981. Early detection of osteoporosis and prevention of hip fractures in elderly women. *Med Times* special section (April), pp. 1s–17s.

33. Gruber, H.; Ivey, J.; Baylink, D.; Matthews, M.; Nelp, W.; Sisom, K.; and Chestnut, C. 1984. Long-term calcitonin therapy in postmenopausal osteoporosis. *Metabolism* 33, 4:295–300.

34. Heaney, R. P. 1962. Radiocalcium metabolism in disuse osteoporosis in man. *Am J Med* 33:188–200.

35. Heaney, R. P.; Recker, R. R.; and Saville, P. D. 1977. Calcium balance and calcium requirements in middle aged women. *Am J Clin Nutr* 30: 1603.

36. Hempel, Von E.; Kriester, A.; Freesmeyer, E.; and Walter, W. 1979. Perspecktive studie zur osteoporose nach bilater ovarektomie mit und ohne postoperative ostregenprophylaxe. *Zentralblatt für Gynakologie* 101: 309–19.

37. Hosie, C. J.; Hart, D. M.; Smith, D. A. S.; and Al-Azzawi, F. 1989. Differential effect of long-term oestrogen therapy on trabecular and cortical bone. *Maturitas* 11:137–45.

38. Hurley, D. L.; Tiegs, R. D.; Barta, J.; Laakso, K.; and Heath, H., III. 1989. Effects of oral contraceptive and estrogen administration on plasma calcitonin in pre- and postmenopausal women. *Journal of Bone and Mineral Research* 4, 1:89–95.

39. Isaia, G.; Bodrato, L.; Carlevatto, V.; Mussetta, M.; Salamano, G.; and Molinatti, G. M. 1988. Osteoporosis in type II diabetes. *Acta Diabetol Lat* 24, 2:305–10.

40. Ireland, P., and Fordtran, J. S. 1973. Effect of dietary calcium on age on jejunal calcium absorption in humans studied by intestinal perfusion. *J Clin Invest* 52:2672–81.

41. Jacobson, P. C.; Beaver, W.; Grubb, S. A.; Taft, T. N.; and Talmage, R. V. 1984. Bone density in women: college athletes and older athletic women. *Journal of Orthopaedic Research* 2:328–32.

42. Krolner, B.; Toft, B.; Nielsen, S. P.; and Tondevold, E. 1983. Physical exercise as prophylaxis against involutional vertebral bone loss: a controlled trial. *Clin Sci* 64:541–46.

43. Lafferty, F. W.; Spencer, G. E.; and Pearson, O. H. 1964. Effects of androgens, estrogens and high calcium intakes on bone formation and resorption in osteoporosis. *Am J Med* 36:514–28.

44. Lee, C. J.; Lawler, G. S.; and Johnson, G. H. 1981. Effects of supplementation of the diets with calcium and calcium rich foods on bone density of elderly females with osteoporosis. *Am J Clin Nutr* 34:819–23.

45. Lindsay, R.; Aitken, J. M.; and Anderson, J. B. 1976. Long term prevention of postmenopausal osteoporosis by estrogen. *Lancet* 1:1038–40.

46. Lindsay, R.; Aitken, J. M.; Hart, D. M.; and Purdie, D. 1978. The effect of ovarian sex steroids on bone mineral status in the oophorectomized rat and in the human. *Postgrad Med J* 54:50–58.

47. Marshall, D. H.; Crilly, R. G.; and Nordin, B. E. 1977. Plasma androstenedione and oestrone levels in normal and osteoporotic postmenopausal women. *Brit Med J* 2:1177–79.

48. Meema, H. E.; Bunker, M. I.; and Meema, S. 1965. Loss of compact bone due to menopause. *Obstet Gynecol* 26:333–38.

49. Meema, S., and Meema, H. E. 1976. Menopausal bone loss and estrogen replacement. *Israel J Med Sci* 12:601–6.

50. Meunier, P.; Courpron, P.; Edourd, C.; Bernard, J.; Bringuier, J.; and Vignon, E. 1973. Physiological senile involution and pathological rarefaction of bone. *Clin Endocrinol Metab* 2:239–56.

51. Minne, H. W.; Leidig, G.; Wuster, C.; Siromachkostov, L.; Baldauf, G.; Bickel, R.; Sauer, P.; Lojen, M.; and Ziegler, G. 1988. A newly developed spine deformity index (SDI) to quantitate vertebral crush fractures in patients with osteoporosis. *Bone Miner* 3, 4:335–49.

52. Nachtigall, L. E.; Nachtigall, R. H.; Nachtigall, R. D.; and Beckman, E. M. 1979. Estrogen replacement therapy I: a 10 year prospective study in the relationship to osteoporosis. *Obstet Gynecol* 53:277–81.

53. Nordin, B. E. C.; Gallagher, J. C.; Aaron, J. E.; and Horsman, H. 1975. Postmenopausal osteopenia and osteoporosis. In *Estrogens in the postmenopause.* Vol. 3 of *Frontiers in hormone research.* Basel: Karger.

54. Nordin, B. E. C.; Horsman, A.; Marshall, D. H.; Simpson, M.; and Waterhouse, G. M. 1979. Calcium requirement and calcium therapy. *Clin Orthop and Rel Res* 140:216–39.

55. Orimo, H.; Shiraki, M.; Hayashi, T.; and Nakamura, T. 1987. Reduced occurrence of vertebral crush fractures in senile osteoporosis treated with 1 alpha (OH)-vitamin Dsub 3. *Bone Miner* 3, 1:47–52.

56. Ott, S. M.; Kilcoyne, R. F.; and Chestnut, C. H., III. 1988. Comparisons among methods of measuring bone mass and relationship to severity of vertebral fractures in osteoporosis. *J Clin Endocrinol Metab* 66, 3:501–7.

57. Overgaard, K.; Riis, B. J.; Christiansen, C.; Podenphant, J.; and Johansen, J. S. 1989. Nasal calcitonin for treatment of established osteoporosis. *Clin Endocrinol* 30, 4:435–42.

58. Pocock, N. A.; Eisman, J. A.; Yeates, M. G.; Sambrook, P. N.; and Eberl, S. 1986. Physical fitness is a major determinant of femoral neck and lumbar spine bone mineral density. *J Clin Invest* 78:618–21.

59. Prince, R. L.; Dick, I. M.; and Price, R. I. 1989. Plasma calcitonin levels are not lower than normal in osteoporotic women. *J Clin Endocrinol Metab* 68, 3:684–87.

59a. Prior, J. C.; Vigna, Y. M.; Schechter, M. T.; and Burgess, A. E. 1990. Spinal bone loss and ovulation disturbances. *NEJM* 323:1221–72.

60. Quigley, M. E. T.; Martin, P. L.; Burnier, A. M.; and Brooks, P. 1987. Estrogen therapy arrests bone loss in elderly women. *Am J Obstet Gynecol* 156, 6:1516–23.

61. Rasmussen, H.; Bordier, P.; Marie, P.; Auguier, L.; Eisinger, J. B.; Kuntz, D.; Caulin, F.; Argemi, B.; Gueris, J.; and Julien, A. 1980. Effect of combined therapy with phosphate and calcitonin on bone volume in osteoporosis. *Metab Bone Dis & Rel Res* 2:107–11.

62. Rawlings, C. E., III; Wilkins, R. H.; Martinez, S.; and Wilkinson, R. H., Jr. 1988. Osteoporotic sacral fractures: a clinical study. *Neurosurgery* 22, 1 I:72–76.

63. Reid, I. R.; Alexander, C. J.; King, A. R.; and Ibbertson, H. K. 1988. Prevention of steroid-induced osteoporosis with (3-amino-1-hydroxy-propylidene)-1, 1-bisphosphonate (APD). *Lancet* 1, 8578:143–46.

64. Reynolds, J. J.; Holick, M. F.; and DeLuca, H. H. F. 1973. The role of vitamin D metabolites in bone resorption. *Calcif Tiss Res* 12:295–301.

65. Riggs, B. L. 1988. Pathogenesis of osteoporosis. *Maturitas* 9:380.

66. Riggs, B. L.; Hodgson, S. F.; Hoffman, D. L.; Kelly, P. J.; Johnson, K. A.; and Taves, D. 1980. Treatment of primary osteroporosis with fluoride and calcium. *JAMA* 243:446.

67. Riggs, B. L.; Seeman, E.; Hodgson, S. F.; Taves, D. R.; and O'Fallon, W. M. 1982. Effect of the fluoride/calcium regimen on vertebral fracture occurrence in postmenopausal osteoporosis. *NEJM* 306:446–50.

68. Riis, B., and Christiansen, C. 1988. Measurement of spinal or peripheral bone mass to estimate early postmenopausal bone loss? *The Am J Med* 84:646–53.

69. Schaadt, O., and Bohr, H. 1988. Different trends of age-related diminution of bone mineral content in the lumbar spine, femoral neck, and femoral shaft in women. *Calcif Tiss Int* 42, 2:71–76.

70. Slemenda, C., and Johnston, C. 1988. Bone mass measurement: which site to measure? *Am J Med* 84, 4:643–45.

71. Smith, D. M.; Khairi, M. R. A.; Norton, J.; and Johnston, C. C., Jr. 1976. Age and activity effects on rate of bone mineral loss. *J Clin Invest* 568:716–21.

72. Sokoll, L. J.; Morrow, F. D.; Quirbach, D. M.; and Dawson-Hughes, B. 1988. Intact parathyrin in postmenopausal women. *Clin Chem* 34, 2:407–10.

73. Sowers, M. F. R.; Wallace, R. B.; and Lemke, J. H. 1986. The relationship of bone mass and fracture history to fluoride and calcium intake: a study of three communities. *Am J Clin Nutr* 44:889–98.

73a. Stall, G.; Harris, S.; Sokoll, L.; and Hughes, B. D. 1990. Accelerated bone loss in hypothyroid patients overtreated with L-thyroxine. *AIM* 113:265–69.

74. Stevenson, J. C. 1987. The use of estrogen replacement therapy on calcitonin in the prevention of postmenopausal bone loss. Fifth International Conference on the Menopause, 6–10 April 1987, Sorrento, Italy.

75. Taelman, P.; Kaufman, J. M.; Janssens, X.; and Vermuelen, A. 1989. Persistence of increased bone resorption and possible role of dehydroepiandrosterone as a bone metabolism determinant in osteoporotic women in late post-menopause. *Maturitas* 11:65–73.

76. Urist, M. R. 1973. Orthopedic management of postmenopausal osteoporosis. *Clin Endocrinol Metab* 2:159–76.

77. Watson, R. C. 1973. Bone growth and physical activity. In *International conference on bone mineral measurements,* 380–85.

78. Yoganandan, N.; Myklebust, J. B.; Cusick, J. R.; Wilson, C. R.; and Sances, A., Jr. 1988. Functional biomechanics of the thoracolumbar vertebral cortex. *Clin Biomech* 3, 1:11–18.

ADDITIONAL RECOMMENDED READINGS

Aitken, J. M.; Hart, D. M.; and Lindsay, R. 1973. Oestrogen replacement therapy for prevention of osteoporosis after oophorectomy. *Brit Med J* 3:515–18.

Brown, D. J.; Spanos, E.; and MacIntyre, I. 1980. Role of pituitary hormones in regulating renal vitamin D metabolism in man. *Brit Med J* 1:277–78.

Cann, C. E.; Genant, H. K.; Ettinger, B.; and Gordan, G. S. 1980. Spinal mineral loss of quantitative computed tomography in oophorectomized women. *JAMA* 244:2056–59.

Crilly, R. G.; Marshall, D. H.; and Nordin, B. E. 1979. Effect of age on plasma androstenedione concentration in oophorectomized women. *Clin Endocrinol (Oxf)* 10:199–201.

Dalen, N., and Olsson, K. E. 1974. Bone mineral content and physical activity. *Acta Orthopaedica Scandinavia* 45:170–74.

Daniell, H. W. 1976. Osteoporosis of the slender smoker. *Arch Intern Med* 136:298 ff.

Deftos, L. J.; Roos, B. A.; Bronzert, D.; and Parthemore, J. G. 1975. Immunochemical heterogeneity of calcitonin in plasma. *Clin Endocrinol Metab* 40:409–12.

Deftos, L. J., and Weisman, M. H. 1980. Influence of age and sex on plasma calcitonin in human beings. *NEJM* 40:409–12.

Gallagher, J. C.; Aaron, J.; Horsman, A.; Marshall, D. H.; Wilkinson, R.; and Nordin, B. E. C. 1973. The crush fracture syndrome in postmenopausal women. *Clin Endocrinol Metab* 2:293.

Gallagher, J. C.; Horsman, A.; and Nordin, B. E. C. 1974. Osteoporosis in the menopause. In *The menopausal syndrome,* ed. R. B. Greenblatt, V. B. Mahesh, and P. G. McDonough. New York: Medcom Press.

Gallagher, J. C.; Melton, L. J.; Riggs, B. L.; and Bergstrath, E. 1980. Epidemiology of fractures of the proximal femur in Rochester, Minnesota, USA. *Clin Orthop* 150:163–71.

Girgis, S. I.; Hillyard, C. J.; MacIntyre, I.; and Szelke, M., eds. 1977. *An immunological comparison of normal circulating calcitonin with calcitonin from medullary carcinoma.* Amsterdam: Elsevier North-Holland Biomedical Press.

Goldsmith, N. F. 1971. Bone-mineral estimation in normal and osteoporotic women: a comparability trial of four methods and seven bone sites. *J Bone Joint Surg (AM)* 53A:83–100.

Heaney, R. P. 1974. Pathophysiology of osteoporosis: implication for treatment. *Tex Med* 70:37–45.

Heath, H., and Sizemore, G. 1977. Plasma calcitonin in normal man. *J Clin Invest* 60:1135–40.

Hillyard, C. J.; Stevenson, J. C.; and MacIntyre, I. 1978. Relative deficiency of plasma-calcitonin in normal women. *Lancet* 961–62.

Horsman, A.; Gallagher, J. C.; Simpson, M.; and Nordin, B. E. C. 1977. Prospective trial of oestrogen and calcium in postmenopausal women. *Brit Med J* 2:789–92.

Horsman, A.; Nordin, B. E. C.; Gallagher, J. C.; Kirby, P. A.; Milner, R. M.; and Simpson, M. 1977. Observations of sequential changes in bone mass in post-menopausal women: a controlled trial of oestrogen and calcium therapy. *Calcif Tiss Res* suppl. 22:217–24.

Hutchinson, T. A.; Polansy, S. M.; and Feinstein, A. R. 1979. Postmenopausal estrogens protect against fractures of hip and distal radius, a case-control study. *Lancet* 2:705–9.

Lindsay, R.; Hart, D. M.; MacLean, A.; Clark, A. C.; Kraszewski, A.; and Garwood, J. 1978. Bone response to termination of oestrogen treatment. *Lancet* 1:1325–27.

Longcope, C.; Jafee, W.; and Griffin, G. 1981. Production rates of androgens and oestrogens in postmenopausal women. *Maturitas* 3:215–23.

MacIntyre, I.; Evans, I. M. A.; Hobitz, H. H. G.; Joplin, G. F.; and Stevenson, J. C. 1980. Chemistry, physiology, and therapeutic applications of calcitonin. *Arthritis and Rheumatism* 23:1139–47.

MacIntyre, I., and Parsons, J. A. 1967. The effect of thyrocalcitonin on blood bone calcium equilibrium in the perfused tibia of the cat. *J Physiol (Lond)* 191:393–405.

Marshall, D. H.; Crilly, R.; and Nordin, B. E. 1978. The relation between plasma androstenedione and oestrone levels in untreated and corticosteroid treated postmenopausal women. *Clin Endocrinol (Oxf)* 9:407–12.

Marshall, D. H., and Nordin, B. E. 1977. The effect of 1 alpha-hydroxyvitamin D3 with and without oestrogens on calcium balance in postmenopausal women. *Clin Endocrinol (Oxf)* 7, suppl.:159s–68s.

Martin, P. 1982. Unpublished data.

Nilson, B. E., and Westlin, N. E. 1971. Bone density in athletes. *Clin Orthop and Rel Res* 77:179–82.

Pak, C. Y. C.; Stewart, A.; Kaplan, R.; Bone, H.; Notz, C.; and Browne, R. 1975. Photon absorptiometric analysis of bone density in primary hyperparathyroidism. *Lancet* 2:7–8.

Rasmussen, H., and Bordier, P. 1974. *The physiological basis of metabolic bone disease.* Baltimore: Williams & Wilkins.

Recker, R. R.; Saville, P. C.; and Heaney, R. P. 1977. Effect of estrogens and calcium carbonate on bone loss in postmenopausal women. *Ann Int Med* 87: 649–55.

Riggs, B. L.; Jowsey, J.; Goldsmith, R. S.; Kelly, P. J.; Hoffman, D. L.; and Arnaud, C. D. 1972. Short and long-term effects of estrogen and synthetic anabolic hormone in postmenopausal osteoporosis. *J Clin Invest* 51:1659–63.

Riggs, B. L.; Jowsey, J.; Kelly, P. J.; Jones, J. D.; and Maher, F. T. 1969. Effect of sex hormones on bone in primary osteoporosis. *J Clin Invest* 48:1065.

Samaan, N., and Anderson, G. D. 1975. Immunoreactive calcitonin in the mother, neonate, child and adult. *Am J Obstet Gynecol* 121:622–25.

Smith, E. L., and Reddan, W. 1976. Physical activity—a modality for bone accretion in the aged: conference on bone mineral measurement. *Am J Roentgenology* 126:1297.

Smith, E. L.; Reddan, W.; and Smith, P. E. 1981. Physical activity and calcium modalities of bone mineral increase in aged women. *Med Sci Sports and Exercise* 13:60–64.

Stevenson, J. C. 1980. The structure and function of calcitonin. *Investigations and Cell Path* 3:187–93.

Stevenson, J. C.; Hillyard, C. J.; Abeyasekara, G.; Phang, K. G.; MacIntyre, I.; Campbell, S.; Young, O.; Townsend, P. T.; and Whitehead, M. I. 1981. Calcitonin and the calcium-regulating hormones in postmenopausal women: effect of estrogens. *Lancet* 693–95.

Stevenson, J. C., and Whitehead, M. I. 1982. Calcitonin secretion and postmenopausal osteoporosis. *Lancet* 804.

Taggart, H.; Ivey, J. L.; Sison, K.; Chestnut, C. H., III; Baylink, D. J.; Huber, M. B.; and Roos, B. A. 1982. Deficient calcitonin response to calcium stimulation in postmenopausal osteoporosis. *Lancet* 475.

Wallach, S., and Henneman, P. H. 1959. Prolonged estrogen therapy in postmenopausal women. *JAMA* 171:1637.

Whyte, M. P.; Bergfeld, M. A.; Murphy, W. A.; Avioli, L. V.; and Teitelbaum, S. L. 1982. Postmenopausal osteoporosis: a heterogeneous disorder as assessed by histomorphometric analysis of iliac crest bone from untreated patients. *Am J Med* 72:193–202.

Wiske, P. S.; Epstein, N. H.; Bell, N. H.; Queener, S. F.; Edmondson, J.; and Johnston, C. C. 1979. Increases in immunoreactive parathyroid hormone with age. *NEJM* 300:1419–21.

CHAPTER 5.   HORMONE REPLACEMENT THERAPY I

1. Abdalla, H. I.; Beastall, G.; Fletcher, D.; Hawthorn, J. S.; Smith, J.; and Hart, D. M. 1987. Sex steroid replacement in post-menopausal women: effects on thyroid hormone status. *Maturitas* 9, 1:49–54.

2. Aedo, A. R.; Le Donne, M.; Landgren, B. M.; and Diczfalusy, E. 1989. Effect of orally administered oestrogens on gonadotropin levels in post-menopausal women. *Maturitas* 11:147–57.

3. Aitken, J. M.; Hart, D. M.; and Lindsay, R. 1973. Oestrogen replacement therapy for prevention of osteoporosis after oophorectomy. *Brit Med J* 3:515–18.

4. Al-Azzawi, F.; Smith, D.; Parkin, D.; Hart, D. M.; and Lindsay, R. 1989. Blood coagulation profile in long-term hormone replacement therapy with mestranol. *Maturitas* 11:95–101.

4a. Alexander, S.; Aksel, S.; Hazelton, J.; Yeoman, R.; and Gilmore, S. 1990. The effect of aging on hypothalamic function in oophorectomized women. *Am J Obstet Gynecol* 162:446–49.

5. Arafat, E. S.; Hargrove, J. T.; Maxson, W. S.; Desiderio, D. M.; Colston Wentz, A.; and Andersen, R. N. 1988. Sedative and hypnotic effects of oral administration of micronized progesterone may be mediated through its metabolites. *Am J Obstet Gynecol* 15, 5:1203–9.

6. Bancroft, J.; Davidson, D. W.; Warner, P.; and Tyrer, G. 1979. Androgens and sexual behavior in women using oral contraceptives. *Clin Endocrinol* 12:327–40.

7. Barrett-Connor, E.; Wingard, D. L.; and Criqui, M. N. 1989. Post-menopausal estrogen use and heart disease risk factors in the 1980's. *JAMA* 261, 14:2095–2100.

8. Bolton, C. H.; Ellwood, M.; Hartog, M.; Martin, R.; Rowe, A. S.; and Wensley, R. T. 1975. Comparison of the effects of ethinyl oestradiol and conjugated equine oestrogens in oophorectomized women. *Clin Endocrinol (Oxf)* 4:131–38.

9. Bradley, D. D.; Wingerd, J.; and Petitti, D. B. 1978. Serum high density lipoprotein cholesterol in women using oral contraceptives, estrogens and progestins. *NEJM* 299:17–20.

10. Brincat, M.; Versi, E.; O'Dowd, T.; Moniz, C. F.; Magos, A.; Kabalan, S.; and Studd, J. W. W. 1987. Skin collagen changes in post-menopausal women receiving oestradiol gel. *Maturitas* 9, 1:1–6.

11. Brown, A. G. 1977. Postmenopausal urinary problems. *Clinics in Obstet & Gynaecol* 4:181–206.

12. Burnier, A. M.; Martin, P. L.; Yen, S. S. C.; and Brooks, P. 1981. Sublingual absorption of micronized 17β estradiol. *Am J Obstet Gynecol* 140: 146–50.

13. Burns, D. D., and Mendels, J. 1979. Serotonin and affective disorders. In *Current developments in psychopharmacology,* ed. W. B. Easman and L. Valzelli, pp. 293–359. Vol 5. New York: SP Medical and Scientific Books.

14. Bush, T. L.; Cowan, L. D.; Barrett-Connor, E.; Criqui, M. H.; Karon, J. M.; Wallace, R. B.; Tyroler, H. A.; and Rifkind, B. M. 1983. Estrogen use and all-cause mortality. *JAMA* 249:903–6.

15. Byrd, B. F.; Burch, J. C.; and Vaughn, W. K. 1977. The impact of long term estrogen support after hysterectomy: a report of 1016 cases. *Ann Surg* 185:574–80.

16. Campbell, S., and Whitehead, M. 1977. Oestrogen therapy and the menopausal syndrome. *Clinics in Obstet & Gynaecol* 4:31–47.

17. Carlstrom, K.; Pschera, H.; and Lunell, N. O. 1988. Serum levels of oestrogens, progesterone, follicle-stimulating hormone and sex-hormone-binding globulin during simultaneous vaginal administration of 17β-oestradiol and progesterone in the pre- and post-menopause. *Maturitas* 10: 307–16.

18. Cutler, W. C.; Davidson, J. M.; and McCoy, N. 1983. Sexual behavior, steroids, and hot flashes during the perimenopause. *Neuroendocrinol* 5, 3:185.

18a. D'Amato, G.; Cavallini, A.; Messa, C.; Mangini, V.; and Misciagna, G. 1989. Serum and bile lipid levels in a postmenopausal woman after percutaneous and oral natural estrogens. *Am J Obstet Gynecol* 160:600–1.

19. Davidson, B. J.; Rea, C. D.; and Valenzuela, G. J. 1988. Atrial natriuretic peptide, plasma renin activity, and aldosterone in women on estrogen therapy and with premenstrual syndrome. *Fertil Steril* 50, 5:743–46.

20. Deghengh, R. 1979. Chemistry and biochemistry of natural estrogens. In *The menopause and post menopause: proceedings of an international symposium,* ed. N. Pasetto, R. Paoletti, and J. L. Ambrus, pp. 3–16. England: MTP Press.

21. Dennerstein, L., and Burrows, G. 1986. Psychological effects of progestogens in the post-menopausal years. *Maturitas* 8:101–6.

22. Dennerstein, L.; Burrows, G. D.; and Hyman, G. 1979. Hormone therapy and affect. *Maturitas* 1:247–59.

23. Deutch, S.; Ossowski, R.; and Benjamin, I. 1981. Comparison between degree of systemic absorption of vaginally and orally administered estrogens at different dose levels in post menopausal women. *Am J Obstet Gynecol* 139:967–68.

24. Englund, D. E., and Johansson, E. D. B. 1980. Endometrial effect of oral estriol treatment in postmenopausal women. *Acta Obstet et Gynecol Scand* 59:449–51.

25. Facchinetti, F.; Martignoni, E.; Petraglia, F.; Sances, M. G.; Nappi, G.; and Genazzani, A. R. 1987. Premenstrual fall of plasma b-endorphin in patients with pre-menstrual syndrome. *Fertil Steril* 47, 4:570–73.

26. Fahraeus, L.; Larsson-Cohn, U.; and Wallentin, L. 1983. L-norgestrel and progesterone have different influences on plasma lipoproteins. *Eur J Clin Invest* 13:447.

27. Fedor-Freybergh, P. 1977. The influence of estrogens on the well-being and mental performance in the climacterica and postmenopausal women. *Acta Obstet et Gynecol Scand* 64, suppl. 1:1–66.

28. Feigen, G. A.; Fraser, R. C.; and Peterson, N. W. 1978. Sex hormones and the immune response II: perturbation of antibody production by estradiol 17β. *Int Arch Allergy Appl Immunol* 57:488–97.

29. Fletcher, C. D.; Farish, E.; Dagen, M. M.; Allam, B. F.; and Hart, D. M. 1988. Effects of conjugated equine oestrogens with and without the addition of cyclical norgestrel on serum and urine electrolytes, and the biochemical indices of bone metabolism and liver function. *Maturitas* 9:347–57.

30. Fraser, D. I.; Padwick, M. L.; Whitehead, M. I.; White, J.; Ryder, T. A.; and Pryse-Davies, J. 1989. The effects of the addition of nomegestrol acetate to post-menopausal oestrogen therapy. *Maturitas* 11:21–34.

31. Gambrell, R. D. 1982. The menopause: benefits and risks of estrogen-progestogen replacement therapy. *Fertil Steril* 4:457–74.

32. García, C.-R., and Drill, V. A. 1977. Contraceptive steroids and liver lesions. *J Toxicol Environ Health* 3:197–206.

33. Genazzani, A. R.; Facchinetti, F.; Ricci-Danero, M. G.; Parini, D.; Petraglia, F.; LaRosa, R.; and D'Antona, N. 1981. Beta-lipotropin and beta-endorphin in physiological and surgical menopause. *J Endocrinol Invest* 4:375–78.

34. Geola, F.; Frumar, A.; Tataryn, I.; Lu, K.; Hershman, J.; Eggena, P.; Sambhi, M.; and Judd, H. 1980. Biological effects of various doses of conjugated equine estrogens in postmenopausal women. *J Clin Endocrinol Metab* 51:620–25.

35. Gordan, W. E.; Herman, H. W.; and Hunter, D. C. 1979. Treatment of

atrophic vaginitis in postmenopausal women with micronized estradiol cream—a follow up study. *J Kentucky Med Assn* 77:337–39.

36. Greenblatt, R. B. 1987. The use of androgens in the menopause and other gynecologic disorders. *Obstet Gynecol Clin NA* 14, 1:251–68.

37. Greene, J. G., and Hart, D. M. 1987. Evaluation of a psychological treatment programme for climacteric women. *Maturitas* 9, 1:41–48.

38. Hargrove, J. T.; Maxson, W. S.; Colston Wentz, A.; and Burnett, L. S. 1989. Menopausal hormone replacement therapy with continuous daily oral micronized estradiol and progesterone. *Obstet Gynecol* 73, 4:606–12.

39. Haspels, A. A.; Bennink, J. H.; VanKeep, P. A.; and Schreurs, W. H. 1975. Estrogens and vitamin B6. *Front Horm Res* 3:199–207.

40. Haspels, A. A.; Coelingh Bennink, H. J. T.; and Schreurs, W. H. P. 1978. Disturbance of tryptophan metabolism and its correction during oestrogen treatment in postmenopausal women. *Maturitas* 1:15–20.

41. Hasselquist, M.; Goldberg, N.; Schroeter, A.; and Spelsbert, T. 1980. Isolation and characterization of the estrogen receptor in human skin. *J Clin Endocrinol Metab* 50:76–82.

42. Henderson, B. E.; Paganini-Hill, A.; and Ross, R. K. 1988. Estrogen replacement therapy and protection from acute myocardial infarction. *Am J Obstet Gynecol* 159, 2:312–17.

43. Hirvonen, E.; Malkonen, M.; and Manninen, V. 1980. Effects of different progestogens on lipoproteins during postmenopausal replacement therapy. *NEJM* 304:560–63.

44. Hirvonen, E.; Stenman, U. H.; Malkonen, M.; Rasi, V.; Vartiainen, E.; and Ylostalo, P. 1988. New natural oestradiol/cyproterone acetate oral contraceptive for pre-menopausal women. *Maturitas* 10:201–13.

45. Holmgren, P. A.; Lindskog, M.; and von Schoultz, B. 1989. Vaginal rings for continuous low-dose release of oestradiol in the treatment of urogenital atrophy. *Maturitas* 11:55–63.

46. Honore, I. H. 1980. Increased incidence of symptomatic cholesterol cholelithiasis in perimenopausal women receiving estrogen replacement therapy. *J Reprod Med* 25:187–90.

47. Hovik, P.; Sundsbak, H. P.; Gaasemyr, M.; and Sandvik, L. 1989. Comparison of continuous and sequential oestrogen-progestogen treatment in women with climacteric symptoms. *Maturitas* 11:75–82.

48. Jasonni, V. M.; Bulletti, C.; Naldi, S.; Ciotti, P.; DiCosmo, D.; Lazzaretto, R.; and Flamigni, C. 1988. Biological and endocrine aspects of transdermal 17β-oestradiol administration in post-menopausal women. *Maturitas* 10:263–70.

49. Jasonni, V. M.; Naldi, S.; Ciotti, P.; Bulletti, C.; and Flamigni, C. 1987. Comparative metabolism of oestrone sulphate after oral and intravenous administration in post-menopausal women. *Maturitas* 9:201–5.

49a. Jensen, J., and Christiansen, C. 1987. Dose-response effects on serum lipids and lipoproteins following combined oestrogen-progestogen therapy in post-menopausal women. *Maturitas* 9:259–66.

50. Jensen, J.; Christiansen, C.; and Rodbro, P. 1986. Oestrogen-progestogen replacement therapy changes body composition in early post-menopausal women. *Maturitas* 8:209–16.

51. Jensen, P. B.; Jensen, J.; Riis, B. J.; Rodbro, P.; Strom, V.; and Christiansen, C. 1987. Climacteric symptoms after oral and percutaneous hormone replacement therapy. *Maturitas* 9:207–15.

52. Jensen, J.; Riis, B. J.; Strom, V.; and Christiansen, C. 1989. Long-term and withdrawal effects of two different oestrogen-progestogen combinations on lipid and lipoprotein profiles in post-menopausal women. *Maturitas* 11:117–28.

53. Johannisson, E.; Landgren, B. M.; and Diczfalusy, E. 1988. Endometrial and vaginal response to three different oestrogen preparations administered by the transdermal and oral routes. *Maturitas* 10:181–92.

54. Kegel, A. M. 1951. Physiologic therapy for urinary stress incontinence. *JAMA* 146:915–17.

55. Kopera, H.; Steffensen, K.; Dieben, T. O. M.; and Assendorp, R. 1988. An oral contraceptive particularly suitable for women over 35. *Maturitas,* suppl. 1:141–54.

56. Kupperman, H. S.; Wetchler, B. B.; and Blatt, M. H. G. 1959. Contemporary therapy for the menopausal syndrome. *JAMA* 171:1627–37.

57. Larsson-Cohn, U.; Johansson, E.; Kagedal, B.; and Wallentin, L. 1977. Serum FSH, LH and oestrone levels in postmenopausal patients on oestrogen therapy. *Br J Obstet Gynaecol* 86:367–72.

58. Lauritzen, C. 1973. The management of the premenopausal and the post-menopausal patient. *Front Horm Res* 2:2–21.

58a. Lindberg, U. B.; Enk, L.; Crona, N.; and Silverstolpe, G. 1988. A comparison of the effects of ethinyl estradiol and estradiol valerate on serum and lipoprotein lipids. *Maturitas* 10:343–52.

59. Magos, A. L.; Brincat, M.; O'Dowd, T.; Wardle, P. J.; Schlesinger, P.; and Studd, J. W. W. 1985. Endometrial and menstrual response to subcutaneous oestradiol and testosterone implants and continuous oral progestogen therapy in post-menopausal women. *Maturitas* 7, 4:297–302.

60. Martin, P.; Yen, S. S. C.; Burnier, A. M.; and Hermann, H. 1979. Systemic absorption and sustained effects of vaginal estrogen creams. *JAMA* 242:2699–2700.

61. Mashchak, C. A.; Lobo, R. A.; Dozono-Takano, R.; Eggena, P.; Nakamura, R. M.; Brenner, P. F.; and Mishell, D. R. 1982. Comparison of pharmacodynamic properties of various estrogen formulations. *Am J Obstet Gynecol* 144:511–18.

62. Mathur, R. S.; Landgrebe, S. C.; Moody, L. O.; Semmens, J. P.; and Williamson, H. O. 1985. The effect of estrogen treatment on plasma concentrations of steroid hormones, gonadotropins, prolactin and sex hormone-binding globulin in post-menopausal women. *Maturitas* 7:129–33.

62a. Molander, U.; Milsom, I.; Ekelund, P.; Mellstrom, D.; and Eriksson, O. 1990. Effect of oral oestriol on vaginal flora and cytology and urogenital symptoms in the post-menopause. *Maturitas* 12:113–20.

63. Moore, B.; Paterson, M.; and Sturdee, D. 1987. Effect of oral hormone replacement therapy on liver function tests. *Maturitas* 9, 1:7–16.

63a. Morris, M.; Salmon, P.; Steinberg, H.; Sykes, E. A.; Bouloux, P.; Newbould, E.; McLoughlin, L.; Besser, G. M.; and Grossman, A. 1990. Endogenous opiods modulate the cardiovascular response to mental stress. *Psychoneuroendocrinology* 15:185–92.

64. Myers, E. R.; Sondheimer, S. J.; Freeman, E. W.; Strauss, J. F., III; and Rickels, K. 1987. Serum progesterone levels following vaginal administration of progesterone during the luteal phase. *Fertil Steril* 47, 1:71–75.

65. Nielson, F. H.; Honore, E.; Kristoffersen, K.; Secher, N. J.; and Pederson, G. T. 1977. Changes in serum lipids during treatment with norgestrel, oestradiol-valerate and cycloprogynon. *Acta Obstet et Gynecol Scand* 56:367–70.

66. Ottoson, U. B.; Johansson, B. G.; and von Schoultz, B. 1985. Subfractions of high density lipoprotein cholesterol during estrogen replacement therapy: comparison between progestogens and natural progesterone. *Am J Obstet Gynecol* 1151:746.

67. Padwick, M. L.; Endacott, J.; Matson, C.; and Whitehead, M. I. 1986. Absorption and metabolism of oral progesterone when administered twice daily. *Fertil Steril* 46, 3:402–7.

68. Padwick, M. L.; Pryse-Davies, J.; Path, F. R. C.; and Whitehead, M. I. 1986. A simple method for determining the optimal dosage of progestin in postmenopausal women receiving estrogens. *NEJM* 315, 15:930–34.

69. Pallas, K. G.; Holzwarth, G. J.; Stern, M. P.; and Lucas, C. P. 1977. The effects of conjugated estrogen on the renin-angiotensin system. *J Clin Endocrinol Metab* 44:1061–68.

70. Petraglia, F.; DiMeo, G.; DeLeo, V.; Nappi, C.; Facchinetti, F.; and Genazzani, A. R. 1986. Plasma B-endorphin levels in anovulatory states: changes after treatments for the induction of ovulation. *Fertil Steril* 45, 2:185–90.

71. Polan, M. L.; Daniele, A.; and Kuo, A. 1988. Gonadal steroids modulate human monocyte interleukin-1 (IL-1) activity. *Fertil Steril* 49, 6:964–68.

72. Punonen, R. 1972. Effect of castration and peroral estrogen therapy on the skin. *Acta Obstet et Gynecol Scand* suppl 21:1–44.

73. Punonen, R.; Lammintausta, R.; Erkkola, R.; Rauramo, L. 1980. Estra-

diol valerate therapy and the renin-aldosterone system in castrated women. *Maturitas* 2:91–94.

74. Punonen, R., and Rauramo, L. 1977. The effect of long-term oral oestriol succinate therapy on the skin of castrated women. *Ann Chir Gynaecol* 66: 214–15.

75. Rigg, L. A.; Hermann, H.; and Yen, S. S. C. 1977. Absorption of estrogens from vaginal creams. *NEJM* 242:2699–2700.

76. Riis, B. J.; Johansen, J.; and Christiansen, C. 1988. Continuous oestrogen-progestogen treatment and bone metabolism in post-menopausal women. *Maturitas* 10:51–88.

77. Riphagen, F. E. 1988. Contraceptive behavior of women aged over 35. *Maturitas* suppl. 1:51–61.

78. Rose, D. P. 1966. Excretion of xanthurenic acid in the urine of women taking progestogen-oestrogen preparations. *Nature* 210:196–97.

79. Schiff, I., and Ryan, K. 1980. Benefits of estrogen replacement. *Obstet Gynecol Survey* 35:400–11.

80. Schiff, I.; Tulchinsky, D.; and Ryan, K. J. 1977. Vaginal absorption of estrogen and 17β estradiol. *Fertil Steril* 23:1063–66.

81. Schiff, I.; Wentworth, B.; Koos, B.; Ryan, K. J.; and Tulchinsky, D. 1978. Effect of estriol administration on the hypogonadal woman. *Fertil Steril* 30:278–82.

82. Schneider, M. A.; Brotherton, P. L.; and Hailes, J. 1977. The effect of exogenous oestrogens on depression in menopausal women. *Med J Aust* 2:162–63.

83. Schwartz, U.; Schneller, E.; Moltz, L.; and Hammerstein, J. 1982. Vaginal administration of ethinyl estradiol: effects on ovulation and hepatic transcortin synthesis. *Contraception* 25:253.

84. Semmens, J. P., and Wagner, G. 1982. Estrogen deprivation and vaginal function in post menopausal women. *JAMA* 248:445–48.

84a. Sherwin, B. 1988. The role of androgens in menopausal women. In *Androgens in the menopause,* ed. Leon Speroff. Marietta, Ga.: Reid-Rowell.

85. Sherwin, B. B., and Gelfand, M. M. 1989. A prospective one-year study of estrogen and progestin in postmenopausal women: effects on clinical symptoms and lipoprotein lipids. *Obstet Gynecol* 73, 5:759–66.

86. Sherwin, B. B.; Gelfand, M. M.; and Brender, W. 1985. Androgen enhances sexual motivation in females: a prospective, crossover study of sex steroid administration in the surgical menopause. *Psychosomatic Medicine* 474:339–51.

87. Silfverstrolpe, G.; Gustafson, A.; Samsioe, G.; and Svanborg, A. 1979. Lipid metabolic studies in oophorectomized women: effects of three different progestogens. *Acta Obstet et Gynecol Scand* suppl. 88:89–95.

88. Shoupe, D.; Mont, F. J.; and Lobo, R. A. 1985. The effects of estrogen

and progestin on endogenous opioid activity in oophorectomized women. *J Clin Endocrinol Metab* 60, 1:178–83.

89. Skouby, S. O. 1988. Oral contraceptives: hormonal dose and effects on carbohydrate metabolism. *Maturitas* suppl. 1:111–15.

90. Sporrong, T.; Samsioe, G.; Larsen, S.; and Mattson, L.-A. 1989. A novel statistical approach to analysis of bleeding patterns during continuous hormone replacement therapy. *Maturitas* 11:209–15.

91. Stark, M.; Adonia, A.; Milwidsky, A.; Gilon, G.; and Palti, Z. 1978. Can estrogens be useful for treatment of vaginal relaxation in elderly women? *Am J Obstet Gynecol* 131:585–86.

92. Studd, J. W. W.; Collins, W. P.; Chakravarti, S.; Newton, J. R.; Oram, D.; and Parsons, A. 1977. Oestradiol and testosterone implants in the treatment of psychosexual problems in the postmenopausal woman. *Br J Obstet Gynaecol* 84:314–16.

93. Teichmann, A. T. 1988. Age, metabolism and oral contraception. *Maturitas* suppl. 1:117–30.

94. Teichmann, A. T.; Wieland, H.; Cremer, P.; Hinney, B.; Kuhn, W.; and Seidel, D. 1985. Effects of medrogestone and conjugated oestrogens on serum lipid and lipoprotein concentrations. *Maturitas* 7:343–50.

94a. Teran, A. Z., and Gambrell, R. D. 1988. Androgens in clinical practice. In *Androgens in the menopause,* ed. Leon Speroff. Marietta, Ga.: Reid-Rowell.

95. Thomson, J.; Maddock, J.; Aylward, M.; and Oswald, I. 1977. Relationship between nocturnal plasma oestrogen concentration and free plasma tryptophan in postmenopausal women. *J Endoc* 72:395–96.

96. Thomson, J., and Oswald, I. 1977. Effect of oestrogen on the sleep, mood and anxiety of menopausal women. *Brit Med J* 2:317–19.

97. VanKeep, P. A.; Serr, D. M.; Greenblatt, R. B.; and Kopera, H. 1978. Effects, side effects, and dosage schemes of various sex hormones in the peri and post menopause. Workshop report in *Female and male climacteric: current opinion 1978.* Baltimore: University Park Press.

98. Veith, J. L.; Anderson, J.; Slade, S. A.; Thompson, P.; Laugel, G. R.; and Getzlaf, S. 1983. Plasma β-endorphin, pain thresholds and anxiety levels across the human menstrual cycle. *Physiol & Behav* 32:31–34.

99. Von Schoultz, B. 1986. Climacteric complaints as influenced by progestogens. *Maturitas* 8:107–12.

99a. Wild, R. A.; Grubb, B.; Hartz, A.; Van Nort, J. J.; Bachman, W.; and Bartholomew, M. 1990. Clinical signs of androgen excess as risk factors for coronary artery disease. *Fertil Steril* 54:255–59.

100. Ylostalo, P.; Kauppila, A.; Kivinen, S.; Tuimala, R.; and Vihko, R. 1983. Endocrine and metabolic effects of low dose estrogen-progestin treatment in climacteric women. *Obstet Gynecol* 62:682–86.

101. Ylostalo, P.; Vartiainen, E.; Stenman, U.-H.; and Widholm, O. 1986.

Ovarian function during oestrogen-progestin replacement treatment in pre-menopausal women. *Maturitas* 8:19–27.

CHAPTER 6. HORMONE REPLACEMENT THERAPY II: THE CANCER RISK

1. Baker, L. 1982. Breast cancer detection demonstration project: Five year summary report. *Cancer* 32:194.
2. Beard, C. M.; Kottke, T. E.; Annegers, J. F.; and Ballard, D. J. 1989. The Rochester coronary heart disease project: Effect of cigarette smoking, hypertension, diabetes, and steroidal estrogen use on coronary heart disease among 40- to 59-year-old women, 1960 through 1982. *Mayo Clin Proc* 64:1471–80.
3. Bergkvist, L.; Adami, H. O.; Persson, I.; Hoover, R.; and Schairer, C. 1989. The risk of breast cancer after estrogen and estrogen-progestin replacement. *NEJM* 321:293–97.
4. Brownson, R. C.; Blackwell, C. W.; Pearson, D. K.; Reynolds, R. D.; Richens, J. W., Jr.; and Papermaster, B. W. 1988. Risk of breast cancer in relation to cigarette smoking. *Arch Intern Med* 148, 1:140–44.
5. Buchman, M. I.; Kramer, E.; and Felman, G. B. 1978. Aspiration curettage for asymptomatic patients receiving estrogen. *Obstet Gynecol* 51:339–41.
6. Budoff, P. W., and Sommers, J. C. 1979. Estrogen progesterone therapy in postmenopausal women. *J Reprod Med* 22:241–47.
7. Campbell, S.; Minardi, J.; McQueen, J.; and Whitehead, M. 1978. Endometrial factors: the modifying effect of progestogen on the response of the postmenopausal endometrium to exogenous estrogens. *Postgrad Med J* 54:59–64.
8. Cooper, R. A. 1989. Mammography. *Clinics in Obstet & Gynaecol* 32, 4:768–84.
9. Creasman, W. T.; Henderson, D.; Hinshaw, W.; and Clarke-Pearson, D. L. 1986. Estrogen replacement therapy in the patient treated for endometrial cancer. *Obstet Gynecol* 67:326–30.
10. Cummings, S. R.; Black, D. M.; and Rubin, S. M. 1989. Lifetime risks of hip, collar, or vertebral fracture and coronary heart disease among white postmenopausal women. *Arch Intern Med* 149:2445–48.
11. Cutler, W. 1988. *Hysterectomy: before and after.* New York: Harper & Row.
12. Denis, R.; Barnett, J. M.; and Forbes, S. E. 1973. Diagnostic suction curettage. *Obstet Gynecol* 42:301–3.
13. *Dorland's illustrated medical dictionary.* 1974. 25th ed. Philadelphia: Saunders.

14. Dupont, W. D., and Page, D. L. 1985. Risk factors for breast cancer in women with proliferative breast disease. *NEJM* 312:146-51.

15. Eddy, D. M.; Hasselblad, V.; McGivney, W.; and Hendee, W. 1988. The value of mammography screening in women under age 50 years. *JAMA* 259, 10:1512-19.

16. Fisher, B.; Redmond, C.; Poisson, R.; Margolese, R.; Wolmark, N.; Wickerham, L.; Fisher, E.; Deutsch, M.; Caplan, R.; Pilch, Y.; Glass, A.; Shibata, H.; Lerner, H.; Terz, J.; and Sidorovich, L. 1989. Eight-year results of a randomized clinical trial comparing total mastectomy and lumpectomy with or without irradiation in the treatment of breast cancer. *NEJM* 320, 13:822-28.

17. Flickinger, G. L.; Elsner, C.; Illingworth, D. V.; Muechler, E. K.; and Mikhail, G. 1977. Estrogen and progesterone receptors in the female genital tract of humans and monkeys. *Ann NY Academy of Sciences* 286:180-89.

18. Fraser, D. I.; Padwick, M. L.; Whitehead, M. I.; White, J.; Ryder, T. A.; and Pryse-Davies, J. 1989. The effects of the addition of nomegestrol acetate to post-menopausal oestrogen therapy. *Maturitas* 11:21-34.

19. Gambrell, R. D. 1987. Use of progestogen therapy. *Am J Obstet Gynecol* 156, 5:1304-13.

20. ———. 1986. Prevention of endometrial cancer with progestogens. *Maturitas* 8:159-68.

21. ———. 1982. The menopause: benefits and risks of estrogen-progestogen replacement therapy. *Fertil Steril* 37:457-74.

22. Gambrell, R. D.; Maier, R. C.; and Sanders, B. I. 1983. Decreased incidence of breast cancer in postmenopausal estrogen-progestogen users. *Obstet Gynecol* 62:435-43.

23. Gambrell, R. D., Jr. 1982. Role of hormones in the etiology and prevention of endometrial and breast cancer. *Acta Obstet et Gynecol Scand* suppl. 106:37-46.

24. ———. 1977. Postmenopausal bleeding. *Clinics in Obstet & Gynaecol* 4:1.

25. Gambrell, R. D., Jr.; Castaneda, T. A.; and Ricci, C. A. 1978. Management of postmenopausal bleeding to prevent endometrial cancer. *Maturitas* 1:99-106.

26. Gambrell, R. D., Jr.; Massey, F. M.; Castaneda, T. A.; Ugenas, A. J.; Ricci, C. A.; and Wright, J. M. 1980. Use of progestogen challenge test to reduce the risk of endometrial cancer. *Obstet Gynecol* 55:732-38.

27. Gordon, J.; Reagan, J. W.; Finkle, W. D.; and Ziel, H. K. 1977. Estrogen and endometrial carcinoma: independent pathology review supporting original risk estimate. *NEJM* 297:570-71.

28. Greenblatt, R. B.; Mahesh, V. B.; and Sullivan, D. 1987. Gross cystic disease of the breast. *Maturitas* 9:171-81.

29. Gurpide, E.; Gusberg, S. B.; and Tseng, L. 1976. Oestradiol binding and

metabolism in human endometrial hyperplasia and adenocarcinoma. *J Steroid Biochem* 7:891–96.

30. Gusberg, S. B. 1976. The individual at high risk for endometrial carcinoma. *Am J Obstet Gynecol* 126:535.

31. ———. 1975. A strategy for the control of endometrial cancer. *Proc Royal Soc of Med* 68:163–68.

32. Guyton, A. C. 1981. *Textbook of medical physiology.* 6th ed. Philadelphia: Saunders.

33. Hammond, C. B. 1980. Progestins with estrogen replacement curb cancer risk. *Ob/Gyn News,* Sept. 15, pp. 4–5.

34. Hammond, C. B.; Jelovsek, F. R.; Lee, K. L.; Creasman, W. T.; and Parker, R. T. 1979. Effects of long term estrogen replacement therapy II: neoplasia. *Am J Obstet Gynecol* 133:537–47.

34a. Hargrove J. T.; Maxson, W. S.; Colston Wentz, A.; and Burnett, L. S. 1989. Menopausal hormone replacement therapy with continuous daily oral micronized estradiol and progesterone. *Obstet Gynecol* 73, 4:606–12.

35. Hayes, H., Jr.; Vandergrift, J.; and Diner, W. C. 1988. Mammography and breast implants. *Plastic and Reconstructive Surgery* 82, 1:1–8.

36. Heinonen, P. K.; Morsky, P.; Aine, R.; Koivula, T.; and Pystynen, P. 1988. Hormonal activity of epithelial ovarian tumours in post-menopausal women. *Maturitas* 9:325–38.

37. Holst, J.; Cajander, S.; and von Schoultz, B. 1986. Endometrial response in postmenopausal women during treatment with percutaneous 17β-oestradiol opposed by oral progesterone. *Maturitas* 8:201–7.

38. Hoover, R.; Gray, L. A.; Cole, P.; and MacMahon, B. 1976. Menopausal estrogens and breast cancer. *NEJM* 295:401–5.

39. Huggins, G. R., and Zucker, P. K. 1987. Oral contraceptives and neoplasia: 1987 update. *Fertil Steril* 47, 4:733–61.

40. Hughes, L. E.; Mansel, R. E.; and Webster, D. J. T. 1989. Chapter 3—aberrations of normal development and involution (ANDI): a concept of benign breast disorders based on pathogenesis. In *Benign disorders and diseases of the breast: concepts and clinical management.* London: Bailliere Tindall.

41. ———. 1989. Chapter 4—the epidemiology of benign breast disease and assessment of cancer risk. In *Benign disorders and diseases of the breast: concepts and clinical management.* London: Bailliere Tindall.

42. Hulka, B. 1980. Effect of exogenous estrogen on postmenopausal women: the epidemiologic evidence. *Obstet Gynecol Surv* 35:389–99.

43. Hutton, J. D.; Morse, A. R.; Anderson, M. C.; and Beard, R. W. 1978. Endometrial assessment with Isaacs Cell Sampler. *Brit Med J* 1:947–49.

44. Jick, S. S.; Walker, A. M.; and Jick, H. 1986. Conjugated estrogens and fibrocystic breast disease. *Am J Epidemiol* 124, 5:746–51.

45. Jones, G. 1966. Sexual difficulties after 50: gynecological comments. *Obstet Gynecol Surv* 21:628.

46. Jordan, J. A. 1980. Is death from cervical cancer avoidable? *Royal Soc of Health J* 100:231–33.

47. Kaizer, L.; Fishell, E. K.; Hunt, J. W.; Foster, F. S.; and Boyd, N. F. 1988. Ultrasonographically defined parenchymal patterns of the breast: relationship to mammographic patterns and other risk factors for breast cancer. *Br J Radiol* 61, 7:118–24.

48. Kay, C. R. 1978. Logistics of study on hormone therapy in the climacteric. *Postgrad Med J* 2:92–94.

49. King, R. J.; Whitehead, M. I.; Campbell, S.; and Minardi, J. 1978. Biochemical studies of endometrium from postmenopausal women receiving hormone replacement therapy. *Postgrad Med J* 54:65–68.

49a. Kistner, R. W. 1977. Estrogens and endometrial cancer. *Obstet Gynecol* 48:479.

50. Kupperman, H. S.; Wetchler, B. B.; and Blatt, M. H. G. 1959. Contemporary therapy for the menopausal syndrome. *JAMA* 171:1627–37.

51. Lais, C. W.; Williams, T. J.; and Gaffey, T. A. 1988. Prevalence of ovarian cancer found at the time of infertility microsurgery. *Fertil Steril* 49, 3:551–53.

52. Larsson-Cohn, U.; Johansson, E.; Kagedal, B.; and Wallentin, L. 1977. Serum FSH, LH and oestrone levels in postmenopausal patients on oestrogen therapy. *Br J Obstet Gynaecol* 85:367–72.

53. London, S. J.; Colditz, G. A.; Stampfer, M. J.; Willett, W. C.; Rosner, B.; and Speizer, F. E. 1989. Prospective study of relative weight, height, and risk of breast cancer. *JAMA* 262, 20:2853–58.

54. Ludwig, N. 1982. The morphologic response of the human endometrium to long-term treatment with progestational agents. *Am J Obstet Gynecol* 142:796–808.

55. McBride, J. M. 1959. Premenopausal cystic glandular hyperplasia and endometrial carcinoma. *J Ob Gyn of the Br Commonwealth* 66:288 ff.

56. McDonald, T. W.; Annegers, J. F.; and O'Fallon, W. M. 1977. Exogenous estrogen and endometrial carcinoma. *Am J Obstet Gynecol* 127:572–80.

57. MacMahon, B. 1974. Risk factors for endometrial cancer. *Gynecol Oncol* 2:122–29.

58. Mango, D.; Scirpa, P.; Liberati, M.; Manna, P.; Ricci, S.; and Mancuso, S. 1989. Gonadotropin response to releasing hormone in post-menopausal patients with ovarian tumors. *Maturitas* 11:129–36.

59. Mauvais-Jarvis, P.; Sitruk-Ware, R.; and Kuttenn, F. 1985. Luteal phase defect and benign breast disease: relationship to breast cancer genesis. *Breast Diseases—Senologia* 1, 1:58–66.

60. Menczer, J.; Modan, M.; Ezra, D.; and Serr, D. M. 1980. Prognosis in

pre- and post-menopausal patients with endometrial adenocarcinoma. *Maturitas* 2:37–44.

61. Mickal, A., and Torres, J. 1974. Adenocarcinoma of endometrium. In *The menopausal syndrome*, ed. R. B. Greenblatt, V. B. Mahesh, and P. G. McDonough. New York: Medcome Press.

62. Ng, A. B. P., and Reagan, J. W. 1970. Incidence and prognosis of endometrial carcinoma by histologic grade and extent. *Obstet Gynecol* 35: 437–42.

63. Ng, A. B. P.; Reagan, J. W.; Storaasli, J. P.; and Wentz, W. B. 1973. Mixed adenosquamos carcinoma of the endometrium, *Am J Clin Pathol* 59:765–81.

64. Nyirjesy, I., and Billingsley, F. S. 1984. Detection of breast carcinoma in a gynecologic practice. *Obstet Gynecol* 64, 6:747–51.

64a. Osmers, R.; Volksen, M.; and Schauer, A. 1990. Vaginosonography for early detection of endometrial carcinoma? *Lancet* 335:1569–71.

65. Paterson, M. E. L.; Wade-Evans, T.; Sturdee, D. W.; Thom, M. H.; and Studd, J. W. W. 1980. Endometrial disease after treatment with oestrogens and progestogens in the climacteric. *Brit Med J* 96:1–8.

66. Reagan, J. W., and Ng, A. B. P. 1973. *The cells of uterine adenocarcinoma*. 2d ed. Basel: Kargel.

67. Rosenfeld, D. L., and García, C.-R. 1975. Endometrial biopsy in the cycle of conception. *Fertil Steril* 26:1088–93.

68. Ross, R. K.; Paganini-Hill, A.; Gerkins, V. R.; Mack, T. M.; *et al.* 1980. A case control study of menopausal estrogen therapy and breast cancer. *JAMA* 243:1635.

69. Schapira, D. V.; Kumar, N. B.; Lyman, G. H.; and Cox, C. E. 1990. Abdominal obesity and breast cancer risk. *Ann Int Med* 112, 3:182–86.

70. Schiff, I., and Ryan, K. 1980. Benefits of estrogen replacement. *Obstet Gynecol Surv* 35:400–11.

71. Schurz, B.; Metka, M.; Heytmanek, G.; Wimmer-Greinecker, G.; and Reinold, E. 1988. Sonographic changes in the endometrium of climacteric women during hormonal treatment. *Maturitas* 9:367–74.

72. Sitruk-Ware, L. R.; Sterkers, N.; Mowszowicz, I.; and Mauvais-Jarvis, P. 1977. Inadequate corpus luteal function in women with benign breast diseases. *J Clin Endocrinol Metab* 44:771–74.

73. Sitruk-Ware, R.; deLignieres, B.; and Mauvais-Jarvis, P. 1986. Progestogen treatment in post-menopausal women. *Maturitas* 8:95–100.

74. Skrabanek, P. 1985. False premises and false promises of breast cancer screening. *Lancet* 316–20.

75. Stahl, N. L. 1974. Hormones and cancer. In *The menopausal syndrome,* ed. R. B. Greenblatt, V. B. Mahesh, and P. G. McDonough. New York: Medcome Press.

76. Sturdee, D. W.; Wade-Evans, T.; Paterson, M. E.; Thon, M.; and Studd,

J. W. 1978. Relations between bleeding pattern, endometrial histology, and oestrogen treatment in menopausal women. *Brit Med J* 1:1575–77.

77. Tseng, L., and Gurpide, E. 1973. Effect of estrone and progesterone on the nuclear uptake of estradiol by slices of endometrium. *Endocrinol* 93: 245–48.

78. Turner, J.; Roy, D.; Irwins, G.; Blaney, R.; Odling-Smee, W.; and Mackenzie, G. 1984. Does a booklet on breast self-examination improve subsequent detection rates? *Lancet* 337–39.

79. Valle, R. F. 1981. Hysteroscopic evaluation of patients with abnormal uterine bleeding. *Surg Gynecol Obstet* 153:521–26.

80. Vanderick, C.; Beernaert, J.; and DeMuylder, E. 1975. Hormonal contraception, sequential formulations and the endometrium. *Contraception* 12: 655–64.

81. VanKeep, P. A.; Serr, D. M.; Greenblatt, R. B.; and Kopera, H. 1978. Effects, side effects, and dosage schemes of various sex hormones in the peri and post menopause. Workshop report in *Female and male climacteric: current opinion 1978.* Baltimore: University Park Press.

82. Verbeek, A. I. M.; Hendriks, J. H. C. L.; Holland, R.; *et al.* 1984. Screening and breast cancer. *Lancet* 690.

83. Vorherr, H. 1987. Endocrinology of breast cancer. *Maturitas* 9:113–22.

84. ———. 1986. Fibrocystic breast disease: pathophysiology, pathomorphology, clinical picture, and management. *Am J Obstet Gynecol* 154:161–79.

85. Waldron, I. 1982. An analysis of causes of sex differences in mortality and morbidity. In *The fundamental connection between nature and nurture,* ed. W. R. Gove and G. R. Carpenter. Lexington, Mass.: Lexington Books.

86. Weiss, N. J. 1975. Risks and benefits of estrogen use. *NEJM* 293:1200–2.

87. Wentz, W. B. 1985. Progestin therapy in lesions of the endometrium. *Seminars in Oncology* 12, 1:23–27.

88. ———. 1974. Progestin therapy in endometrial hyperplasia. *Gynecol Oncol* 2:362–67.

89. Whitehead, M. I.; McQueen, J.; Minardi, J.; and Campbell, S. 1978. Clinical considerations in the management of the menopause: the endometrium. *Postgrad Med J* 54:69–73.

90. Whitehead, M. I.; Townsend, P. T.; Pryse-Davies, J.; Ryder, T. A.; and King, R. J. B. 1981. Effects of estrogens and progestins on the biochemistry and morphology of the postmenopausal endometrium. *NEJM* 305: 1599–1605.

91. Whitehead, M. I.; Townsend, P. T.; Pryse-Davies, J.; Ryder, T.; Lane, G.; Soddle, N.; and King, R. J. B. 1982. Actions of progestins on the morphology and biochemistry of the endometrium of postmenopausal women receiving low-dose estrogen therapy. *Am J Obstet Gynecol* 142:791–95.

92. Wile, A. G., and DiSaia, P. J. 1989. Hormones and breast cancer. *Am J Surg* 157, 4:438–42.
93. Wynder, E. L.; Eschjer, G. C.; and Matnel, N. 1966. An epidemiological investigation of cancer of the endometrium. *Cancer* 19:489–520.
94. Ziel, H. K., and Finkle, W. D. 1975. Increased risk of endometrial carcinoma among users of conjugated estrogens. *NEJM* 293:1167–70.

ADDITIONAL RECOMMENDED READINGS

Abramson, D., and Driscoll, S. G. 1966. Endometrial aspiration biopsy. *Obstet Gynecol* 27:381–91.

Botella Llusia, J.; Oriol-Bosch, A.; Sanchez-Garrido, F.; and Tresquerres, J. A. F. 1980. Testosterone and 17β oestradiol secretion of the human ovary, II: normal postmenopausal women, postmenopausal women with endometrial hyperplasia and postmenopausal women with adenocarcinoma of the endometrium. *Maturitas* 2:7–12.

Callantine, M. R.; Martin, P. L.; Bolding, O. T.; Warner, P. O.; and Greaney, M. O., Jr. 1975. Micronized 17 beta estradiol for oral estrogen therapy in menopausal women. *Obstet Gynecol* 46:37–41.

Campbell, S., and Whitehead, M. 1977. Oestrogen therapy and the menopausal syndrome. *Clinics in Obstet & Gynaecol* 4:31–47.

Centaro, A.; Ceci, G.; de Laurentis, G.; and de Salvia, D. 1974. Epidemiologic studies of postmenopausal endometrial adenocarcinoma. In *The menopausal syndrome,* ed. R. B. Greenblatt, V. B. Mahesh, and P. G. McDonough, pp. 133–38. New York: Medcome Press.

Horwitz, R. I., and Feinstein, A. R. 1978. Alternative analytic methods for case control studies of estrogens and endometrial cancer. *NEJM* 299:1089–94.

Horwitz, R. I.; Feinstein, A. R.; Horwitz, S. M.; and Robboy, S. J. 1981. Necropsy diagnosis of endometrial cancer and detection bias in case/control studies. *Lancet* 66–67.

Tseng, L.; Stolee, A.; and Gurpide, E. 1972. Quantitative studies on the uptake and metabolism of estrogens and progesterone by human endometrium. *Endocrinol* 90:390–404.

Van Campehout, J.; Choquette, P.; and Vauclair, P. 1980. Endometrial pattern in patients with primary hypoestrogenic amenorrhea receiving estrogen replacement therapy. *Obstet Gynecol* 56:349–55.

CHAPTER 7.   HORMONE REPLACEMENT THERAPY AND COEXISTING DISEASE

1. Bhatia, N. N.; Bergman, A.; and Karram, M. M. 1989. Effects of estrogen on urethral function in women with urinary incontinence. *Am J Obstet Gynecol* 160, 1:176–81.

2. Coutinho, E. M., and Goncalves, M. T. 1989. Long-term treatment of leiomyomas with gestrinone. *Fertil Steril* 51, 6:939–46.

3. Dlugi, A.; Rufo, S.; D'Amico, J.; and Seibel, M. 1988. A comparison of the effects of Buserelin versus danazol on plasma lipoproteins during treatment of pelvic endometriosis. *Fertil Steril* 49, 5:913–16.

4. Donnez, J.; Schrurs, B.; Gillerot, S.; Sandow, J.; and Clerckx, F. 1989. Treatment of uterine fibroids with implants of gonadotropin-releasing hormone agonist: assessment by hysterography. *Fertil Steril* 51, 6:947–50.

5. Friedman, A. J. 1989. Treatment of leiomyomata uteri with short-term leuprolide followed by leuprolide plus estrogen-progestin hormone replacement therapy for 2 years: a pilot study. *Fertil Steril* 51, 3:526–28.

6. Friedman, A. J.; Barbieri, R. L.; Benacerraf, B. R.; and Schiff, I. 1987. Treatment of leiomyomata with intranasal or subcutaneous leuprolide, a gonadotropin-releasing hormone agonist. *Fertil Steril* 48, 4:560–64.

7. Friedman, A. J.; Barbieri, R. L.; and Doubilet, P. M. 1988. A randomized, double-blind trial of a gonadotropin releasing-hormone agonist (leuprolide) with or without medroxyprogesterone acetate in the treatment of leiomyomata uteri. *Fertil Steril* 49, 3:404–9.

8. Friedman A. J.; Harrison-Atlas, D.; Barbieri, R. L.; Benacerraf, B.; Gleason, R.; and Schiff, I. 1989. A randomized, placebo-controlled, double-blind study evaluating the efficacy of leuprolide acetate depot in the treatment of uterine leiomyomata. *Fertil Steril* 51, 2:251–56.

9. Karram, M. M., and Bhatia, N. N. 1989. Management of coexistent stress and urge urinary incontinence. *Obstet Gynecol* 73, 1:4–7.

10. Kawaguchi, K.; Fujii, S.; Konishi, I.; Nanbu, Y.; Nonogaki, H.; and Mori, T. 1989. Mitotic activity in uterine leiomyomas during the menstrual cycle. *Am J Obstet Gynecol* 160:637–41.

11. Lemay, A.; Sandow, J.; Quesnel, G.; Bereron, J.; and Merat, P. 1988. Escape from the down-regulation of the pituitary-ovarian axis following decreased infusion of luteinizing hormone-releasing hormone agonist. *Fertil Steril* 49, 5:802–8.

12. Letterie, G. S.; Coddington, C. C.; Winkel, C. A.; Shawker, T. H.; Loriaux, D. L.; and Collins, R. L. 1989. Efficacy of a gonadotropin-releasing hormone agonist in the treatment of uterine leiomyomata: long-term follow-up. *Fertil Steril* 51, 6:951–56.

13. Mathur, S.; Chihal, H. J.; Homm, R. J.; Garza, D. E.; Rust, P. F.; and Williamson, H. O. 1988. Endometrial antigens involved in the autoimmunity of endometriosis. *Fertil Steril* 50, 6:860–63.

14. Matta, W. H. M.; Stabile, I.; Shaw, R.; and Campbell, S. 1988. Doppler assessment of uterine blood flow changes in patients with fibroids receiving the gonadotropin-releasing hormone agonist Buserelin. *Fertil Steril* 49, 6:1083–85.

15. Nash, J. D.; Ozols, R. F.; Smyth, J. F.; and Hamilton, T. C. 1989. Estrogen and anti-estrogen effects on the growth of human epithelial ovarian cancer in vitro. *Obstet Gynecol* 73, 6:1009–16.
16. Stewart, F.; Guest, F.; Stewart, G.; and Hatcher, R. 1987. *Understanding Your Body.* New York: Bantam.
17. Wild, R. A., and Bartholomew, M. J. 1988. The influence of body weight on lipoprotein lipids in patients with polycystic ovary syndrome. *Am J Obstet Gynecol* 159, 2:423–27.

CHAPTER 8. SEXUALITY IN THE MENOPAUSAL YEARS

1. Abramov, L. 1976. Sexual life and frigidity among women developing acute myocardial infarction. *Psychosomatic Medicine* 38:418–25.
2. Adamopoulos, D. A.; Georgiacodis, F.; and Abrahamian-Michalakis, A. 1988. Effects of antiandrogen-estrogen treatment on sexual and endocrine parameters in hirsute women. *Arch Sex Beh* 17, 5:421–29.
3. Adams, D. B.; Gold, A. R.; and Burt, A. D. 1978. Rise in female-initiated sexual activity at ovulation and its suppression by oral contraceptives. *NEJM* 299:1145–50.
3a. Alzate, H. 1990. Vaginal erogeneity, the "G spot," and female ejaculation. *Journal of Sex Education and Therapy* 16, 2:137–40.
3b. ———. 1989. Sexual behavior of unmarried Colombian university students: a follow-up. *Arch Sex Beh* 18, 3:239–50.
3c. ———. 1985. Letter to the editor: a clarification to Perry. *Journal of Sex and Marital Therapy* 11, 1:67–68.
3d. ———. 1985. Vaginal eroticism: a replication study. *Arch Sex Beh* 14, 6:529–37.
3e. ———. 1985. Vaginal eroticism and female orgasm: a current appraisal. *Journal of Sex and Marital Therapy* 11, 4:271–84.
3f. Alzate, H., and Hoch, Z. 1988. Letter to the editor: a reply to Zaviacic. *Journal of Sex and Marital Therapy* 14, 4:299–301.
3g. ———. 1986. The "G-spot" and "female ejaculation": a current appraisal. *Journal of Sex and Marital Therapy* 12, 3:211–20.
3h. Alzate, H., and Londono, M. L. 1987. Subjects' reactions to a sexual experimental situation. *J Sex Res* 23, 3:362–400.
3i. ———. 1984. Vaginal erotic sensitivity. *Journal of Sex and Marital Therapy* 10, 1:49–56.
4. Bancroft, J.; Davidson, D. W.; Warner, P.; and Tyrer, G. 1979. Androgens and sexual behavior of women using oral contraceptives. *Clin Endocrinol* 12:327–40.

5. Bancroft, J., and Skakkeback, N. S. 1978. Androgens and human sexual behavior. 209–20. In *CIBA Foundation symposium, 62: Sex, hormones and behavior.* Amsterdam: Excerpta Medica.

6. Batra, S.; Bjellin, L.; Losif, S.; Martensson, L.; and Sjorgren, C. 1985. Effect of oestrogen and progesterone on the blood flow in the lower urinary tract of the rabbit. *Acta Physiol Scand* 123, 2:191–94.

7. Bretschneider, J. G., and McCoy, N. L. 1988. Sexual interest and behavior in healthy 80- to 102-year olds. *Arch Sex Beh* 17, 2:109–29.

8. Christenson, C. V., and Johnson, A. B. 1973. Sexual patterns in a group of older never-married women. *J Geriatr Psychiatry* 7:80–98.

9. Cutler, W. 1988. *Hysterectomy: before and after.* New York: Harper & Row.

10. Cutler, W. B.; Davidson, J. M.; and McCoy, N. 1983. Sexual behavior frequency and hot flashes. *Neuroendocrinol* 5, 3:185.

11. Darling, C. A.; Davidson, J. K.; and Conway-Welch, C. 1990. Female ejaculation: perceived signs, the Gräfenberg spot/area, and sexual responsiveness. *Arch Sex Behav* 19:29–37.

12. Davidson, J. M.; Chen, J.; Crapo, L.; Gray, G.; Greenleaf, W. J.; and Catania, J. A. 1983. Hormonal changes and sexual function in aging men. *J Clin Endocrinol Metab.* 57, 1:71–77.

13. Dennerstein, L.; Burrows, G.; Wood, C.; and Hyman, G. 1980. Hormones and sexuality: effect of estrogen and progestogen. *Obstet Gynecol* 56:316–22.

14. Easley, E. B. 1978. Sex problems after the menopause. *Clinics in Obstet & Gynecol* 21:269–77.

15. Erickson, B. E. 1979. Emotional, sexual and hormonal differences in women with long and short menses. In *The Eastern Conference on Reproductive Behavior.* New Orleans: Tulane University.

16. Fedor-Freybergh, P. 1977. The influence of oestrogens on the well being and mental performance in climacteric and postmenopausal women. *Acta Obstet et Gynecol Scand* suppl. 64:1–64.

17. Gonzalez, E. R. 1980. Vitamin E report. *JAMA* Sept. 5, 1077–78.

18. Gooren, L. J. G. 1987. Androgen levels and sex functions in testosterone-treated hypogonadal men. *Arch Sex Beh* 16, 6:463–73.

19. Greenblatt, R. B. 1987. The use of androgens in the menopause and other gynecologic disorders. *Obstet Gynecol Clin NA* 14:251–68.

20. Gruis, M. L., and Wagner, N. N. 1979. Sexuality during the climacteric. *Postgrad Medicine* 65:197–207.

21. Hallstrom, T. 1977. Sexuality in the climacteric. *Clinics in Obstet & Gynaecol* 4:227–39.

22. Harman, S. M., and Tsitouras, P. D. 1980. Reproductive hormones in aging men, I: measurement of sex steroids, basal luteinizing hormone, and Leydig cell response to human chorionic gonadotropin. *J Clin Endocrinol Metab* 51:35–40.

23. Henker, F. C. 1977. A male climacteric syndrome: sexual, psychic and physical complaints in 50 middle-aged men. *Psychosomatics* 18:23–27.

24. Hite, S. 1976. *The Hite report.* New York: Macmillan.

25. Keverne, E. B.; Martensz, N. D.; and Tuite, B. 1989. Beta-endorphin concentrations in cerebrospinal fluid of monkeys are influenced by grooming relationships. *Psychoneuroendocrinology* 14, 1 and 2:155–61.

26. Kinsey, A.; Pomeroy, W.; and Martin, C. 1953. *Sexual behavior in the human female.* Philadelphia: Saunders.

27. Leiblum, S.; Bachmann, G.; Kemmann, E.; Colburn, D.; and Swartzman, L. 1983. Vaginal atrophy in the postmenopausal woman: the importance of sexual activity and hormones. *JAMA* 249:2195–98.

28. McCoy, N.; Cutler, W.; and Davidson, J. M. 1985. Relationships among sexual behavior, hot flashes and hormone levels in peri-menopausal women. *Arch Sex Beh* 14:385–94.

29. Masters, W., and Johnson, V. 1970. *Human sexual inadequacy.* Boston: Little Brown.

30. ———. 1966. *Human sexual response.* Boston: Little Brown.

31. Mathur, R. S.; Landgrebe, S. C.; Moody, L. O.; Semmens, J. P.; and Williamson, H. O. 1985. The effect of estrogen treatment on plasma concentrations of steroid hormones, gonadotropins, prolactin and sex hormone–binding globulin in post-menopausal women. *Maturitas* 7:129–33.

32. Neugarten, B. L.; Wood, V.; Kraines, R. J.; and Loomis, B. 1963. Women's attitudes toward the menopause. *Vita Humana* 6:140–51.

33. Notelovitz, M. 1978. Gynecologic problems of menopausal women, part 3: Changes in extragenital tissues and sexuality. *Geriatrics* 78:51–58.

33a. Perry, J. D., and Whipple, B. 1981. Pelvic muscle strength of female ejaculators: evidence in support of a new theory of orgasm. *J Sex Res* 17: 22–39.

34. Pfeiffer, E.; Verwoerdt, A.; and Davis, G. 1972. Sexual behavior in middle life. *Am J Psychiat* 128:1262–67.

35. Rosen, R. C.; Kostis, J. B.; and Jekelis, A. W. 1988. Beta-blocker effects on sexual function in normal males. *Arch Sex Beh* 17, 3:241–55.

36. Schover, L. R.; Evans, R. B.; and von Eschenbach, A. D. 1987. Sexual rehabilitation in a cancer center: diagnosis and outcome in 384 consultations. *Arch Sex Beh* 16, 6:445–61.

37. Schultz, W. C. M. W.; van de Wiel, H. B. M.; Klatter, J. A.; Sturm, B. E.; and Nauta, J. 1989. Vaginal sensitivity to electric stimuli: theoretical and practical implications. *Arch Sex Beh* 18, 2:87–95.

38. Semmens, J. P. 1983. In reply to Wulf Utian's letter to the editor. *JAMA* 249:195.

39. Semmens, J. P., and Wagner, G. 1982. Estrogen deprivation and vaginal function in postmenopausal women. *JAMA* 248:445–48.

40. Sherwin, B. B., and Gelfand, M. M. 1985. Sex steroids and affect in the

surgical menopause: a double-blind, cross-over study. *Psychoneuroendocrinology* 10, 3:325-35.

41. Sherwin, B. B.; Gelfand, M. M.; and Brender, W. 1985. Androgen enhances sexual motivation in females: a prospective, crossover study of sex steroid administration in the surgical menopause. *Psychosomatic Medicine* 474:339-51.

42. Stanislaw, H., and Rice, F. J. 1988. Correlation between sexual desire and menstrual cycle characteristics. *Arch Sex Beh* 17, 6:499-508.

43. Studd, J. W. W.; Collins, W. P.; Chakravarti, S.; Newton, J. R.; Oram, D.; and Parsons, A. 1977. Oestradiol and testosterone implants in the treatment of psychosexual problems in the postmenopausal woman. *Br J Obstet Gynaecol* 84:314-16.

44. Tsai, C. C.; Semmens, J. P.; Curtis Semmens, E.; Lam, C. F.; and Lee, F. S. 1987. Vaginal physiology in postmenopausal women: pH value, transvaginal electropotential difference, and estimated blood flow. *South Med J* 80, 8:987-90.

45. Utian, W. H. S. 1972. The true clinical features of postmenopause and oophorectomy and their response to oestrogen therapy. *S Afr Med J* 46: 732-37.

46. Weizman, R., and Hart, J. 1987. Sexual behavior in healthy married elderly men. *Arch Sex Beh* 16, 1:39-44.

47. Wincze, J. P.; Malhotra, C.; Susset, J. G.; Bansal, S.; Balko, A.; and Malamud, M. 1988. A comparison of nocturnal penile tumescence during waking states in comprehensively diagnosed groups of males experiencing erectile difficulties. *Arch Sex Beh* 17, 4:333-48.

Chapter 9.   Hysterectomy

1. Amias, A. G. 1975. Sexual life after gynaecological operations. *Brit Med J* 2:608-9.

2. Andrews, M. C., and Wentz, A. C. 1975. The effects of danazol on gonadotropins and steroid blood levels in normal and anovulatory women. *Am J Obstet Gynecol* 121:817-28.

3. Annegers, J. F.; Strom, H.; Decker, D. G.; Dockerty, H. B.; and O'Fallon, W. 1979. Ovarian cancer: incidence and case-control study. *Cancer* 43:723-29.

4. Azziz, R.; Steinkampf, M. P.; and Murphy, A. 1989. Postoperative recuperation: relation to the extent of endoscopic surgery. *Fertil Steril* 51, 6:1061-64.

5. Backstrom, T., and Boyle, H. 1980. Persistence of premenstrual tension symptoms in hysterectomized women. Unpublished ms.

6. Ballinger, C. B. 1975. Psychiatric morbidity and the menopause: screening of general population sample. *Brit Med J* 3:344–46.

7. Barker, M. C. 1968. Psychiatric illness after hysterectomy. *Brit Med J* 2:91–95.

8. Barrett-Connor, E.; Wingard, D. L.; and Criqui, M. H. 1989. Postmenopausal estrogen use and heart disease risk factors in the 1980's. *JAMA* 261, 14:2095–2100.

9. Blauer, K. L., and Colins, R. L. 1988. The effect of intraperitoneal progesterone on postoperative adhesion formation in rabbits. *Fertil Steril* 49, 1:144–49.

10. Boyers, S.; Diamond, M.; and DeCherney, A. 1988. Reduction of postoperative pelvic adhesions in the rabbit with Gore-Tex surgical membrane. *Fertil Steril* 49, 6:1066–69.

10a. Brooks, P.; DeCherney, A.; Loffer, F.; and Neuwirth, R. 1989. Resectoscopy: mastering the challenges. *Contem OB/GYN* 32:131–48.

10b. Brooks, P.; Loffer, F.; and Serden, S. 1989. Resectoscopic removal of symptomatic intrauterine lesions. *J Reprod Med* 34:435–37.

11. Bunker, J. P. 1976. Elective hysterectomy—pro and con: public-health rounds at the Harvard School of Public Health. *NEJM* 295:264–68.

12. Burch, J. C.; Byrd, B. F.; and Vaughn, W. K. 1975. The effects of long-term estrogen administration to women following hysterectomy. *Front Horm Res* 3:208–14.

13. Byrd, B. F., Jr.; Burch, J. C.; and Vaughn, W. K. 1977. The impact of long term estrogen support after hysterectomy: a report of 1016 cases. *Ann Surg* 185:574–80.

14. Callantine, M. R., and Martin, P. L. 1975. Micronized 17 beta estradiol for oral estrogen therapy in menopausal women. *Obstet Gynecol* 46:37–41.

15. Centerwall, B. S. 1981. Premenopausal hysterectomy and cardiovascular disease. *Am J Obstet Gynecol* 139:58–61.

16. Coppen, A.; Bisshop, M.; Beard, R. J. H.; Barnard, G. J. R.; and Collins, W. P. 1981. Hysterectomy, hormones, and behavior. *Lancet* 126–28.

17. Craig, G. A., and Jackson, P. 1975. Letter: sexual life after vaginal hysterectomy. *Brit Med J* 3:97.

18. Cutler, W. 1990. *Hysterectomy: before and after.* New York: Harper & Row.

20. Dalton, K. 1957. Discussion on the aftermath of hysterectomy and oophorectomy. *Proc Royal Soc of Med* 50:415–18.

21. DeNeef, J. C., and Hollenbeck, Z. J. R. 1966. The fate of ovaries preserved at the time of hysterectomy. *Am J Obstet Gynecol* 96:1088–97.

22. Dennerstein, L.; Wood, D.; and Burrows, G. 1977. Sexual response following hysterectomy and oophorectomy. *Obstet Gynecol* 49:92–96.

23. Dicker, R. C.; Scally, M. J.; Greenspan, J. R.; Layde, P. M.; and Maze, J. M. 1982. Hysterectomy among women of reproductive age. *JAMA* 248:323–27.

24. Donahue, V. C. 1976. Elective hysterectomy: pro and con. *NEJM* 295: 264.

25. Doyle, L. I.; Barclay, D. L.; Duncan, G. W.; and Kirton, K. T. 1971. Human luteal function as assessed by plasma progestin. *Am J Obstet Gynecol* 110:92–97.

26. Forney, J. P. 1980. The effect of radical hysterectomy on bladder physiology. *Am J Obstet Gynecol* 138:374–82.

27. Gambone, J. C.; Lench, J. B.; Slessinski, M. J.; Reiter, R. C.; and Moore, J. G. 1989. Validation of hysterectomy indications and the quality assurance process. *Obstet Gynecol* 6:1045–49.

28. Gambrell, R. D.; Castaneda, T. A.; and Ricci, C. A. 1978. Management of postmenopausal bleeding to prevent endometrial cancer. *Maturitas* 1:99–106.

29. García C.-R., and Rosenfeld, D. L. 1977. *Human fertility: the regulation of reproduction.* Philadelphia: F. A. Davis.

30. Gath, D. H. 1980. Psychiatric aspects of hysterectomy. In *The social consequences of non-psychiatric illness.* New York: Bruner/Mazel.

31. Greenberg, M. 1981. Hysterectomy, hormones and behavior: letter to the editor. *Lancet* 449.

32. Hasselquist, M.; Goldberg, N.; Schroeter, A.; and Spelsberg, T. 1980. Isolation and characterization of the estrogen receptors in human skin. *J Clin Endocrinol Metab* 50:76–82.

33. Hempel, Von E.; Kriester, A.; Freesmeyer, E.; and Walter, W. 1979. Prospektive studie zur osteoporose nach bilater ovarektomie mit und ohne postoperative ostrogenprophylaxe. *Zentralblatt für gynakologie* 101:309–19.

34. Hunter, D. J.; Julier, D.; Franklin, M.; and Green, E. 1977. Plasma levels of estrogen, luteinizing hormone, and follicle stimulating hormone following castration and estradiol implant. *Obstet Gynecol* 49:180–85.

35. Janson, P. O., and Jansson, I. 1977. The acute effect of hysterectomy on ovarian blood flow. *Am J Obstet Gynecol* 127:349–52.

36. Jick, H.; Dinan, B.; and Rotheman, K. 1978. Noncontraceptive estrogens and nonfatal myocardial infarctions. *JAMA* 239:1407–8 and subsequent personal communication.

37. Johnson, J. 1982. Tubal sterilization and hysterectomy. *Family Planning Perspectives* 14:28–30.

38. Kilkku, P. 1983. Supravaginal uterine amputation vs. hysterectomy: effects on coital frequency and dyspareunia. *Acta Obstet et Gynecol Scand* 62:141–45.

39. Kilkku, P.; Gronroos, M.; Hirvonen, T.; and Rauramo, L. 1983. Supravaginal uterine amputation vs. hysterectomy: effects on libido and orgasm. *Acta Obstet et Gynecol Scand* 62:147–52.

40. Knapp, R. C.; Donahue, V. C.; and Friedman, E. A. 1973. Dissection of paravesical and pararectal spaces in pelvic operations. *Surg Gynecol Obstet* 137:758–62.

41. Laros, R. K., and Work, B. A. 1975. Female sterilization, III: vaginal hysterectomy. *Am J Obstet Gynecol* 122:693–97.

42. Lewis, E., and Bourne, S. 1981. Hysterectomy, hormones and behavior: letter to the editor. *Lancet* 324–25.

43. Loffer, F. D. 1989. Hysteroscopy with selective endometrial sampling compared with D & C for abnormal uterine bleeding: the value of a negative hysteroscopic view. *Obstet Gynecol* 73, 1:16–20.

44. Longcope, C.; Hunter, R.; and Franz, C. 1980. Steroid secretion by the postmenopausal ovary. *Am J Obstet Gynecol* 138:564–68.

45. Lyon, L. J., and Gardner, J. W. 1977. The rising frequency of hysterectomy: its effect on uterine cancer rates. *Am J Epidemiol* 105:439–43.

46. MacManon, B., and Worcester, J. 1966. National Center for Health Statistics: age at menopause, US 1960–1962. Washington, D.C., USPHS publication 1000, series 11, no. 19.

47. McNatty, K. P.; Makris, A.; DeGrazia, C.; Osathanondh, R.; and Ryan, K. J. 1979. The production of progesterone, androgens, and estrogens by granulosa cells, thecal tissue and stromal tissue by human ovaries in vitro. *J Clin Endocrinol Metab* 49:687–99.

48. Mikhail, G. 1970. Hormone secretion by the human ovaries. *Gynec Invest* 1:5–20.

49. Monroe, S. E., and Menon, K. M. J. 1977. Changes in reproductive hormone secretion during the climacteric and postmenopausal periods. *Clinics in Obstet & Gynaecol* 20:113–22.

50. Moore, J., and Tolley, D. 1976. Depression following hysterectomy. *Psychosomatics* 17:86–89.

51. Morgan, S. 1980. Sexuality after hysterectomy and castration. Published in offpress collection of women's writings.

52. Morizaki, N.; Morizaki, J.; Hayashi, R. H.; and Garfield, R. E. 1989. A functional and structural study of the innervation of the human uterus. *Am J Obstet Gynecol* 160:218–28.

53. Nakano, R.; Shima, K.; Yamoto, M.; Kobayashi, M.; Nishimori, K.; and Hiroaka, J. T. 1989. Binding sites for gonadotropins in human postmenopausal ovaries. *Obstet Gynecol* 73:196–200.

54. Perry, J. D., and Whipple, B. 1981. Pelvic muscle strength of female ejaculators: evidence in support of a new theory of orgasm. *J Sex Res* 17:22–39.

55. Polivy, J. 1974. Psychological reactions to hysterectomy. *Am J Obstet Gynecol* 118:417–26.

56. Punonen, R., and Rauramo, L. 1977. The effect of long-term oral oestriol

succinate therapy on the skin of castrated women. *Ann Chir Gynaecol* 66: 214–15.

57. Randall, C. L. 1963. Ovarian conservation. In *Progress in gynecology,* ed. J. V. Meigs and S. H. Sturgis, pp. 457–64. New York: Grune & Stratton.

58. Ranney, B., and Abu-Ghazaleh, S. 1977. The future function and control of ovarian tissue which is retained in vivo during hysterectomy. *Am J Obstet Gynecol* 128:626–34.

59. Reynoso, R. L.; Aznar, R. R.; Bedolla, T. N.; and Cortes Gallego, V. 1975. Cyclic concentration of estradiol and progesterone in hysterectomized women. *Reproduction* 2:45–49.

60. Richards, B. C. 1978. Hysterectomy: from women to women. *Am J Obstet Gynecol* 131:446–49.

61. Richards, D. H. 1973. Depression after hysterectomy. *Lancet* 2:430–33.

62. ———. 1974. A post-hysterectomy syndrome. *Lancet* 983–85.

63. Ritterband, A. B.; Jaffe, I. A.; Densen, P. M.; Magagna, J. F.; and Reed, E. 1963. Gonadal function and the development of coronary heart disease. *Circulation* 27:237–44.

64. Rivin, A. U., and Dimitroff, S. P. 1954. The incidence and severity of atherosclerosis in estrogen-treated males and in females with a hypoestrogenic or hyperestrogenic state. *Circulation* 9:533–39.

65. Robinson, R. W.; Higano, N.; and Coehn, W. D. 1959. Increased incidence of coronary heart disease in women castrated prior to menopause. *Arch Intern Med* 104:908–11.

66. Rodriguez, M. H.; Platt, L. D.; Medearis, A. L.; Lacarra, M.; and Lobo, R. A. 1988. The use of transvaginal sonography for evaluation of postmenopausal ovarian size and morphology. *Am J Obstet Gynecol* 159, 4:810–14.

67. Rosenberg, L.; Hennekens, C. H.; Rosner, B.; Belanger, C.; Rothman, K. J.; and Speizer, R. E. 1981. Early menopause and the risk of myocardial infarction. *Am J Obstet Gynecol* 139:47–51.

67a. Saarikoski, S.; Yliskoski, M.; and Penttila, I. 1990. Sequential use of norethisterone and natural progesterone in pre-menopausal bleeding disorders. *Maturitas* 12:89–97.

68. Shafik, A., and Mohi-el-Din, M. 1988. Pelvic organ venous communications. *Am J Obstet Gynecol* 159:347–51.

68a. Sherwin, B. 1988. Estrogen and/or androgen replacement therapy and cognitive functioning in surgically menopausal women. *Psychoneuroendocrinology* 13:345–57.

69. Sherwin, B. B., and Gelfand, M. M. 1985. Sex steroids and affect in the surgical menopause: a double-blind, cross-over study. *Psychoneuroendocrinology* 10, 3:325–35.

70. Sherwin, B. B.; Gelfand, M. M.; and Brender, W. 1985. Androgen en-

hances sexual motivation in females: a prospective, crossover study of sex steroid administration in the surgical menopause. *Psychosomatic Medicine* 474:339–51.

70a. Sherwin, B. B., and Phillips, S. 1990. Estrogen and cognitive functioning in surgically menopausal women. *Ann NY Academy of Sciences* 592:474–75.

71. Siegler, A. M., and Valle, R. F. 1988. Therapeutic hysteroscopic procedures. *Fertil Steril* 50, 5:685–701.

72. Simon, J. A., and di Zerega, G. S. 1982. Physiologic estradiol replacement following oophorectomy: failure to maintain precastration gonadotropin levels. *Obstet Gynecol* 59:511–13.

73. Stadel, B. V., and Weiss, N. 1975. Characteristics of menopausal women: a survey of King and Pierce Counties in Washington, 1973–1974. *Am J Epidemiol* 102:209–16.

74. Steinleitner, A.; Lambert, H.; Montoro, L.; Kelly, E.; Swanson, J.; and Sueldo, C. 1988. The use of calcium channel blockage for the prevention of postoperative adhesion formation. *Fertil Steril* 50, 5:818–21.

75. Stone, S. C.; Dickey, R. P.; and Mickal, A. 1975. The acute effect of hysterectomy on ovarian function. *Am J Obstet Gynecol* 121:193–97.

75a. Stuart, C. A., and Nagamani, M. 1990. Insulin infusion acutely augments ovarian androgen production in normal women. *Fertil Steril* 54:788–92.

76. Studd, J. W. W.; Chakravarti, S.; and Collins, W. P. 1978. Plasma hormone profiles after the menopause and bilateral oophorectomy. *Postgrad Med J* 54:25–30.

77. Tobachman, J. K.; Tucker, M. A.; Kase, R.; Greene, M. K.; Costa, J.; and Fraumeni, J. F., Jr. 1982. Intra-abdominal carcinomatosis after prophylactic oophorectomy in ovarian cancer prone families. *Lancet* 795–97.

78. Treloar, A. 1981. Menstrual cyclicity and the pre-menopause. *Maturitas* 3:249–64.

79. Utian, W. H. 1975. Definitive symptoms of postmenopause—incorporating use of vaginal parabasal cell index. *Front Horm Res* 3:74–93.

80. ———. 1975. Effect of hysterectomy, oophorectomy and estrogen therapy on libido. *Int J Obstet Gyn* 13:97–100.

81. Waldron, I. 1982. An analysis of causes of sex differences in mortality and morbidity. In *The fundamental connection between nature and nurture,* eds. W. R. Gove and G. R. Carpenter. Lexington, Mass.: Lexington Books.

82. ———. 1980. Employment and women's health: an analysis of causal relationships. *Int J Health Services* 10:435–54.

83. White, S. C.; Wartel, L. J.; and Wade, M. E. 1971. Comparison of abdominal and vaginal hysterectomies: a review of 600 operations. *Obstet Gynecol* 37:530–37.

84. Wright, R. C. 1969. Hysterectomy: past, present and future. *Obstet Gynecol* 33:560–63.

85. Wuest, J. H.; Dry, T. J.; and Edwards, J. E. 1953. The degree of atherosclerosis in bilaterally oophorectomized women. *Circulation* 7:801–9.

86. Zussman, L.; Zussman, S.; Sunley, R.; and Bjornson, E. 1981. Sexual
response after hysterectomy-oophorectomy: recent studies and reconsideration of psychogenesis. *Am J Obstet Gynecol* 140:725–29.

CHAPTER 10. CARDIOVASCULAR HEALTH

1. Adams, M. R.; Clarkson, T. B.; Koritnik, D. R.; and Nash, H. A. 1987.
Contraceptive steroids and coronary artery atherosclerosis in cynomolgus
macaques. *Fertil Steril* 47:1010–18.

2. Aitken, J. M.; Lorimer, A. R.; Hart, D. M.; Lawrie, T. D. V.; and Smith,
D. A. 1971. The effects of oophorectomy and long term mestranol therapy on the serum lipids of middle aged women. *Clin Sci* 41:597–603.

3. Akljaersing, N., *et al.* 1988. Blood coagulation in postmenopausal women
given estrogen treatment: comparison of transdermal and oral administration. *J Lab Clin Med* 111, 2:224–28.

4. Allen, T., and Adler, N. T. 1978. Localized uptake of (14) deogyglucose
by the preoptic area of female rats in response to vaginocervical stimulation. *Neuroscience Abstracts* 4.

5. Avogaro, P.; Cazzalato, G.; Bittolo, B. G.; and Quinci, G. B. 1979. Are
apolipoproteins better discriminators than lipids for atherosclerosis? *Lancet* 1:901–3.

6. Aylward, M. 1978. Coagulation factors in opposed and unopposed oestrogen treatment at the climacteric. *Postgrad Med J* 54:31–37.

7. Barrett-Connor, E.; Brown, W. V.; Turner, J.; Austin, M.; and Criqui,
M. H. 1979. Heart disease risk factors and hormone use in postmenopausal women. *JAMA* 241:2167–69.

8. Blair, S. N.; Kohl, H. W.; Paffenbarger, R. S.; Clark, D. G.; Cooper,
K. H.; and Gibbons, L. W. 1989. Physical fitness and all-cause mortality: a
prospective study of healthy men and women. *JAMA* 262:2395–2401.

9. Bolton, C. H.; Ellwood, M.; Hartog, M.; Martin, R.; Rowe, A. S.; and
Wensley, R. T. 1975. Comparison of the effects of ethinyl oestradiol and
conjugated equine oestrogens in oophorectomized women. *Clin Endocrinol (Oxf)* 4:131–38.

10. Boston Collaborative Drug Surveillance Program. 1974. Surgically confirmed gallbladder disease, venous thromboembolism, and breast tumors
in relation to postmenopausal estrogen therapy: a report from Boston
University Medical Center. *NEJM* 290:15–19.

11. Bradby, G. V. H.; Valente, A. J.; and Walton, K. W. 1978. Serum high-
density lipoproteins in peripheral vascular disease. *Lancet* 2:1271–74.

12. Bradley, D. B.; Wingerd, J.; Petitti, D. B.; Krauss, R. M.; and Ramcharan, S. 1978. Serum high density lipoprotein cholesterol in women using oral contraceptives, estrogens and progestins. *NEJM* 299:17–20.

13. Castelli, W.; Garrison, R.; Wilson, P.; Abbott, R.; Kalousdian, S.; and Kannel, W. 1986. Incidence of coronary heart disease and lipoprotein cholesterol levels: the Framingham Study. *JAMA* 256:2835–38.

14. Chetkowski, R. M., Meldrum, D. R.; Steingold, K. A.; Randle, D.; Lu, J. K.; Eggena, P.; Hershman, J. M.; Alkjaersig, N. K.; Fletcher, A. P.; and Judd, H. L. 1986. Biologic effects of transdermal estradiol. *NEJM* 314: 25:1615–20.

15. Crane, M. G.; Harris, J. J.; and Winsor, W., III. 1971. Hypertension, oral contraceptive agents, and conjugated estrogens. *Ann Int Med* 74:13–21.

16. Crews, D. E. 1988. Body weight, blood pressure and the risk of total and cardiovascular mortality in an obese population. *Human Biology* 60, 3:417–33.

17. Cutler, W., and García, C.-R. 1984. *The medical management of menopause and pre-menopause.* Philadelphia: Lippincott.

18. Drygas, W.; Jegler, A.; and Kunski, H. 1988. Study on threshold dose of physical activity in coronary heart disease prevention, part 1: relationship between leisure time, physical activity and coronary risk factors. *International Journal of Sports Medicine* 9:275–78.

19. Fahraeus, L., and Wallentin, L. 1983. High density lipoprotein subfractions during oral and cutaneous administration of 17β estradiol to menopausal women. *J Clin Endocrinol Metab* 56:797.

20. Farish, E.; Fletcher, C. D.; Dagen, M. M.; Hart, D. M.; Al-Azzawi, F.; Parkin, D. E.; and Howie, C. A. 1989. Lipoprotein and apolipoprotein levels in postmenopausal women on continuous oestrogen/progestogen therapy. *Br J Obstet Gynaecol* 96, 3:358–64.

21. Gordon, T.; Castelli, W. P.; Hjortland, M. P.; Kannel, W. B.; and Dawber, T. R. 1977. The Framingham study: high density lipoprotein as a protective factor against coronary heart disease. *Am J Med* 62:707–14.

22. Gustafson, A., and Svanborg, A. 1972. Gonadal steroid effects on plasma lipoproteins and individual phospholipids. *J Clin Endocrinol Metab* 35: 203–7.

23. Henderson, B. E.; Paganini-Hill, A.; and Ross, R. K. 1988. Estrogen replacement therapy and protection from acute myocardial infarction. *Am J Obstet Gynecol* 159, 2:312–17.

24. Higano, N.; Cohen, W. D.; and Robinson, R. W. 1959. Effects of sex steroids on lipids. *Ann NY Academy of Sciences* 72:970–79.

25. Hirvonen, E.; Malknonen, M.; and Nanninen, V. 1980. Effects of different progestogens on lipoproteins during postmenopausal replacement therapy. *NEJM* 304:560–63.

26. Houston, M. C. 1986. Review: sodium and hypertension. *Arch Intern Med* 146:179–85.

27. Jensen, J., and Christiansen, C. 1988. Effects of smoking on serum lipoproteins and bone mineral content during postmenopausal hormone replacement therapy. *Am J Obstet Gynecol* 159, 4:820–25.

28. Jick, H.; Dinan, B.; and Rothman, K. 1978. Noncontraceptive estrogens and nonfatal myocardial infarctions. *JAMA* 239:1407–8.

29. Kannel, W. B.; Castelli, W. P.; Gordon, T.; and McNamara, P. 1971. Serum cholesterol, lipoproteins and the risk of coronary heart disease. *Ann Int Med* 174:1–12.

30. Knopp, R. H.; Walden, C. E.; Wahl, P. W.; and Hoover, J. J. 1982. Effects of oral contraceptives on lipoprotein triglycerides and cholesterol: relationships to estrogen and progestin potency. *Am J Obstet Gynecol* 1421:725–31.

31. Lapidus, L. 1986. Ischemic heart disease, stroke and total mortality in women—results from a prospective population study in Gothenburg, Sweden. *Acta Med Scand [Suppl]* 219:1–42.

31a. Lapidus, L.; Andersson, H.; Bengtsson, C.; and Bosaeus, I. 1986. Dietary habits in relation to incidence of cardiovascular disease and death in women: a 12-year follow-up of participants in the population study of women in Gothenburg, Sweden. *Am J Clin Nutr* 44:444–48.

32. Lauritzen, C. 1973. The management of the premenopausal and the postmenopausal patient. *Front Horm Res* 2:2–21.

33. Lind, T.; Cameron, E. C.; Hunter, W. M.; Leon, C.; Moran, P. F.; Oxley, A.; Gerrard, J.; and Lind, U. C. G. 1979. A prospective controlled trial of six forms of hormone replacement therapy given to postmenopausal women. *Br J Obstet Gynaecol* 86, 3:1–29.

34. Lindberg, U. B.; Crona, N.; Stigendal, L.; Teger-Nilsson, A. C.; and Silfverstolpe, G. 1989. A comparison between effects of estradiol and low dose ethinyl estradiol on haemostasis parameters. *Thromb Haemostasis* 61, 1:65–69.

35. Marmorston, J.; Madgson, O.; Lewis, J. J.; Mehl, J.; Moore, F. J.; and Bernstein, J. 1958. Effect of small doses of estrogen on serum lipids in female patients with myocardial infarction. *NEJM* 258, 583–86.

36. Noma, A.; Yokosuka, T.; and Kitamura, K. 1983. Plasma lipids and apolipoproteins as discriminators for presence and severity of angiographically defined coronary artery disease. *Atherosclerosis* 49:1–7.

37. Notelovitz, M. 1977. Coagulation, oestrogen and the menopause. *Clinics in Obstet & Gynaecol* 4:107–28.

38. Notelovitz, M., and Southwood, B. 1974. Metabolic effect of conjugated oestrogens (USP) on lipids and lipoproteins. *S A Med J* 48:2552–56.

39. Paffenbarger, R.; Hyde, R.; Wiag, L.; and Steinmetz, C. 1984. A natural history of athleticism and cardiovascular health. *JAMA* 252:491–95.

40. Pfeffer, R. I.; Whipple, G. H.; Kurosaki, T. T.; and Chapman, J. M. 1978. Coronary risk and estrogen use in postmenopausal women. *Am J Epidemiol* 107:479–87.

41. Plunkett, E. R. 1982. Contraceptive steroids, age and the cardiovascular system. *Am J Obstet Gynecol* 142:747–51.

42. Punnonen, R., and Rauramo, L. 1976. The effect of castration and oral estrogen therapy on serum lipids. In *Consensus on menopause research,* ed. P. van Keep, R. B. Greenblatt, and M. Albeaux-Fernet, pp. 132–38. Proceedings of the First International Congress on the Menopause, France, 1976. Baltimore: University Park Press.

43. Pyorala, T. 1976. The effect of synthetic and natural estrogens on glucose tolerance, plasma insulin and lipid metabolism in postmenopausal women. In *The management of the menopause and postmenopausal years,* ed. S. Campbell, pp. 195–210. Lancaster, Eng.: MTP Press.

44. Robinson, R. W.; Cohen, W. D.; and Higano, N. 1958. Estrogen replacement therapy in women with coronary atherosclerosis. *Ann Int Med* 48:95–101.

45. Robinson, R. W.; Higano, N.; and Cohen, W. 1960. Effects of long-term administration of estrogens on serum lipids of postmenopausal women. *NEJM* 263:828–31.

46. Rosenberg, L.; Armstrong, B.; and Jick, H. 1976. Myocardial infarction and estrogen therapy in postmenopausal women. *NEJM* 294:1256–59.

47. Ross, R. K.; Paganini-Hill, A.; Mack, T. M.; Arthur, M.; and Henderson, B. 1981. Menopausal oestrogen therapy and protection from death from ischaemic heart disease. *Lancet* 1:858–60.

48. Saunders, D. M.; Hunter, J. C.; Shutt, D. A.; and O'Neill, B. J. 1978. The effect of oestradiol valerate therapy on coagulation factors and lipid and oestrogen levels in oophorectomized women. *Aust N Z J Obstet Gynaecol* 18, 3:198–201.

49. Shaffer, C. F. 1970. Ascorbic acid and atherosclerosis. *Am J Clin Nutr* 23:127–30.

50. Silverstolpe, G.; Gustafson, A.; Samsioe, G.; and Svanborg, A. 1979. Lipid metabolic studies in oophorectomized women: effects of three different progestogens. *Acta Obstet et Gynecol Scand* suppl. 88:89–95.

51. Sniderman, A.; Shapiro, S.; Marpole, D.; Skinner, B.; Teng, B.; and Kwiterovich, P. 1980. Association of coronary atherosclerosis with hyperapobetalipoproteinaemia (increased protein but normal cholesterol levels in human low density (B) lipoproteins). *Proc Natl Acad Sci USA* 77:604–8.

52. Stangel, J. J.; Innerfield, I.; and Reyniak, J. V. 1976. The effects of conjugated estrogens on hh coagulability in menopausal women. *Obstet Gynecol* 49:314–16.

53. Studd, J.; Dubiel, M.; Kakkar, V. V.; Thom, M.; and White, P. J. 1978.

The effect of hormone replacement therapy on glucose tolerance, clotting factors, fibrinolysis and platelet behavior in postmenopausal women. In *The Role of Estrogen/Progestogen in the Management of the Menopause,* ed. I. D. Cooke, pp. 41–60. Baltimore: University Park Press.

54. Tikkanen, M. J.; Kuusi, T.; Vartianien, E.; and Nikkila, E. A. 1979. Treatment of post-menopausal hypercholesterolaemia with estradiol. *Acta Obstet et Gynecol Scand* suppl. 88:83–88.

55. Tikkanen, M. J., and Nikkila, E. A. 1978. Natural oestrogen as an effective treatment for type-11 hyperlipoproteinaemia in postmenopausal women. *Lancet* 490–91.

56. Toy, J. L.; Davies, J. A.; and McNicol, G. P. 1978. The effects of long term therapy with oestriol succinate on the haemostatic mechanism in postmenopausal women. *Br J Obstet Gynaecol* 85:363–66.

57. Villecco, A. S.; de Aloysio, D.; Pilati, G.; Mauloni, M.; Roncuzzi, A.; Bottiglioni, F.; and Pisi, E. 1987. Non-invasive 24-hour monitoring of high blood pressure in climacteric outpatients. *Maturitas* 9:267–74.

58. Wahl, P.; Walden, C.; Knopp, R.; Hoover, J.; Wallace, R.; Heiss, G.; and Rifkind, B. 1983. Effect of estrogen/progestin potency on lipid/lipoprotein cholesterol. *NEJM* 308:862–67.

59. Wallace, R. B.; Hoover, J.; Barrett-Conner, E.; Rifkind, B. M.; Hunninghake, D. B.; Mackenthun, A.; and Heiss, G. 1979. Altered plasma lipid and lipo-protein levels associated with oral contraceptives and oestrogen use. *Lancet* 2:112–14.

60. Wallentin, L., and Larsson-Cohn, U. 1977. Metabolic and hormonal effects of postmenopausal oestrogen replacement treatment, II: plasma lipid. *Acta Endocrinol* 86:597–607.

61. Walter, S., and Jensen, H. K. 1977. The effect of treatment with oestradiol and oestriol on fasting serum cholesterol and triglyceride levels in postmenopausal women. *Br J Obstet Gynaecol* 84, 11:869–72.

62. Whayne, T. F.; Alaupovic, P.; Curry, M. D.; Lee, E. T.; Anderson, P. S.; and Schecter, E. 1981. Plasma apolipoprotein B and VLDL-, LDL-, and HDL-cholesterol as risk factors in the development of coronary artery disease in male patients examined by angiography. *Atherosclerosis* 39:411–24.

63. Wilson, P. W. F.; Garrison, R. J.; and Castelli, W. P. 1985. Post-menopausal estrogen use, cigarette smoking and cardiovascular morbidity in women over 50. *NEJM* 313, 17:1038–43.

64. Yancey, M. K.; Hannan, C. J.; Plymate, S. R.; Stone, I. K.; Friedl, K. E.; and Wright, J. R. 1990. Serum lipids and lipoproteins in continuous or cyclic medroxyprogesterone acetate treatment in postmenopausal women treated with conjugated estrogens. *Fertil Steril* 54:778–82.

CHAPTER 11.   NUTRITION

1. Allen, L. H.; Oddoye, E. A.; and Margen, S. 1979. Protein-induced hypercalciurea: a longer term study. *Am J Clin Nutr* 32:741–49.
2. Anand, C. R., and Linkswiler, H. M. 1974. Effect of protein intake on calcium balance of young men given 500 mg. calcium daily. *J Nutr* 104: 695–700.
3. Bendich, A., and Langseth, L. 1989. Safety of vitamin A. *Am J Clin Nutr* 49:358–71.
4. Berry, E. M.; Hirsch, J.; Most, J.; McNamara, D. J.; and Thornton, J. 1986. The relationship of dietary fat to plasma lipid levels as studied by factor analysis of adipose tissue fatty acid composition in a free-living population of middle-aged American men. *Am J Clin Nutr* 44:220–31.
5. Blacklock, N. 1985. Renal stone. In *Dietary fibre, fibre-depleted foods and disease,* ed. H. Trowell, D. Burkett, and K. Heaton, ch. 21, pp. 345–59. New York: Academic Press.
6. Bowes, A., and Church, C. 1970. *Food values of portions commonly used,* rev. 11th ed., ed. C. F. Church and H. N. Church, pp. 1–80. Philadelphia: Lippincott.
7. Burkitt, D. 1985. Varicose veins, haemorrhoids, deep-vein thrombosis and pelvic phleboliths. In *Dietary fibre, fibre-depleted foods and disease,* ed. H. Trowell, D. Burkett, and K. Heaton, ch. 19, pp. 317–29. New York: Academic Press.
8. Callaway, C. W. 1986. Nutrition. *JAMA* 256, 15:2097–99.
9. Cameron, E.; Pauling, L.; and Lebowitz, B. 1979. Ascorbic acid and cancer. *Cancer Res* 29:663–81.
10. Castelli, W.; Garrison, R.; Wilson, P.; Abbott, R.; Kalousdian, S.; and Kannel, W. 1986. Incidence of coronary heart disease and lipoprotein cholesterol levels: the Framingham Study. *JAMA* 256:2835–38.
11. Castelli, W. P.; Doyle, J. T.; and Gordon, T. 1977. HDL cholesterol and other lipids in coronary heart disease. *Circulation* 55:767–72.
12. Chatham, M. D.; Eppler, J. H.; Sauder, L. R.; Green, D.; and Kulle, T. J. 1987. Evaluation of the effects of vitamin C on ozone-induced broncho-constriction in normal subjects. Third conference on vitamin C. *Ann NY Academy of Sciences* 498:269–79.
13. Chu, J. Y.; Margen, S.; and Costa, F. M. 1975. Studies in calcium metabolism: effects of low calcium and variable intake on human calcium metabolism. *Am J Clin Nutr* 28:1028–35.
14. Chu, S. Y.; Lee, N. C.; Wingo, P. A.; and Webster, L. A. 1989. Alcohol consumption and the risk of breast cancer. *Am J Epidemiol* 130, 5:867–77.
15. Counseller, V. S.; Hunt, W.; and Haigler, F. H. 1955. Carcinoma of the ovary following hysterectomy. *Am J Obstet Gynecol* 69:538–42.

16. Crofton, R. W.; Gvozdanovic, D.; Gvosdanovic, S.; Khin, C. C.; Brunt, P. W.; Mowat, N. A. G.; and Aggett, P. J. 1989. Inorganic zinc and the intestinal absorption of ferrous iron. *Am J Clin Nutr* 50:141–44.

17. Cummings, J. 1985. Cancer of the large bowel. In *Dietary fibre, fibre-depleted foods and disease,* ed. H. Trowell, D. Burkitt, and K. Heaton, ch. 9, pp. 161–89. New York: Academic Press.

18. Cummings, J. H. 1978. Nutritional implications of dietary fiber. *Am J Clin Nutr* 31, 10 (suppl.):S21–S29.

19. Cummings, J. H.; Hill, M. J.; Jivraj, T.; Houston, H.; Branch, W. J.; and Jenkins, D. J. A. 1979. The effect of meat protein and dietary fiber on colonic function and metabolism: changes in bowel habit, bile acid excretion, and calcium absorption. *Am J Clin Nutr* 32:2086–93.

20. Cutler, W. B. 1988. *Hysterectomy: before and after.* New York: Harper & Row.

21. Dawson-Hughes, B.; Seligson, F. H.; and Hughes, V. A. 1986. Effects of calcium carbonate and hydroxyapatite on zinc and iron retention in post-menopausal women. *Am J Clin Nutr* 44:83–88.

21a. Dreon, D. M.; Vranizan, K. M.; Krauss, R.; Austin, M. A.; and Wood, P. D. 1990. The effects of polyunsaturated fat vs. monounsaturated fat on plasma lipoproteins. *JAMA* 263:2461–66.

22. Edington, J. D.; Geekie, M.; Carter, R.; Benfield, L.; Ball, M.; and Mann, J. 1989. Serum lipid response to dietary cholesterol in subjects fed a low-fat, high-fiber diet. *Am J Clin Nutr* 50:58–62.

23. Fahey, P. J.; Boltri, J. M.; and Monk, J. S. 1987. Key issues in nutrition. *Postgrad Med* 81, 6:123–28.

24. Freudenheim, J. L.; Johnson, N. E.; and Smith, E. L. 1986. Relationships between usual nutrient intake and bone-mineral content of women 35–65 years of age: longitudinal and cross-sectional analysis. *Am J Clin Nutr* 44:863–76.

24a. Gey, K. F.; Stahelin, H. B.; Puska, P.; and Evans, A. 1987: Relationship of plasma level of vitamin C to mortality from ischemic heart disease. Third conference on vitamin C. *Ann NY Academy of Sciences* 498:110–23.

25. Glembotski, C. C. 1987. The role of ascorbic acid in the biosynthesis of the neuroendocrine peptides a-MSH and TRH. Third conference on vitamin C. *Ann NY Academy of Sciences* 498:54–62.

26. Glueck, C. J.; Gordon, D. J.; Nelson, J. J.; Davis, C. E.; and Tyroler, H. A. 1986. Dietary and other correlates of changes in total and low density lipoprotein cholesterol in hypercholesterolemic men: the lipid research clinics coronary primary prevention trial. *Am J Clin Nutr* 44:489–500.

27. Goldin, B. R., *et al.* 1982. Estrogen excretion patterns and plasma levels in vegetarian and omnivorous women. *NEJM* 307:1542–47.

28. Griessen, M.; Cochet, B.; Infante, F.; Jung, A.; Bartholdi, P.; Donath,

A.; Loizeau, C.; and Courvoisier, B. 1989. Calcium absorption from milk in lactase-deficient subjects. *Am J Clin Nutr* 49:377–84.

29. Hadley, E. C. 1986. Bladder training and related therapies for urinary incontinence in older people. *JAMA* 256, 3:372–79.

30. Hallberg, L.; Brune, M.; and Rossander, L. 1989. Iron absorption in man: ascorbic acid and dose-dependent inhibition by phytate. *Am J Clin Nutr* 49:140–44.

31. Hallberg, L.; Brune, M.; and Rossander-Hulthen, L. 1987. Is there a physiological role of vitamin C in iron absorption? Third conference on vitamin C. *Ann NY Academy of Sciences* 498:324–32.

32. Heaney, R. P.; Gallagher, J. C.; Johnston, C. C.; Neer, R.; Parfitt, A. M.; Chir, E.; and Wheldon, G. D. 1982. Calcium nutrition and bone health in the elderly. *Am J Clin Nutr* 36:986–1013.

33. Heaney, R. P., and Recker, R. R. 1982. Effects of nitrogen, phosphorus and caffeine on calcium balance in women. *J Lab Clin Med* 99:46–56.

34. Heaney, R. P.; Weaver, C. M.; and Recker, R. R. 1988. Calcium absorbability from spinach. *Am J Clin Nutr* 47:707–9.

35. Heaton, K. 1985. Gallstones. In *Dietary fibre, fibre-depleted foods and disease,* ed. H. Trowell, D. Burkett, and K. Heaton, ch. 17, pp. 289–304. New York: Academic Press.

36. Hegsted, D. M. 1986. Serum-cholesterol response to dietary cholesterol: a re-evaluation. *Am J Clin Nutr* 44:299–305.

37. Hegsted, M., and Linkswiler, H. M. 1981. Long-term effects of level of protein intake on calcium metabolism in young adult women. *J Nutr* 3:244–51.

38. Hegsted, M.; Schuette, S. A.; Zemel, M. B.; and Linkswiler, H. M. 1981. Urinary calcium and calcium balance in young men as affected by level of protein and phosphorous intake. *J Nutr* 3:553–62.

39. Herold, E.; Mottin, J.; and Sabry, Z. 1979. Effect of vitamin E on human sexual functioning. *Arch Sex Beh* 8:397–403.

40. Herold, P. M., and Kinsella, J. E. 1986. Fish oil consumption and decreased risk of cardiovascular disease: a comparison of findings from animal and human feeding trials. *Am J Clin Nutr* 43:566–98.

41. Holbrook, J. T.; Smith, Jr.; J. C.; and Reiser, S. 1989. Dietary fructose or starch: effects on copper, zinc, iron, manganese, calcium, and magnesium balances in humans. *Am J Clin Nutr* 49:1290–94.

42. Jacques, P. F.; Hartz, S. C.; McGandy, R. B.; Jacob, R. A.; and Russell, R. M. 1987. Vitamin C and blood lipoproteins in an elderly population. Third conference on vitamin C. *Ann NY Academy of Sciences* 498:100–9.

43. Kato, I.; Tominaga, S.; and Terao, C. 1989. Alcohol consumption and cancers of hormone-related organs in females. *Jpn J Clin Oncol* 19, 3:202–7.

44. Kestin, M.; Clifton, P. M.; Rouse, I. L.; and Nestel, P. J. 1989. Effect of

dietary cholesterol in normolipidemic subjects is not modified by nature and amount of dietary fat. *Am J Clin Nutr* 50:528–32.

45. Keys, A. 1986. Serum cholesterol response to dietary cholesterol. *Am J Clin Nutr* 44:309–11.

46. Komindr, S.; Nichoalds, G. E.; and Kitabchi, A. E. 1987. Bimodal effects of megadose vitamin C on adrenal steroid production in man: an in vivo study. Third conference on vitamin C. *Ann NY Academy of Sciences* 498: 487–90.

47. Krasinski, S. D.; Russell, R. M.; Otradovec, C. L.; Sadowski, J. A.; Hartz, S. C.; Jacob, R. A.; and McGandy, R. B. 1989. Relationship of vitamin A and vitamin E intake to fasting plasma retinol, retinol-binding protein, retinyl esters, carotene, β-tocopherol, and cholesterol among elderly people and young adults: increased plasma retinyl esters among vitamin A-supplement users. *Am J Clin Nutr* 49:112–20.

47a. Kritchevsky, D. 1985. Lipid metabolism and coronary heart disease. In *Dietary fibre, fibre-depleted foods and disease,* ed. H. Trowell, D. Burkett, and K. Heaton, ch. 18, pp. 305–15. New York: Academic Press.

48. Kupperman, H. S.; Wetchler, B. B.; and Blatt, M. H. G. 1959. Contemporary therapy of the menopausal syndrome. *JAMA* 171:1627–37.

49. Leuchtenberger, L., and Leuchtenberger, R. 1977. Protection of hamster lung culture of L-cysteine or vitamin C against carcinogenic effects of fresh smoke from tobacco or marijuana cigarettes. *Br J Exp Pathol* 58:625–34.

50. Levine, M., and Hartzell, W. 1987. Ascorbic acid: the concept of optimum requirements. Third conference on vitamin C. *Ann NY Academy of Sciences* 498:424–44.

51. Licata, A. A.; Bori, E.; Bartter, F. C.; and West, F. 1976. Acute effects on dietary protein on calcium metabolism in patients with osteoporosis. *J Geron* 36, 1:14–19.

52. Lohmann, W. 1987. Ascorbic acid and cancer. Third conference on vitamin C. *Ann NY Academy of Sciences* 498:402–17.

53. Lowerfels, A. B., and Zevola, S. A. 1989. Alcohol and breast cancer: an overview. *Alcoholism (NY)* 13, 1:109–11.

54. Lubin, F.; Wax, Y.; Ron, E.; Black, M.; Chetrit, A.; Rosen, N.; Alfandary, E.; and Modan, B. 1989. Nutritional factors associated with benign breast disease etiology: a case-control study. *Am J Clin Nutr* 50:551–56.

55. Mann, J. 1985. Diabetes mellitus: some aspects of aetiology and management of non-insulin-dependent diabetes. In *Dietary fibre, fibre-depleted foods and Disease,* ed. H. Trowell, D. Burkett, and K. Heaton, ch. 16, pp. 263–87. New York: Academic Press.

55a. Margen, S.; Chu, J. Y.; Kaufmann, N. A.; and Calloway, D. H. 1974. Studies in calcium metabolism: the calciuretic effect of dietary protein. *Am J Clin Nutr* 27:584–89.

56. Margetts, B. M. 1986. Recent developments in the etiology and treatment of hypertension: dietary calcium, fat and magnesium. *Am J Clin Nutr* 44:704.

57. Meara, J.; McPherson, K.; Roberts, M.; Jones, L.; and Vessey, M. 1989. Alcohol, cigarette smoking and breast cancer. *Br J Cancer* 60, 1:70–73.

58. Michael, R. P., and Zumpe, D. 1976. Environmental and endocrine factors influencing annual changes in sexual potency in primates. *Psychoneuroendocrinology* 1:303–13.

59. Mohsenin, V., and DuBois, A. B. 1987. Vitamin C and airways. Third conference on vitamin C. *Ann NY Academy of Sciences* 498:259–68.

60. Morse, D. R.; Schacterle, G. R.; Furst, L.; Zaydenberg, M.; and Pollack, R. L. 1989. Oral digestion of a complex-carbohydrate cereal: effects of stress and relaxation on physiological and salivary measures. *Am J Clin Nutr* 49:97–105.

61. Nestel, P. J. 1986. Fish oil attenuates the cholesterol induced rise in lipoprotein cholesterol. *Am J Clin Nutr* 43:752–57.

62. Nielsen, F. H.; Hunt, C. D.; Mullen, L. M.; and Hunt, J. R. 1987. Effect of dietary boron on mineral, estrogen, and testosterone metabolism in postmenopausal women. *FASEB J* 1, 5:394–97.

63. Oh, S. Y., and Miller, L. T. 1985. Effect of dietary egg on variability of plasma cholesterol levels and lipoprotein cholesterol. *Am J Clin Nutr* 42: 421–31.

64. Oh, S. Y., and Monaco, P. A. 1985. Effect of dietary cholesterol and degree of fat unsaturation on plasma lipid levels, lipoprotein composition and fecal steroid excretion in normal young adult men. *Am J Clin Nutr* 42:399–413.

65. Omaye, S. T.; Skala, J. H.; and Jacob, R. A. 1986. Plasma ascorbic acid in adult males: effects of depletion and supplementation. *Am J Clin Nutr* 44:257–64.

66. Painter, N. 1985. Diverticular disease of the colon. In *Dietary fibre, fibre-depleted foods and disease,* ed. H. Trowell, D. Burkett, and K. Heaton, ch. 8, pp. 145–59. New York: Academic Press.

67. Pauling, L. 1986. *How to live long and feel better.* New York: Freeman.

68. Reiser, R.; Probstfield, J. L.; Silvers, A.; Scott, L. W.; Shorney, M. L.; Wood, R. D.; O'Brien, B. C.; Gotto, A. M.; Phil, D.; and Insull, W. 1985. Plasma lipid and lipoprotein response of humans to beef fat, coconut oil and safflower oil. *Am J Clin Nutr* 42:190–97.

69. Richardson, S.; de Vincenzi, I.; Pujol, H.; and Gerber, M. 1989. Alcohol consumption in a case-control study of breast cancer in southern France. *Int J Cancer* 44, 1:84–89.

70. Ringsdorf, W. M., and Cheraskin, E. 1982. Vitamin C and human wound healing. *Oral Surgery* 53:231–36.

70a. Rivers, J. M. 1987. Safety of high-level vitamin C ingestion. Third conference on vitamin C. *Ann NY Academy of Sciences* 498:445–54.

71. Robinson, R. W.; Higano, N.; and Cohen, W. D. 1959. Increased incidence of coronary heart disease in women castrated prior to menopause.
Arch Intern Med 104:908–13.

72. Romney, S. L.; Duttagupta, C.; Basu, J.; Palan, P. R.; Karp, S.; Slagle, S.;
Dwyer, A.; Wassertheil-Smoller, S.; and Wylie-Rosett, J. 1985. Plasma
vitamin C and uterine cervical dysplasia. *Am J Obstet Gynecol* 151:976–80.

73. Romney, S. L., *et al.* 1981. Retinoids and the prevention of cervical dysplasia. *Am J Obstet Gynecol* 141:890–94.

74. Rosenberg, L.; Palmer, J. R.; Miller, D. R.; Clarke, E. A.; and Shapiro, S.
1990. A case-control study of alcoholic beverage consumption and breast
cancer. *Am J Epidemiol* 131, 1:6–14.

75. Schatzkin, A.; Carter, C. L.; Green, S. B.; Kreger, B. E.; Splansky, G. L.;
Anderson, K. M.; Helsel, W. E.; and Kannel, W. B. 1989. Is alcohol
consumption related to breast cancer?: results from the Framingham Heart
Study. *J Natl Cancer Inst* 81, 1:31–35.

76. Schatzkin, A.; Piantadosi, S.; Miccozzi, M.; and Bartee, D. 1989. Alcohol consumption and breast cancer: a cross-national correlation study. *Int
J Epidemiol* 18, 1:28–31.

77. Schuette, S. A., and Linkswiler, H. M. 1982. Effects of Ca and P metabolism in humans by adding meat, meat plus milk, or purified proteins plus
Ca and P to a low protein diet. *J Nutr* 112:338–49.

78. Scrimshaw, N. S., and Murray, E. B. 1988. Chapter 12, summary and
conclusions. *Am J Clin Nutr* 48:1140.

79. Segal, I. 1985. Hiatal hernia and gastro-oesophageal reflux. In *Dietary
fibre, fibre-depleted foods and disease,* ed. H. Trowell, D. Burkett, and K.
Heaton, ch. 14, pp. 241–47. New York: Academic Press.

80. Shaffer, C. F. 1970. Ascorbic acid and atherosclerosis. *Am J Clin Nutr* 23,
1:27–30.

81. Shanmugasundaram, K. R.; Visvanathan, A.; Dhandapani, K.; Srinivasan,
N.; Rasappan, P.; Gilbert, R.; Alladi, S.; Kancharla, S.; and Vasanthi, N.
1986. Effect of high-fat diet on cholesterol distribution in plasma lipoproteins, cholesterol esterifying activity in leucocytes and erythrocyte
membrane components studied: importance of body weight. *Am J Clin
Nutr* 44:805–15.

82. Shultz, T. D., and Leklem, J. E. 1983. Nutrient intake and hormonal
status of premenopausal vegetarian Seventh Day Adventists and premenopausal nonvegetarians. *Nutr Cancer* 4:247–59.

83. Simpson, H. C. R., and Mann, J. I. 1982. Effect of high-fibre diet on
hemostatic variables in diabetes. *Brit Med J* 284:1608.

84. Sirtori, C. R.; Tremoli, E.; Gatti, E.; Montanari, G.; Sirtori, M.; Colli,

S.; Gianfranceschi, G.; Maderna, P.; Dentone, C. Z.; Testolin, G.; and Galli, C. 1986. Controlled evaluation of fat intake in the Mediterranean diet: comparative activities of olive oil and corn oil on plasma lipids and platelets in high-risk patients. *Am J Clin Nutr* 44:635–42.

85. Smith, J. L., and Hodges, R. E. 1987. Serum levels of vitamin C in relation to dietary and supplemental intake of vitamin C in smokers and non-smokers. Third conference on vitamin C. *Ann NY Academy of Sciences* 498: 144–52.

86. Southgate, D., and Englyst, H. 1985. Dietary fibre: chemistry, physical properties and analysis. In *Dietary fibre, fibre-depleted foods and disease,* ed. H. Trowell, D. Burkett, and K. Heaton, ch. 3, pp. 31–55. New York: Academic Press.

87. Spencer, H.; Kramer, L.; DeBartol, M.; Norris, C.; and Osis, D. 1983. Further studies of the effect of a high protein diet as meat on calcium metabolism. *Am J Clin Nutr* 37:924–29.

88. Spencer, I.; Kramer, L.; Osis, D.; and Norris, C. 1978. Effect of a high protein (meat) intake on calcium metabolism in man. *Am J Clin Nutr* 31:2167–80.

89. Tannenbaum, S. R., and Wishnok, J. S. 1987. Inhibition of nitrosamine formation by ascorbic acid. Third conference on vitamin C. *Ann NY Academy of Sciences* 498:354–63.

90. Thuesen, L.; Henriksen, L. B.; Diet, C.; and Engby, B. 1986. One-year experience with a low-fat, low-cholesterol diet in patients with coronary heart disease. *Am J Clin Nutr* 44:212–19.

91. Toniolo, P.; Riboli, E.; Protta, F.; Charrel, M.; and Cappa, A. P. 1989. Breast cancer and alcohol consumption: a case-control study in northern Italy. *Cancer Res* 49, 18:5203–6.

92. Trowell, H.; Burkett, D.; and Heaton, K. 1985. Definitions of dietary fibre and fibre-depleted foods. In *Dietary fibre, fibre-depleted foods and disease,* ed. H. Trowell, D. Burkett, and K. Heaton, ch. 2, pp. 23–29. New York: Academic Press.

93. Vallance, S. 1977. Relationships between ascorbic acid and serum proteins of the immune system. *Brit Med J* 2:437–38.

94. vant Veer, P.; Kok, F. J.; Hermus, R. J.; and Sturmans, F. 1989. Alcohol dose, frequency and age at first exposure in relation to the risk of breast cancer. *Int J Epidemiol* 18, 3:511–17.

95. Walker, A. 1985. Mineral metabolism. In *Dietary fibre, fibre-depleted foods and disease,* ed. H. Trowell, D. Burkett, and K. Heaton, ch. 22, pp. 361–75. New York: Academic Press.

96. Wassertheil-Smoller, S., *et al.* 1981. Dietary vitamin C and uterine cervical dysplasia. *Am J Epidemiol* 114:714.

96a. Whelan, E., and Stare, F. 1990. Nutrition. *JAMA* 263:2661–63.

97. Whiting, S. J., and Draper, H. H. 1980. The role of sulfate in the calciuria of high protein diets in adult rats. *J Nutr* 110:212–22.

98. Williams, P. T.; Krauss, R. M.; Kindel-Joyce, S.; Dreon, D. M.; Vranizan, K. M.; and Wood, P. D. 1986. Relationship of dietary fat, protein, cholesterol and fiber intake to atherogenic lipoproteins in men. *Am J Clin Nutr* 44:788–97.

99. Wylie-Rosett, J. A., *et al.* 1984. Influence of vitamin A on cervical dysplasia and carcinoma in situ. *Nutr Cancer* 6:49–57.

100. Young, T. B. 1989. A case-control study of breast cancer and alcohol consumption habits. *Cancer* 64, 2:552–58.

101. Zannoni, V. G.; Brodfuehrer, J. I.; Smart, R. C.; and Susick, R. L. 1987. Ascorbic acid, alcohol, and environmental chemicals. Third conference on vitamin C. *Ann NY Academy of Sciences* 498:364–88.

102. Zemel, M. B.; Schuette, S. A.; Hegsted, M.; and Linkswiler, H. M. 1981. Role of the sulfur-containing amino acids in protein-induced hypercalciuria in men. *J Nutr* 3:545–52.

CHAPTER 12.   SMOKING AND OBESITY

1. Bowes, A., and Church, C. 1970. *Food values of portions commonly used,* 11th ed., rev. Charles F. Church and Helen N. Church, pp. 1–80. Philadelphia: Lippincott.

2. Callaway, C. W. 1986. Nutrition. *JAMA* 256, 15:2097–99.

3. Daniell, H. W. 1976. Osteoporosis in the slender smoker. *Arch Intern Med* 136:298–304.

4. ———. 1980. Estrogen receptors, breast cancer and smoking. *NEJM* 302:1478.

5. Eastwood, M., and Brydon, W. G. 1985. Physiological effects of dietary fibre on the alimentary tract. In *Dietary fibre, fibre-depleted foods and disease,* ed. H. Trowell, D. Burkett, and K. Heaton, ch. 6, pp. 105–32. New York: Academic Press.

6. Elliot, D. L.; Goldberg, L.; Kuehl, K. S.; and Bennett, W. M. 1989. Sustained depression of the resting metabolic rate after massive weight loss. *Am J Clin Nutr* 49:93–96.

7. Gusberg, S. B. 1975. A strategy for the control of endometrial cancer. *Proc Royal Soc of Med* 68:163–68.

8. Hammer, R. L.; Barrier, C. A.; Roundy, E. S.; Bradford, J. M.; and Fisher, A. G. 1989. Calorie-restricted low-fat diet and exercise in obese women. *Am J Clin Nutr* 49:77–85.

9. James, P. 1985. Obesity: the interaction of environment and genetic predisposition. In *Dietary fibre, fibre-depleted foods and disease,* ed. H. Trowell,

D. Burkett, and K. Heaton, ch. 15, pp. 249–61. New York: Academic Press.

10. Jensen, J.; Christiansen, C.; and Rodbro, P. 1985. Cigarette smoking, serum estrogens and bone loss during hormone-replacement therapy after early menopause. *NEJM* 313, 16:973–75.

11. Judd, H. L.; Davidson, B. J.; Frumar, A. M.; Shamonki, I. M.; Lagasse, L. D.; and Ballon, S. C. 1980. Serum androgens and estrogens in post-menopausal women with and without endometrial cancer. *Am J Obstet Gynecol* 135:859–71.

12. Lindsay, R. 1981. The influence of cigarette smoking on bone mass and bone loss. In *Osteoporosis: recent advances in pathogenesis and treatment,* ed. H. F. DeLuca *et al.,* p. 481. Baltimore: University Park Press.

13. Lindsay, R.; Coutts, J. R.; and Hart, D. M. 1977. The effect of endogenous oestrogen on plasma and urinary calcium and phosphate in oophorectomized women. *Clin Endocrinol (Oxf)* 6, 2:87–93.

14. MacDonald, P. C.; Edman, C. D.; Hemsell, D. L.; Porter, J. C.; and Siiteri, P. K. 1978. Effect of obesity on conversion of plasma and androstenedione to estrone in postmenopausal women with and without endometrial cancer. *Am J Obstet Gynecol* 130, 4:448–55.

15. Pelleter, O. 1968. Smoking and vitamin C levels in humans. *Am J Clin Nutr* 21:1259–67.

16. Pirke, K. M.; Schweiger, U.; Laessle, R.; Dickaut, B.; Schweiger, M.; and Waechteler, M. 1986. Dieting influences the menstrual cycle: vegetarian vs. nonvegetarian diet. *Fertil Steril* 46:1083–88.

17. Pirke, K. M.; Schweiger, U.; Strowitzki, T.; Tuschl, R.; Laessle, R. G.; Broocks, A.; Huber, B.; and Middendorf, R. 1989. Dieting causes menstrual irregularities in normal weight young women through impairment of episodic luteinizing hormone secretion. *Fertil Steril* 51, 2:263–68.

18. Sarles, H.; Gerolami, A.; and Cros, R. C. 1978. Diet and cholesterol gallstones: a further study. *Digestion* 17:128–34.

18a. Schlemmer, A.; Jensen, J.; Riis, B. J.; and Christiansen, C. 1990. Smoking induces increased androgen levels in early post-menopausal women. *Maturitas* 12:99–104.

19. Schweiger, U.; Laessle, R.; Pfister, H.; and Hoehl, C. 1987. Diet-induced menstrual irregularities: effects of age and weight loss. *Fertil Steril* 48, 5:746–51.

20. Stamford, B. A.; Matter, S.; Fell, R. D.; and Papanek, P. 1986. Effects of smoking cessation on weight gain, metabolic rate, caloric consumption and blood lipids. *Am J Clin Nutr* 43:486–94.

21. Thallasinos, N. C.; Gutteridge, D. H.; Joplin, G. F.; and Fraser, T. R. 1982. Calcium balance in osteoporotic patients on long-term oral calcium therapy with and without sex hormones. *Clin Sci* 62:221–26.

22. Van Dale, D., and Saris, W. H. M. 1989. Repetitive weight loss and

weight regain: effects on weight reduction, resting metabolic rate, and lipolytic activity before and after exercise and/or diet treatment. *Am J Clin Nutr* 49:409–16.

23. Williams, A. R.; Weiss, N. S.; Ure, C. L.; Ballard, J.; and Daling, J. R. 1982. Effect of weight, smoking, and estrogen use on the risk of hip and forearm fractures in postmenopausal women. *Obstet Gynecol* 60:695–99.

24. Wynder, E. L.; Escher, G. C.; and Mantel, N. 1966. An epidemiological investigation of cancer of the endometrium. *Cancer* 19:489–520.

CHAPTER 13.   EXERCISES

1. Brehm, B. A. 1988. Elevation of metabolic rate following exercise—implications for weight loss. *Sports Medicine* 6:72–78.

2. Carr, D. B.; Bullen, B. A.; Skrinar, G. S.; Arnold, M. A.; Rosenblatt, M.; Beitens, I. Z.; Martin, J. B.; and McArthur, J. W. 1981. Physical conditioning facilitates the exercise-induced secretion of beta endorphin and beta-lipotropin in women. *NEJM* 305:560–63.

3. Cordain, L., and Stager, J. 1988. Pulmonary structure and function in swimmers. *Sports Medicine* 6:271–78.

4. Friden, J.; Sfakianos, P. N.; and Hargens, A. R. 1986. Muscle soreness and intramuscular fluid pressure: comparison between eccentric and concentric load. *American Physiological Society* 61:2175–79.

5. Garrick, J. G., and Requa, R. K. 1988. Aerobic dance: a review. *Sports Medicine* 6:169–179.

6. Glass, A. R.; Deuster, P. A.; Kyle, S. B.; Yahiro, J. A.; Vigersky, R. A.; and Shoomaker, E. B. 1987. Amenorrhea in Olympic marathon runners. *Fertil Steril* 48, 5:740–45.

7. Gossard, D., and DeBusk, R. F. 1986. Effects of low- and high-intensity homebased exercise training on functional capacity in healthy middle-aged men. *JAMA* 256, 3:401.

8. Heyden, S., and Fodor, G. J. 1988. Does regular exercise prolong life expectancy? *Sports Medicine* 6:63–71.

9. Hohtari, H.; Elovainio, R.; Salminen, K.; and Laatikainen, T. 1988. Plasma corticotropin-releasing hormone, corticotropin, and endorphins at rest and during exercise in eumenorrheic and amenorrheic athletes. *Fertil Steril* 50:233–38.

10. Howlett, T.; Tomlin, S.; Ngahfoong, L.; Bullen, B. A.; Skrinar, G. S.; McArthur, J.; and Rees, L. 1984. Exercise-induced release of met-enkephalin and beta endorphins. In *Central and peripheral endorphins,* ed. E. Muller and A. Genazzani, pp. 285–88. New York: Raven.

11. Keast, D.; Cameron, K.; and Morton, A. R. 1988. Exercise and the immune response. *Sports Medicine* 5:248–67.

12. Lazarus, N. B.; Kaplan, G. A.; Cohen, R. D.; and Leu, D.-J. 1989. Smoking and body mass in the natural history of physical activity: prospective evidence from the Alameda County Study, 1965–1974. *Am J Prev Med* 5:127–35.

13. McMurray, R. G.; Forsythe, W. A.; Mar, M. H.; and Hardy, C. J. 1987. Exercise intensity-related responses of beta-endorphin and catecholamines. *Med Sci Sports and Exercise* 19:570–74.

14. McPhillips, J. B.; Pellettera, K. M.; Barrett-Connor, E.; Wingard, D. L.; and Criqui, M. H. 1989. Exercise patterns in a population of older adults. *Am J Prev Med* 2:65–72.

15. Morehouse, L. E.; and Miller, A. T. 1959. *Physiology of exercise.* St. Louis: Mosby.

16. Rahkila, P.; Hakala, E.; Alen, M.; Salminen, K.; and Laatikainen, T. 1988. Beta-endorphin and corticotropin release is dependent on a threshold intensity of running exercise in male endurance athletes. *Life Sciences* 43:551–58.

17. Rahkila, P.; Hakala, E.; Salminen, K.; and Laatikainen, T. 1987. Response of plasma endorphins to running exercises in male and female endurance athletes. *Med Sci Sports and Exercise* 19, 5:451–55.

18. Schutz, Y.; Bessard, T.; and Jequier, E. 1987. Exercise and postprandial thermogenesis in obese women before and after weight loss. *Am Soc Clin Nutr* 45:1424–32.

19. Schweiger, U.; Herrmann, F.; Lawssle, R.; Riedel, W.; Schweiger, M.; and Pirke, K.-L. 1988. Caloric intake, stress, and menstrual function in athletes. *Fertil Steril* 49, 3:447–50.

20. Seidell, J. C.; Cigolini, M.; Deurenberg, P.; Oosterlee, A.; and Doornbos, G. 1989. Fat distribution, androgens, and metabolism in nonobese women. *Am J Clin Nutr* 50:269–73.

21. Sforzo, G. A. 1988. Opiods and exercise. *Sports Medicine* 7:110–24.

22. Van Dam, S.; Gillespy, M.; Notelovitz, M.; and Martin, A. D. 1988. Effect of exercise on glucose metabolism in postmenopausal women. *Am J Obstet Gynecol* 159, 1:82–86.

23. Viswanathan, M.; VanDijk, J. P.; Graham, T. E.; Bonen, A.; and George, J. C. 1987. Exercise- and cold-induced changes in plasma β-endorphin and β-lipotropin in men and women. *J Appl Physiol* 62, 2:622–27.

24. Weissman, C.; Goldstein, S.; Askanazi, J.; Rosenbaum, S. H.; Milic-Emilii, J.; and Kinney, J. M. 1986. Semistarvation and exercise. *Am Physiol Soc* 5:2035–39.

25. Williford, H. N.; Blessing, D. L.; Olson, M. S.; and Smith, F. H. 1989. Is low-impact aerobic dance an effective cardiovascular workout? *Physician and Sports Medicine* 17, 3:95–109.

CHAPTER 14.   ALTERNATIVES TO HORMONE REPLACEMENT THERAPY

1. Alexander, S.; Aksel, S.; Hazelton, J.; Yeoman, R.; and Gilmore, S. 1990. The effect of aging on hypothalamic function in oophorectomized women. *Am J Obstet Gynecol* 162:446–49.

1a. Batra, S., and Losif, S. 1987. Progesterone receptors in vaginal tissue of post-menopausal women. *Maturitas* 9, 1:87–94.

2. Bergmans, M. G. M.; Merkus, J. M. W. M.; Corbey, R. S.; Schellekens, L. A.; and Ubachs, J. M. H. 1987. Effect of Bellergal Retard on climacteric complaints: a double-blind, placebo-controlled study. *Maturitas* 9:227–34.

2a. Brooks, P.; DeCherney, A.; Loffer, F.; and Neuwirth, R. 1989. Resectoscopy: mastering the challenges. *Contem OB/GYN* 34:131–48.

2b. Brooks, P.; Loffer, F.; and Serden, S. 1989. Resectoscopic removal of symptomatic intrauterine lesions. *J Reprod Med* 34:435–37.

3. Bullock, J. L.; Massey, F. M.; and Gambrell, Jr., R. D. 1975. Use of medroxyprogesterone acetate to prevent menopausal symptoms. *Obstet Gynecol* 46, 2:165–68.

4. Chestnut, C. H.; Baylink, D. J.; and Nelp, W. B. 1979. Calcitonin therapy in postmenopausal osteoporosis: preliminary results. *Clin Res* 27:85A, abstract.

5. Claydon, J. R.; Bell, J. Y.; and Pollard, P. 1974. Menopausal flushing: double-blind trial of a non-hormonal medication. *Brit Med J* 1:409–12.

6. Coope, J.; Williams, S.; and Patterson, J. S. 1978. A study of the effectiveness of propanolol in menopausal hot flushes. *Br J Obstet Gynaecol* 85, 6:472–75.

7. Cutler, W. B. 1988. *Hysterectomy: before and after.* New York: Harper & Row.

8. D'Amato, G.; Cavallini, A.; Messa, C.; Mangini, V.; and Misciagna, G. 1989. Serum and bile lipid levels in a postmenopausal woman after percutaneous and oral natural estrogens. *Am J Obstet Gynecol* 160:600–1.

8a. Dreon, D. M.; Vranizan, K. M.; Krauss, R.; Austin, M. A.; and Wood, P. D. 1990. The effects of polyunsaturated fat vs. monounsaturated fat on plasma lipoproteins. *JAMA* 263:2461–66.

8b. Genant, H.; Baylink, D.; Gallagher, J. C.; Harris, S.; Steiger, P.; and Herbert, M. 1990. Effect of estrone sulfate on postmenopausal bone loss. *Obstet Gynecol* 76:579–84.

9. Gennari, C. 1987. The rationale for the use of calcitonin in osteoporotic women. Fifth International Congress on the Menopause, Sorrento, Italy, 6–10 April 1987.

10. Greenspan, E. M. 1983. Ginseng and vaginal bleeding. *JAMA* 249:2018.

11. Gruber, H. E.; Ivey, J. L.; Baylink, D. J.; Matthews, M.; Nelp, W. B.; Sisom, K.; and Chestnut, C. H. 1984. Long-term calcitonin therapy in postmenopausal osteoporosis. *Metab Clin Exper* 33, 4:295–303.

12. Hopkins, M. P.; Androff, L. A.; and Benninghoff, A. S. 1988. Ginseng face cream and unexplained vaginal bleeding. *Am J Obstet Gynecol* 159: 1121–22.

13. Kicovic, P. M.; Cortes-Prieto, J.; Milojevic, S.; Haspels, A. A.; and Aljinovic, A. 1980. The treatment of postmenopausal vaginal atrophy with ovestin vaginal cream or suppositories: clinical, endocrinological and safety aspects. *Maturitas* 2:275–82.

14. Laurian, L. 1987. Calcitonin: an analgesic for osteoporotic women. Fifth International Congress on the Menopause, Sorrento, Italy, 6–10 April 1987.

15. Lindsay, R. 1981. The influence of cigarette smoking on bone mass and bone loss. *Osteoporosis: recent advances in pathogenesis and treatment,* ed. H. L. DeLuca *et al.,* p. 481. Baltimore: University Park Press.

16. Lindsay, R., and Hart, D. M. 1978. Failure of response of menopausal vasomotor symptoms to clonidine. *Maturitas* 1:21–25.

17. Lobo, R. A.; McCormick, M.; Singer, F.; and Roy, S. 1984. Depo-medroxyprogesterone acetate compared with conjugated estrogens for the treatment of postmenopausal women. *Obstet Gynecol* 63:1–5.

17a. Molander, U.; Milsom, I.; Ekelund, P.; Mellstrom, D.; and Eriksson, O. 1990. Effect of oral oestriol on vaginal flora and cytology and urogenital symptoms in the post-menopause. *Maturitas* 12:113–20.

17b. Morris, M.; Salmon, P.; Steinberg, H.; Sykes, E. A.; Bouloux, P.; Newbould, E.; McLoughlin, L.; Besser, G. M.; and Grossman, A. 1990. Endogenous opiods modulate the cardiovascular response to mental stress. *Psychoneuroendocrinology* 15:186–92.

18. Morrison, J. C., *et al.* 1980. The use of medroxyprogesterone acetate (DepoProvera) for relief of climacteric symptoms. *Am J Obstet Gynecol* 138:99–104.

18a. Osmers, R.; Volksen, M.; and Schauer, A. 1990. Vaginosonography for early detection of endometrial carcinoma? *Lancet* 335:1569–71.

19. Overgaard, K.; Riis, B. J.; Christiansen, C.; Podenphant, J.; and Johansen, J. S. 1989. Nasal calcitonin for treatment of established osteoporosis. *Clin Endocrinol* 30, 4:435–42.

20. Punnonen, R., and Lukola, A. 1980. Estrogen-like effect of ginseng. *Brit Med J* 281:1110.

21. Rud, T. 1980. The effects of estrogens & gestagens on the urethral pressure profile in urinary continent & stress incontinent women. *Acta Obstet et Gynecol Scand* 59:265–70.

21a. Saarikoski, S.; Yliskoski, M.; and Penttila, I. 1990. Sequential use of nor-ethisterone and natural progesterone in pre-menopausal bleeding disorders. *Maturitas* 12:89–97.

22. Schiff, I.; Tulchinsky, D.; and Cramer, D. 1980. Oral medroxyprogesterone in the treatment of postmenopausal symptoms. *JAMA* 244:1443–45.

23. Schiff, I.; Wentworth, B.; Koos, B.; Ryan, K. J.; and Tulchinsky, D. 1978. Effect of estriol administration on the hypogonadal woman. *Fertil Steril* 30:278–82.

23a. Schlemmer, A.; Jensen, J.; Riis, B. J.; and Christiansen, C. 1990. Smoking induces increased androgen levels in early post-menopausal women. *Maturitas* 12:99–104.

23b. Sherwin, B. 1988. Estrogen and/or androgen replacement therapy and cognitive functioning in surgically menopausal women. *Psychoneuroendocrinology* 13:345–57.

23c. ———. 1988. The role of androgens in menopausal women. In *Androgens in the menopause,* ed. Leon Speroff. Marietta, Ga.: Reid-Rowell.

23d. Sherwin, B., and Phillips, S. 1990. Estrogen and cognitive functioning in surgically menopausal women. *Ann NY Academy of Sciences* 592:474–75.

23e. Stall, G.; Harris, S.; Sokoll, L.; and Hughes, B. D. 1990. Accelerated bone loss in hypothyroid patients overtreated with L-thyroxine. *AIM* 113:265–69.

24. Stevenson, J. C. 1987. The use of estrogen replacement therapy on calcitonin in the prevention of postmenopausal bone loss. Fifth International Congress on the Menopause, Sorrento, Italy, 6–10 April 1987.

25. ———. 1980. The structure and function of calcitonin. *Invest and Cell Path* 3:187–93.

26. Stevenson, J. C.; Hillyard, C. J.; Abeyasekara, G.; Phang, K. G.; MacIntyre, I.; Campbell, S.; Young, O.; Townsend, P. T.; and Whitehead, M. I. 1981. Calcitonin and the calcium-regulating hormones in postmenopausal women: effect of estrogens. *Lancet* 1:693–95.

26a. Stuart, C. A., and Nagamani, M. 1990. Insulin infusion acutely augments ovarian androgen production in normal women. *Fertil Steril* 54:788–92.

27. Taggart, H.; Ivey, J. L.; Sison, K.; Chesnut, C. H., III; Baylink, D. J.; Huber, M. B.; and Roos, B. A. 1982. Deficient calcitonin response to calcium stimulation in postmenopausal osteoporosis. *Lancet* 2:475–78.

28. Teichmann, A. T.; Cremer, P.; Wieland, H.; Kuhn, W.; and Seidel, D. 1988. Lipid metabolic changes during hormonal treatment of endometriosis. *Maturitas* 10:27–30.

28a. Teran, A. Z., and Gambrell, R. D. 1988. Androgens in clinical practice. In *Androgens in the menopause,* ed. Leon Speroff. Marietta, Ga.: Reid-Rowell.

29. Tulandi, T., and Lal, S. 1985. Menopausal hot flush. *Obstet Gynecol Surv* 40, 9:553–63.

30. Verbeke, K.; Dhont, M.; and Vandekerckhove, D. 1988. Clinical and hormonal effects of long-term veralipride treatment in post-menopausal women. *Maturitas* 10:225–30.
31. Whelan, E., and Stare, F. 1990. Nutrition. *JAMA* 263:2661–63.
32. Wild, R. A.; Grubb, B.; Hartz, A.; Van Nort, J. J.; Bachman, W.; and Bartholomew, M. 1990. Clinical signs of androgen excess as risk factors for coronary artery disease. *Fertil Steril* 54:255–59.
33. Yancey, M. K.; Hannan, C. J.; Plymate, S. R.; Stone, I. K.; Friedl, K. E.; and Wright, J. R. 1990. Serum lipids and lipoproteins in continuous or cyclic medroxyprogesterone acetate treatment in postmenopausal women treated with conjugated estrogens. *Fertil Steril* 54:778–82.

APPENDIX 1

1. Bye, P. B. 1978. Review of the status of oestrogen replacement therapy. *Postgrad Med J* 54:7–10.
2. Callantine, M. R.; Martin, P. L.; Bolding, O. T.; Warner, P. O.; and Greaney, M. O., Jr. 1975. Micronized 17 beta estradiol for oral estrogen therapy in menopausal women. *Obstet Gynecol* 46:37–41.
3. Campbell, S., and Whitehead, M. 1977. Oestrogen therapy and the menopausal syndrome. *Clinics in Obstet & Gynaecol* 4:31–47.
4. Claydon, J. R.; Bell, J. Y.; and Pilard, P. 1974. Menopausal flushing: double blind trial of a non hormonal medication. *Brit Med J* 1:409–12.
5. Dennerstein, L.; Burrow, G.; and Hyman, G. 1978. Menopausal hot flushes: a double blind comparison of placebo, ethinyl oestradiol and norgestrel. *Br J Obstet Gynaecol* 85:852–56.
6. Hunter, D. J.; Julier, D.; Franklin, M.; and Green, E. 1977. Plasma levels of estrogen, luteinizing hormone, and follicle stimulating hormone following castration and estradiol implant. *Obstet Gynecol* 49:180–85.
7. Kupperman, H. S.; Wetchler, B. B.; and Blatt, M. H. G. 1959. Contemporary therapy of the menopausal syndrome. *JAMA* 171:1627–37.
8. Larsson-Cohn, U.; Johansson, E. D.; Kagedal, B.; and Wallentin, L. 1977. Serum FSH, LH, and oestrone levels in postmenopausal patients on oestrogen therapy. *Br J Obstet Gynaecol* 85:367–72.
9. Lauritzen, C. 1973. The management of the premenopausal and the postmenopausal patient. *Front Horm Res* 2:2–21.
10. Lind, T.; Cameron, E. C.; Hunter, W. M.; Leon, C.; Moran, P. F.; Oxley, A.; Gerrard, J.; and Lind, U. C. G. 1979. A prospective controlled trial of six forms of hormone replacement therapy given to postmenopausal women. *Br J Obstet Gynaecol* 86, suppl. 3:1–29.

11. Lindsay, R., and Hart, D. M. 1978. Failure of response of menopausal vasomotor symptoms to clonidine. *Maturitas* 1:21–25.
12. Martin, P.; Yen, S. S. C.; Burnier, A. M.; and Hermann, H. 1979. Systemic absorption and sustained effects of vaginal estrogen creams. *JAMA* 242:2699–2700.
13. Tzingounis, V.; Aksu, M.; and Greenblatt, R. 1978. Estriol in the management of the menopause. *JAMA* 239:1638–41.

APPENDIX 2

1. Aylward, M. 1978. Coagulation factors in opposed and unopposed oestrogen treatment at the climacteric. *Postgrad Med J* 54:31–37.
2. Barret-Conner, E.; Brown, W. V.; Turner, J.; Austin, M. S.; and Criqui, M. H. 1979. Heart disease risk factors and hormone use in postmenopausal women. *JAMA* 241:2167–69.
3. Bolton, C. H.; Ellwood, M., Hartog, M.; Martin, R.; Rowe, A. S.; and Wensley, R. T. 1975. Comparison of the effects of ethinyl oestradiol and conjugated equine oestrogens in oophorectomized women. *Clin Endocrinol (Oxf)* 4:131–38.
4. Bradley, D. B.; Wingerd, J.; Petitti, D. B.; Krauss, R. M.; and Ramcharan, S. 1978. Serum high density lipoprotein cholesterol in women using oral contraceptives, estrogens and progestins. *NEJM* 299:17–20.
5. Burch, J. C.; Byrd, B. F.; and Vaughn, W. K. 1975. The effects of long-term estrogen administration to women following hysterectomy. *Front Horm Res* 3:208–14.
6. Campbell, S., and Whitehead, M. 1977. Oestrogen therapy and the menopausal syndrome. *Clinics in Obstet & Gynaecol* 4:31–47.
7. Christiansen, C.; Christensen, M. S.; Hagen, C.; Stocklund, K. E.; and Transbol, I. 1981. Effects of natural estrogen/gestagen and thiazide on coronary risk factors in normal postmenopausal women. *Acta Obstet et Gynecol Scand* 60:407–12.
8. Crane, M. G.; Harris, J. J.; and Winsor, W., III. 1971. Hypertensions, oral contraceptive agents and conjugated estrogens. *Ann Int Med* 74:13–21.
9. Fedor-Freybergh, P. 1977. The influence of estrogens on the well-being and mental performance in the climacterica and postmenopausal women. *Acta Obstet et Gynecol Scand* 64, suppl. 1:1–64.
10. Gordon, T.; Kanel, W.; Hjortland, M.; and McNamara, P. 1978. Menopause and coronary heart disease: the Framingham Study. *Ann Int Med* 89:157–61.

11. Hirvonen, E.; Malknonen, M.; and Nanninen, V. 1980. Effects of different progestogens on lipoproteins during postmenopausal replacement therapy. *NEJM* 304:560–63.

12. Jick, H.; Dinan, B.; and Rothman, K. 1978. Noncontraceptive estrogens and nonfatal myocardial infarctions. *JAMA* 239:1407–8.

13. Kannel, W. B.; Castelli, W. P.; Gordon, T.; and McNamara, P. 1971. Serum cholesterol, lipoproteins and the risk of coronary heart disease. *Ann Int Med* 174:1–12.

14. Lauritzen, C. 1973. The management of the premenopausal and the postmenopausal patient. *Front Horm Res* 2:2–21.

15. Lind, T.; Cameron, E. C.; Hunter, W. M.; Leon, C.; Moran, P. F.; Oxley, A.; Gerrard, J.; and Lind, U. C. G. 1979. A prospective controlled trial of six forms of hormone replacement therapy given to postmenopausal women. *Br J Obstet Gynaecol* 86, 3:1–29.

16. MacMahon, B. 1978. Oestrogen replacement therapy and the vascular risk. In *Coronary heart disease in young women*, pp. 197–207. Edinburgh: Churchill Livingstone.

17. Maddock, J. 1978. Effects of progestogens on serum lipids in the postmenopause. *Postgrad Med J* 54:367–70.

18. Miller, N. E. 1979. The evidence for the antiatherogenicity of high density lipoprotein in man. *Lipids* 13:914–19.

19. Nielson, F. H.; Honore, E.; Kristoffersen, K.; Secher, N. J.; and Pederson, G. T. 1977. Changes in serum lipids during treatment with norgestrel, oestradiol-valerate and cycloprogynon. *Acta Obstet et Gynecol Scand* 56:367–70.

20. Notelovitz, M. 1977. Coagulation, oestrogen and the menopause. *Clinics in Obstet & Gynaecol* 4:107–28.

21. Notelovitz, M., and Southwood, B. 1974. Metabolic effect of conjugated oestrogens (USP) on lipids and lipoproteins. *S A Med J* 48:2552–56.

22. Pfeffer, R. I., and van den Noort, S. S. 1976. Estrogen use and stroke risk in postmenopausal women. *Am J Epidemiol* 103:445–56.

23. Pfeffer, R. I.; Whipple, G. H.; Kurosaki, T. T.; and Chapman, J. M. 1978. Coronary risk and estrogen use in postmenopausal women. *Am J Epidemiol* 107:479–87.

24. Plunkett, E. R. 1982. Contraceptive steroids, age and the cardiovascular system. *Am J Obstet Gynecol* 142:747–51.

25. Punnonen, R., and Rauramo, L. 1976. The effect of castration and oral estrogen therapy on serum lipids. In *Concensus on menopause research*, ed. P. van Keep, R. B. Greenblatt, and M. Albeaux-Fernet, pp. 132–38. Proceedings of the First International Congress on the Menopause, France, 1976. Baltimore: University Park Press.

26. Pyorala, T. 1976. The effect of synthetic and natural estrogens on glucose

tolerance, plasma insulin and lipid metabolism in postmenopausal women. In *The management of the menopause and postmenopausal years,* ed. S. Campbell, pp. 195–210. Lancaster, Eng.: MTP Press.

27. Rosenberg, L.; Armstrong, B.; and Jick, H. 1976. Myocardial infarction and estrogen therapy in postmenopausal women. *NEJM* 294:1256–59.

28. Ross, R. K.; Paganini-Hill, A.; Mack, T. M.; Arthur, M.; and Henderson, B. 1981. Menopausal oestrogen therapy and protection from death from ischaemic heart disease. *Lancet* 1:858–60.

29. Saunders, D. M.; Hunter, J. C.; Shutt, D. A.; and O'Neill, B. J. 1978. The effect of oestradiol valerate therapy on coagulation factors and lipid and oestrogen levels in oophorectomized women. *Aust N Z J Obstet Gynaecol* 18, 3:198–201.

30. Silverstolpe, G.; Gustafson, A.; Samsioe, G.; and Svanborg, A. 1979. Lipid metabolic studies in oophorectomized women: effects of three different progestogens. *Acta Obstet et Gynecol Scand* suppl. 88:89–95.

31. Tikkanen, M. J.; Kuusi, T.; Vartianien, E.; and Nikkila, E. A. 1979. Treatment of post-menopausal hypercholesterolaemia with estradiol. *Acta Obstet et Gynecol Scand* suppl. 88:83–88.

32. Tikkanen, M. J., and Nikkila, E. A. 1978. Natural oestrogen as an effective treatment for type-11 hyperlipoproteinaemia in postmenopausal women. *Lancet* 490–501.

33. Toy, J. L.; Davies, J. A.; and McNicol, G. P. 1978. The effects of long term therapy with oestriol succinate on the haemostatic mechanism in postmenopausal women. *Br J Obstet Gynaecol* 85:363–66.

34. Utian, W. H. 1978. Effect of postmenopausal estrogen therapy on diastolic blood pressure and bodyweight. *Maturitas* 1:3–8.

35. Wallace, R. B.; Hoover, J.; Barrett-Connor, E.; Rifkind, B. M.; Hunninghake, D. B.; Mackenthun, A.; and Heiss, G. 1979. Altered plasma lipid and lipo-protein levels associated with oral contraceptive and oestrogen use. *Lancet* 2:111–15.

36. Wallentin, L., and Larsson-Cohn, U. 1977. Metabolic and hormonal effects of postmenopausal oestrogen replacement treatment, II: plasma lipid. *Acta Endocrinol* 86:597–607.

37. Walter, S., and Jensen, H. K. 1977. The effect of treatment with oestradiol and oestriol on fasting serum cholesterol and triglyceride levels in postmenopausal women. *Br J Obstet Gynaecol* 84, 11:869–72.

GLOSSARY

adenomatous hyperplasia: a disease of the uterus in which glands are abnormal, swollen, and enlarged. This condition, if left untreated, could lead to cancer.

adenomyosis: a benign condition, asymptomatic or symptomatic, that is characterized by abnormal endometrial growth into the uterine muscle.

adnexal mass: a lump or mass in the uterine tubes and/or ovaries.

adrenaline, noradrenaline: hormones produced in the adrenal gland and certain nerve endings that release substances related to stress.

analog: a chemical compound whose structure is similar to that of the original produced in the body.

androgen: a class of male sex hormones that both men and women have, although men have more.

androstenedione: a weak androgen that menopausal ovaries secrete abundantly, as do the adrenals. This hormone becomes a major source of menopausal estrogens because it is changed into estrogens by the fat cells of the body.

anemia: an abnormally low amount of iron in the blood.

apolipoprotein: a protein that is derived from the lipoproteins. Different classes, such as apolipoprotein A and apolipoprotein B, can be measured using certain blood tests; the levels of the various classes predict the risks for different aspects of cardiovascular disease.

apoprotein: a substance found in the blood that is related to cholesterol and has been associated with cardiovascular health. The A and B classes are distinguished by the lipids to which they bind.

ascorbic acid: vitamin C. This water-soluble vitamin is present in certain citrus fruits and vegetables.

391

assay: a test to measure the concentration of a substance contained inside a fluid or other substance.

atherosclerosis: hardening of the arteries.

atrophic: deteriorating cells.

atypical hyperplasia: a precancerous condition of the endometrial lining of the uterus.

autoimmune endocrine disease: an allergic reaction to one's own hormones.

autonomic nervous system: the system that controls our emotions.

benign breast disease: a confusing term that seems to suggest lack of cancer (benign) and that is usually associated with fibrocystic breast changes. Some professionals argue that the term should be changed to *benign breast changes*.

beta blockers: drugs used to control a variety of conditions, particularly those related to cardiovascular health.

beta-endorphins: a class of internally produced substances that have a variety of calming effects on the nervous system and physical functions.

bilateral salpingo ovariectomy: surgical removal of both ovaries and oviducts.

biopsy: the surgical removal of a piece of body tissue for subsequent testing in the laboratory.

calcitonin: a hormone related to metabolic bone function.

calcitriol: a compound of the vitamin-D class.

calorie: a measure of energy consumed or burned by metabolic function.

cancer cell line: a laboratory term describing the growth of cancer cells in the laboratory in order to study them. A single cancer cell can be copied—or cloned—so that the "offspring" of the cancer cells carry with them similar genetic traits for study.

cardiovascular system: the heart muscle and vessels associated with the pumping and circulation of blood.

case/control study: one of the research methods in which individuals with a particular condition are compared to others who are presumably matched for age, location, and other nondisease variables in order to test for incidence of characteristics that are associated with having a disease.

cervix: the neck of the uterus, which sits on the internal end of the vagina.

cholesterol: a pearly, fatlike steroid alcohol commonly found in a variety of foods as well as circulating within the blood stream.

clonidine: a drug used principally as an antihypertensive but that has been tested in menopausal women for other effects.

coitus: sexual connection per vagina between male and female.

conjugated estrogens: a form of estrogen therapy. These most frequently refer to estrogens that are derived from the urine of pregnant mares.

corpus luteum: the "yellow body" seen in the ovary after ovulation. Its cells produce progesterone and estrogen (in the human) as well as other hormones.

corticosteroids: hormones of the steroid class that are normally manufactured by the adrenal gland's outer region. Drugs that are manufactured to mimic these effects appear to have a strong negative influence on bone tissue.

cystic hyperplasia: a condition of the endometrial lining of the uterus in which the glands become progressively more swollen and enlarged.

D & C: dilatation and curettage. The process by which a physician opens (dilates) the entry to the uterus and then scrapes away the lining (endometrium) of the uterus.

detumescence: loss of swelling as in loss of penile erection.

diverticular disease of the colon: a disease in which the colon forms pouches as a result of chronic constipation.

double-blind study: a study in which neither the experimenter nor the subject knows who is getting what treatment until all the results are in.

dual-photon absorptiometer: a machine that tests bone density.

dyspareunia: difficult or painful coitus. A common condition when the vagina is not able to produce adequate lubrication, as during menopausal estrogen deficiency.

ectopic pregnancy: a pregnancy that occurs in the Fallopian tubes rather than in the uterus.

edema: fluid-filled swelling of body tissues.

embolism: the sudden blocking of an artery by a clot or foreign material.

endocrine gland: *see* gland (endocrine).

endometriosis: a disease in which endometrial tissue is found where it does not belong—that is, on the surface of the uterus, in the Fallopian tubes, in the ovaries, or in other body regions.

endometrium: the lining portion of the uterus. A complex tissue that changes in size and composition throughout the menstrual cycle each month, forming a thick and cushiony mass of cells in preparation for a potential fertilized egg. Should none arrive, the endometrium itself sloughs off and is washed away with the menstrual flow. With estrogen deficiencies, the endometrium becomes thin and atrophic.

epinephrine, norepinephrine: *see* adrenaline, noradrenaline.

ERT: estrogen replacement therapy.

estradiol: the strongest of the natural estrogens.

estriol: the weakest commonly found natural estrogen.

estrogen: a class of female sex hormones that both men and women have, although women have more.

estrogen replacement therapy (ERT):   estrogen treatments that are intended to support tissues with levels of estrogen adequate for the maintenance of good health.

estrone: a natural estrogen weaker than estradiol.

Fallopian tubes: the two tubes that connect the ovaries with the uterus and through which sperm enter to fertilize an egg and an egg travels to reach the uterus.

fibrocystic breast disease: a benign condition of the breast characterized by fibrous and cystic tissue, which causes lumps and sometimes pain.

fibrocystic changes: similar to fibrocystic breast disease but reflecting change in the characteristics of the tissue from the previous baseline. It is probably a more accurate term for fibrocystic breast disease.

functional aerobic age: one's biologic age based on the body's capacity to consume oxygen.

gland (endocrine):   a part of the body (for example, adrenals, ovaries) that manufactures hormones and releases them into the blood stream.

glucocorticoids: hormones produced by the adrenal gland that affect carbohydrate metabolism. Cortisol is the most important natural glucocorticoid. Hydrocortisone is the drug derivative.

GnRH analogs: drugs that control the pituitary gland by mimicking the gonadotropin-releasing hormones that are normally produced at the base of the brain.

gonadotropins: hormones produced in the pituitary gland that travel in the blood stream and affect the gonads (ovaries in women). (FSH and LH are two gonadotropins.) The release of the gonadotropins are triggered by secretion of the releasing hormones—GnRH.

gross obesity: extreme fatness.

G spot (Gräfenberg spot):   named after Dr. Ernst Grafenberg, who first discovered it. In some women, this mound of tissue, located in the vagina usually about 1½ inches inside the external opening at "12:00 o'clock high," contracts to form a small lump when appropriately stimulated.

hemoglobin: the oxygen-carrying pigment of red blood cells found in the blood stream and made up of tiny pieces of iron *(hemo)* attached to globules *(globin).*

hemorrhage: abnormal internal or external bleeding.

high-density lipoprotein (HDL):   formed of protein coupled to a fat droplet, this molecule, which travels in the blood stream, protects against heart disease.

hormone: a substance produced in a gland that can travel in the blood stream and exert action on cells in a different part of the body than where it was produced.

hormone replacement therapy: *see* HRT.

hot flush, hot flash: a sudden and quickly passing sensation of intense internal heat, followed by sweating and possibly a brief chill. Common at the menopause.

HRT: hormone replacement therapy (generally includes progesterone that is given with estrogen).

hyperplasia: an increased *(hyper)* growth of cells *(plasia)*.

hyperplastic disease: a disease characterized by an abnormal increase in the number and size of cells.

hypertension: high blood pressure, usually more than 140/90.

hypertrophy: excessive swelling or increased size of tissue.

hysterectomy: removal of the uterus (not the ovary).

immune substances: blood-borne particles produced by the body to protect itself against disease.

incontinent: unable to control urine retention.

IU (International Units):   a term that describes internationally accepted standards for measurement, commonly used with hormone-level concentrations. Somewhat like *inch* or *mile,* the IU has set standards against which it can be checked.

jaundice: yellow skin produced by a dysfunction in the liver.

Kegel exercises: a set of exercises originally developed by Dr. A. M. Kegel to build up the strength of the PC muscles—that is, the sheet of muscles that extends between the pubic bone and the coccyx and that is responsible for urinary continence.

Kupperman Menopausal Index: a written instrument developed by Dr. Herbert Kupperman that a woman could use to evaluate her level of menopausal distress and associated estrogen deficiency. The scoring test has been validated independently by other researchers.

lactic acid: an acidic substance found in the blood stream that is increased after metabolic energy is expended by muscles. It is also found in, among other places, the vagina.

lactose intolerance: the inability to digest comfortably one of the molecules in milk. This leads to gastric distress.

laser ablation: *see* endometrial ablation in the index.

leiomyomas: fibroid tumors of uterine-muscle origin.

LH: *see* luteinizing hormone.

LH RH analogs: *see* GnRH analogs.

libido: sexual appetite.

lipid: fatty substances that can't dissolve in blood.

lipoprotein: a substance traveling in the blood stream that is part lipid and part protein.

low-density lipoprotein (LDL):   a lipoprotein with less protein and more lipid, as compared to the high-density lipoprotein. High concentrations of this substance appear to promote heart disease.

luteal phase: that part of the human menstrual cycle that begins after ovulation and continues until menstruation and that is characterized by the presence of a corpus luteum in one of the ovaries.

luteal-phase deficiency: an inability of the luteal-phase ovary to produce enough hormones for a sufficient amount of time to insure the adequate development of the endometrial lining which would allow a viable pregnancy to take place. The term is used to describe a type of infertility in which fertilization may or may not take place; when it does, however, the subsequent development of the fetus in the uterus may be aborted.

luteinizing hormone: a hormone produced in the pituitary. A large surge of this hormone precedes ovulation by twelve to twenty-four hours each cycle.

menarche: the first menstrual period of a girl's life.

menopause: the time that follows the last menstrual period of a woman's life.

mestranol: an estrogen-replacement drug.

metabolic rate: the rate at which the body burns calories.

metastasis: the spread of cancer cells via the circulatory system from the site of a tumor to other, distant sites.

micronized estrogen: a form of oral estrogen replacement therapy in which the estrogen substance is first reduced to a fine powder in order to enhance its absorption through the gastrointestinal tract into the body.

multiple myomectomy: a surgical procedure in which fibroid tumors from more than one site in the uterus are surgically removed but the uterus proper is preserved.

myocardial infarction: heart attack.

myomectomy: the surgical removal of one or more uterine fibroid tumors while preserving the uterus.

natural estrogens: manufactured estrogens that mimic the natural ones produced by the body and have a structural configuration similar or identical to the ones produced by the body.

natural hormones: hormones that are chemically identical to those that occur in nature. (In contrast, *see* synthetic hormones.)

neurogenic: of nerve origin.

neurogenic bladder difficulty: a loss of nerve-mediated control with consequent difficulties in urinating.

nulliparous: never having borne a child.

obesity: a condition of fat overgrowth that is deleterious to the health.

oophorectomy: removal of the ovary. Also called ovariectomy.

opposed estrogen: a form of hormone replacement therapy in which the hormone (such as progesterone, progestin, or testosterone) is administered to balance, or oppose, the effects of estrogen.

os: an opening to a body cavity.

osteoporosis: increased porosity of bones. A disease found in estrogen-deficiency states, which leads to bone fractures.

ovariectomy: *see* oophorectomy.

ovary: one of two female organs that contain the eggs and the cells that produce the female hormones estrogen and progesterone.

parenteral: refers to the entry of foodstuffs or drugs by a route other than the digestive tract, such as an intramuscular or intravenous injection.

pelvic phlebitis: inflammation of the pelvic veins.

perimenopause: the time "around" the menopause during which menstrual cycles become irregular and menopausal distress symptoms may appear.

perineal area: the region between the thighs that is bounded by the anus and the vagina.

phleboliths: stony-like substances found in the body.

pituitary gland: a glandular structure, located at the base of the brain, that produces a variety of protein-derived hormones which circulate in the blood stream and affect other glands and body functions throughout the body.

placebo: a pill that has no active ingredients.

polycystic ovary disease (polycystic ovary syndrome): a hormonally induced fibrocystic alteration of the ovary associated with the production of androgens in excess of what is normally found circulating in a woman's body.

polycystic ovary syndrome: *see* polycystic ovary disease.

progestagen: our preferred term for what is sometimes called *progestin* or *progestogen*. We prefer this term because it reflects the "progestational"-like effects—that is, effects that mimic natural progesterone.

proliferative disease: a disease characterized by the abnormal multiplication of cells.

psychotropic: that which exerts an effect on the mind. The term usually describes a drug that can produce such effects.

PUFA oil: polyunsaturated fatty acid oil.

RDA: the Food and Drug Administration's Recommended Daily Allowance for a vitamin or mineral.

retrospective study: a study in which subjects must remember what happened because records have not been kept.

sickle cell anemia: a disorder of the blood cells found principally in blacks.

single-photon densitometer: a machine for measuring bone density usually of the wrist or forearm.

stroke: a blood clot in or hemorrhage of a blood vessel leading to the brain.

subtotal hysterectomy: removal of the uterus except for the cervix.

synthetic estrogens: estrogen drugs that are structurally different from that which is normally produced by the body.

synthetic hormones: hormones that are chemically different from those that occur in nature.

testosterone: the strongest of the male sex hormones. Women also produce testosterone, though much less than men.

thromboembolic disease: obstruction of a blood vessel by a blood clot.

thrombophlebitis: inflammation of a vein by a blood clot.

thrombosis: the formation of a clot.

titration: varying the dosage in small increments until the correct balance is achieved.

total abdominal hysterectomy: removal of the total uterus by abdominal surgery. Does not include oophorectomy.

total hysterectomy: removal of the total uterus.

transdermally: across the skin. The term is applied to a method of delivery of drugs by means of a Band-Aid or other agent applied to the skin until the drug is absorbed.

triglyceride: a blood-borne lipid.

tumor: an abnormal swelling.

type-A personality: a personality characteristic that is ascribed to an individual who is explosive, easily angry, high-pressured.

ultrasonography: visualization of body structures using sound waves.

unopposed estrogen: estrogen treatment without progestin opposition, which is usually recommended.

uterine fibroid tumors (uterine myomas):   fibroid tumors, often benign, of the uterus.

uterine myomas: *see* uterine fibroid tumors.

uterus: a complex female organ composed of smooth muscle and glandular lining.

vagina: a muscular canal in the female that extends from the vulva to the cervix. It is very responsive to estrogen and becomes atrophied during menopausal estrogen-deficiency states.

vaginal transudate: a "sweating," or lubricating, response of the vaginal walls to increased blood flow to the region.

vaginitis: inflammation of the vagina. It is marked by pain, discharge, and itchiness.

venous thrombosis: a blood clot in a vein.

VLDL-cholesterol: very low-density lipoprotein-cholesterol

vulva: the genital organs of a woman. The region includes the outer and inner lips, mons pubis, and vestibule and opening of the vagina.

womb: the uterus.

ANNUAL HEALTH CHARTS

The pages that follow may be used as a personal diary for recording the facts about your passage through and beyond the change of life. By documenting your days of menstruation, symptoms, treatments, and other medical history, you will provide yourself with useful diagnostic tools.

If you are methodical and orderly in keeping an accurate record of your health habits and needs, you will begin a journey into awareness that will help detect problems earlier and will aid you in achieving a happier, healthier, and more productive life. The seven years before your last period are generally characterized by a number of changes in menstrual pattern. It helps to record days of bleeding in order to see the change over time. Beginning at about age forty-three, changes generally become apparent. Figure 26 presents a sample Menstrual Record Chart. If you decide to use it, it will help future diagnoses if you note the character of the blood flow. If other forms than those designated in the code occur (for example, clots), make up your own code letter and add that code letter when appropriate.

Space is provided in the following pages to allow a permanent record, one page for each year—starting now. This record will help you as well as your daughters and granddaughters. It is easy to jot things down as they happen but difficult to remember them accurately after time has passed.

NAME:

AGE: CURRENT YEAR:

MENSTRUAL RECORD CHART

MONTH	1	2	3	4	5	6	7	8	9	10	11	12	13	14	15	16	17	18	19	20	21	22	23	24	25	26	27	28	29	30	31
JAN.																															
FEB.																															
MAR.																															
APR.																															
MAY																															
JUNE																															
JULY																															
AUG.																															
SEPT.																															
OCT.																															
NOV.																															
DEC.																															

Don't forget to have this chart with you when you call or visit your doctor.

TYPE OF FLOW: Normal ☒   Light ◉   Heavy ■   Stain ⊡

FIGURE 26

ANNUAL HEALTH CHART

FOR THE YEAR:

	JAN.	FEB.	MARCH	APRIL	MAY	JUNE	JULY	AUG.	SEPT.	OCT.	NOV.	DEC.
ILLNESSES:												
SURGERIES:												
INJURIES:												
MEDICATIONS AND IMMUNIZATIONS:												
SYMPTOMS:												

NAME:

AGE: CURRENT YEAR:

MENSTRUAL RECORD CHART

MONTH	1	2	3	4	5	6	7	8	9	10	11	12	13	14	15	16	17	18	19	20	21	22	23	24	25	26	27	28	29	30	31
JAN.																															
FEB.																															
MAR.																															
APR.																															
MAY																															
JUNE																															
JULY																															
AUG.																															
SEPT.																															
OCT.																															
NOV.																															
DEC.																															

Don't forget to have this chart with you when you call or visit your doctor.

TYPE OF FLOW: Normal ☒   Light ☐   Heavy ■   Stain ⊡

ANNUAL HEALTH CHART

FOR THE YEAR:

	JAN.	FEB.	MARCH	APRIL	MAY	JUNE	JULY	AUG.	SEPT.	OCT.	NOV.	DEC.
ILLNESSES:												
SURGERIES:												
INJURIES:												
MEDICATIONS AND IMMUNIZATIONS:												
SYMPTOMS:												

NAME:

AGE: CURRENT YEAR:

MENSTRUAL RECORD CHART

MONTH	1	2	3	4	5	6	7	8	9	10	11	12	13	14	15	16	17	18	19	20	21	22	23	24	25	26	27	28	29	30	31
JAN.																															
FEB.																															
MAR.																															
APR.																															
MAY																															
JUNE																															
JULY																															
AUG.																															
SEPT.																															
OCT.																															
NOV.																															
DEC.																															

Don't forget to have this chart with you when you call or visit your doctor.

TYPE OF FLOW: Normal ☒   Light ◯   Heavy ▮   Stain ▪

ANNUAL HEALTH CHART

FOR THE YEAR:

	JAN.	FEB.	MARCH	APRIL	MAY	JUNE	JULY	AUG.	SEPT.	OCT.	NOV.	DEC.
ILLNESSES:												
SURGERIES:												
INJURIES:												
MEDICATIONS AND IMMUNIZATIONS:												
SYMPTOMS:												

NAME:

AGE:　　　CURRENT YEAR:

MENSTRUAL RECORD CHART

MONTH	1	2	3	4	5	6	7	8	9	10	11	12	13	14	15	16	17	18	19	20	21	22	23	24	25	26	27	28	29	30	31
JAN.																															
FEB.																															
MAR.																															
APR.																															
MAY																															
JUNE																															
JULY																															
AUG.																															
SEPT.																															
OCT.																															
NOV.																															
DEC.																															

Don't forget to have this chart with you when you call or visit your doctor.

TYPE OF FLOW:　Normal ☒　Light ⊡　Heavy ■　Stain ⊡

ANNUAL HEALTH CHART

FOR THE YEAR:

	JAN.	FEB.	MARCH	APRIL	MAY	JUNE	JULY	AUG.	SEPT.	OCT.	NOV.	DEC.
ILLNESSES:												
SURGERIES:												
INJURIES:												
MEDICATIONS AND IMMUNIZATIONS:												
SYMPTOMS:												

NAME:

AGE: CURRENT YEAR:

MENSTRUAL RECORD CHART

MONTH	1	2	3	4	5	6	7	8	9	10	11	12	13	14	15	16	17	18	19	20	21	22	23	24	25	26	27	28	29	30	31
JAN.																															
FEB.																															
MAR.																															
APR.																															
MAY																															
JUNE																															
JULY																															
AUG.																															
SEPT.																															
OCT.																															
NOV.																															
DEC.																															

Don't forget to have this chart with you when you call or visit your doctor.

TYPE OF FLOW: Normal [x]   Light [o]   Heavy ■   Stain [•]

ANNUAL HEALTH CHART

FOR THE YEAR: _____

	JAN.	FEB.	MARCH	APRIL	MAY	JUNE	JULY	AUG.	SEPT.	OCT.	NOV.	DEC.
ILLNESSES:												
SURGERIES:												
INJURIES:												
MEDICATIONS AND IMMUNIZATIONS:												
SYMPTOMS:												

NAME:

AGE: CURRENT YEAR:

MENSTRUAL RECORD CHART

MONTH	1	2	3	4	5	6	7	8	9	10	11	12	13	14	15	16	17	18	19	20	21	22	23	24	25	26	27	28	29	30	31
JAN.																															
FEB.																															
MAR.																															
APR.																															
MAY																															
JUNE																															
JULY																															
AUG.																															
SEPT.																															
OCT.																															
NOV.																															
DEC.																															

Don't forget to have this chart with you when you call or visit your doctor.

TYPE OF FLOW: Normal x   Light o   Heavy ■   Stain •

ANNUAL HEALTH CHART

FOR THE YEAR:

	JAN.	FEB.	MARCH	APRIL	MAY	JUNE	JULY	AUG.	SEPT.	OCT.	NOV.	DEC.
ILLNESSES:												
SURGERIES:												
INJURIES:												
MEDICATIONS AND IMMUNIZATIONS:												
SYMPTOMS:												

NAME:

AGE: CURRENT YEAR:

MENSTRUAL RECORD CHART

MONTH	1	2	3	4	5	6	7	8	9	10	11	12	13	14	15	16	17	18	19	20	21	22	23	24	25	26	27	28	29	30	31
JAN.																															
FEB.																															
MAR.																															
APR.																															
MAY																															
JUNE																															
JULY																															
AUG.																															
SEPT.																															
OCT.																															
NOV.																															
DEC.																															

Don't forget to have this chart with you when you call or visit your doctor.

TYPE OF FLOW: Normal [x]   Light [o]   Heavy [■]   Stain [•]

ANNUAL HEALTH CHART

FOR THE YEAR:

	JAN.	FEB.	MARCH	APRIL	MAY	JUNE	JULY	AUG.	SEPT.	OCT.	NOV.	DEC.
ILLNESSES:												
SURGERIES:												
INJURIES:												
MEDICATIONS AND IMMUNIZATIONS:												
SYMPTOMS:												

NAME:

AGE: CURRENT YEAR:

MENSTRUAL RECORD CHART

MONTH	1	2	3	4	5	6	7	8	9	10	11	12	13	14	15	16	17	18	19	20	21	22	23	24	25	26	27	28	29	30	31
JAN.																															
FEB.																															
MAR.																															
APR.																															
MAY																															
JUNE																															
JULY																															
AUG.																															
SEPT.																															
OCT.																															
NOV.																															
DEC.																															

Don't forget to have this chart with you when you call or visit your doctor.

TYPE OF FLOW: Normal ☒   Light ◉   Heavy ■   Stain ●

ANNUAL HEALTH CHART

FOR THE YEAR:

	JAN.	FEB.	MARCH	APRIL	MAY	JUNE	JULY	AUG.	SEPT.	OCT.	NOV.	DEC.
ILLNESSES:												
SURGERIES:												
INJURIES:												
MEDICATIONS AND IMMUNIZATIONS:												
SYMPTOMS:												

NAME:

AGE: CURRENT YEAR:

MENSTRUAL RECORD CHART

MONTH	1	2	3	4	5	6	7	8	9	10	11	12	13	14	15	16	17	18	19	20	21	22	23	24	25	26	27	28	29	30	31
JAN.																															
FEB.																															
MAR.																															
APR.																															
MAY																															
JUNE																															
JULY																															
AUG.																															
SEPT.																															
OCT.																															
NOV.																															
DEC.																															

Don't forget to have this chart with you when you call or visit your doctor.

TYPE OF FLOW: Normal ☒   Light ☉   Heavy ■   Stain ⊡

ANNUAL HEALTH CHART

FOR THE YEAR:

	JAN.	FEB.	MARCH	APRIL	MAY	JUNE	JULY	AUG.	SEPT.	OCT.	NOV.	DEC.
ILLNESSES:												
SURGERIES:												
INJURIES:												
MEDICATIONS AND IMMUNIZATIONS:												
SYMPTOMS:												

NAME:

AGE: CURRENT YEAR:

MENSTRUAL RECORD CHART

MONTH	1	2	3	4	5	6	7	8	9	10	11	12	13	14	15	16	17	18	19	20	21	22	23	24	25	26	27	28	29	30	31
JAN.																															
FEB.																															
MAR.																															
APR.																															
MAY																															
JUNE																															
JULY																															
AUG.																															
SEPT.																															
OCT.																															
NOV.																															
DEC.																															

Don't forget to have this chart with you when you call or visit your doctor.

TYPE OF FLOW: Normal [x]   Light [o]   Heavy [■]   Stain [•]

ANNUAL HEALTH CHART

FOR THE YEAR:

	JAN.	FEB.	MARCH	APRIL	MAY	JUNE	JULY	AUG.	SEPT.	OCT.	NOV.	DEC.
ILLNESSES:												
SURGERIES:												
INJURIES:												
MEDICATIONS AND IMMUNIZATIONS:												
SYMPTOMS:												

NAME:

AGE: CURRENT YEAR:

MENSTRUAL RECORD CHART

MONTH	1	2	3	4	5	6	7	8	9	10	11	12	13	14	15	16	17	18	19	20	21	22	23	24	25	26	27	28	29	30	31
JAN.																															
FEB.																															
MAR.																															
APR.																															
MAY																															
JUNE																															
JULY																															
AUG.																															
SEPT.																															
OCT.																															
NOV.																															
DEC.																															

Don't forget to have this chart with you when you call or visit your doctor.

TYPE OF FLOW: Normal [x]   Light [o]   Heavy ■   Stain [•]

INDEX